J. McDuncan, MD

11/94

ADVANCES IN

Vascular Surgery

VOLUME 2

ADVANCES IN

Vascular Surgery

VOLUME 1

ADVANCES IN

Vascular Surgery

VOLUME 2

Editor-in-Chief
Anthony D. Whittemore, M.D.
Associate Professor Surgery, Harvard University Medical School; Chief,
Division of Vascular Surgery, Brigham and Women's Hospital, Boston,
Massachusetts

Associate Editors
Dennis F. Bandyk, M.D.
Professor of Surgery, University of South Florida College of Medicine; Director,
Vascular Surgery Division, Chief of Vascular Surgery, Tampa General Hospital,
Tampa, Florida

Jack L. Cronenwett, M.D.
Professor of Surgery, Dartmouth Medical School; Chief, Section of Vascular
Surgery, Dartmouth–Hitchcock Medical Center, Lebanon, New Hampshire

Norman R. Hertzer, M.D.
Chairman, Department of Vascular Surgery, Cleveland Clinic Foundation,
Cleveland, Ohio

Rodney A. White, M.D.
Professor of Surgery, University of California at Los Angeles School of
Medicine; Chief of Vascular Surgery, Associate Chairman, Department of
Surgery, Harbor–University of California at Los Angeles Medical Center, Los
Angeles, California

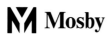 Mosby

St. Louis Baltimore Boston Chicago London Madrid Philadelphia Sydney Toronto

M Mosby

Vice President and Publisher, Continuity Publishing: Kenneth H. Killion
Director, Editorial Development: Gretchen C. Murphy
Developmental Editor: Kris Baumgartner
Sr. Project Editor: Jill C. Waite
Project Supervisor: Maria Nevinger
Proofreading Supervisor: Barbara M. Kelly
Vice President, Professional Sales and Marketing: George M. Parker
Marketing and Circulation Manager: Barry J. Bowlus
Marketing Coordinator: Lynn Stevenson

Printed in the United States of America
Composition by The Clarinda Company
Printing/binding by The Maple-Vail Book Manufacturing Company

Mosby–Year Book, Inc.
11830 Westline Industrial Drive
St. Louis, Missouri 63146

Editorial Office:
Mosby–Year Book, Inc.
200 North LaSalle Street
Chicago, Illinois 60657

International Standard Serial Number: 1069-7292
International Standard Book Number: 0-8151-9406-4

Contributors

George Andros, M.D.
Medical Director, Vascular Laboratory, St. Joseph Medical Center, Burbank, California

Stefano Bartoli, M.D.
Visiting Assistant Professor, Baylor College of Medicine, Houston, Texas

Benjamin B. Chang, M.D.
Assistant Professor of Surgery, Department of Vascular Surgery, Albany Medical College, Albany, New York

David V. Cossman, M.D.
Medical Director, Vascular Laboratory; Attending, Division of Vascular Surgery, Cedars-Sinai Medical Center, Los Angeles, California

Mark A. Creager, M.D.
Vascular Medicine and Atherosclerosis Unit of the Cardiovascular Division of Brigham and Women's Hospital, Boston, Massachusetts

R. Clement Darling III, M.D.
Assistant Professor of Surgery, Department of Vascular Surgery, Albany Medical College, Albany, New York

Hugh A. Gelabert, M.D.
Assistant Professor of Surgery, Section of Vascular Surgery, University of California, Los Angeles, UCLA School of Medicine, Los Angeles, California

Marie D. Gerhard, M.D.
Vascular Medicine and Atherosclerosis Unit of the Cardiovascular Division of Brigham and Women's Hospital, Boston, Massachusetts

Robert W. Harris, M.D.
Private Practice, Burbank, California

Maria G.M. Hunink, M.D., Ph.D.
Associate Professor of Health Sciences, Department of Health Sciences, Faculty of Medicine, University of Groningen; Decision Office for Medical Technology Assessment, Academic Hospital Groningen, Groningen, The Netherlands; Department of Health Policy and Management, Harvard Medical School of Public Health, Boston, Massachusetts

Robert P. Leather, M.D.
Professor of Surgery, Department of Vascular Surgery, Albany Medical College, Albany, New York

Frank W. LoGerfo, M.D.
Professor of Surgery, Harvard Medical School; Chief, Division of Vascular Surgery, Department of Surgery, New England Deaconess Hospital, Boston, Massachusetts

Ross T. Lyon, M.D.
Assistant Professor of Surgery, Jack D. Weiler Hospital of the Albert Einstein College of Medicine, Bronx, New York

John A. Mannick, M.D.
Surgeon-in-Chief, Harvard Medical School/Brigham and Women's Hospital, Boston, Massachusetts

Michael L. Marin, M.D.
Division of Vascular Surgery, Department of Surgery, Albert Einstein College of Medicine, Montefiore Medical Center, Bronx, New York

Walter J. McCarthy, M.D.
Assistant Professor of Surgery, Division of Vascular Surgery, Northwestern University Medical School, Northwestern Memorial Hospital, Chicago, Illinois

Michael F. Meyerovitz, M.D.
Associate Professor of Radiology, Department of Radiology Harvard Medical School; Co-Director, Cardiovascular and Interventional Radiology, Brigham and Women's Hospital, Boston, Massachusetts

Wesley S. Moore, M.D.
Professor of Surgery, Chief, Section of Vascular Surgery, University of California, Los Angeles, UCLA School of Medicine, Los Angeles, California

Thomas F. O'Donnell, Jr., M.D.
Chief, Vascular Surgery Section, Tufts University School of Medicine, New England Medical Center Hospitals, Boston, Massachusetts

Frank B. Pomposelli, Jr., M.D.
Assistant Professor of Surgery, Harvard Medical School; Vascular Surgeon, New England Deaconess Hospital, Boston, Massachusetts

Agustin A. Rodriquez, M.D.
Vascular Surgery Fellow, Tufts University School of Medicine, New England Medical Center Hospitals, Boston, Massachusetts

Hazim J. Safi, M.D.
Associate Professor of Surgery, Baylor College of Medicine, Houston, Texas

Peter A. Schneider, M.D.
Private Practice, Burbank, California

Dhiraj M. Shah, M.D.
Professor of Surgery, Department of Vascular Surgery, Albany Medical College, Albany, New York

Paula K. Shireman, M.D.
General Surgery Resident, Department of Surgery, Northwestern University Medical School, Northwestern Memorial Hospital, Chicago, Illinois

Jonathan B. Towne, M.D.
Professor and Chairman, Department of Vascular Surgery/Surgery, Medical College of Wisconsin, Milwaukee, Wisconsin

Richard L. Treiman, M.D.
Clinical Professor of Surgery, University of Southern California School of Medicine; Senior Attending, Division of Vascular Surgery, Cedars-Sinai Medical Center, Los Angeles, California

Frank J. Veith, M.D.
Professor of Surgery, Albert Einstein College of Medicine; Chief of Vascular
Surgery, Montefiore Medical Center, Bronx, New York

Willis H. Wagner, M.D.
Clinical Assistant Professor of Surgery, University of Southern California
School of Medicine; Chief, Division of Vascular Surgery, Cedars-Sinai Medical
Center, Los Angeles, California

Kurt R. Wengerter, M.D.
Assistant Professor of Surgery, Albert Einstein College of Medicine, Montefiore
Medical Center, Bronx, New York

Preface

Advances in management of the ischemic lower extremity have yielded vastly improved results, even for limbs with the most severely compromised distal vasculature. During the past decade, routine autogenous reconstruction to the level of the pedal arteries has salvaged the majority of threatened limbs, and results have been further optimized with alternative sources of vein using more distal origins for bypass. This second volume of *Advances in Vascular Surgery* focuses on this progress of infrainguinal reconstruction from the perspective of those individuals responsible for many of the underlying contributions. In addition, balloon angioplasty for infrainguinal disease has established a more predictable role in our collective armamentarium, and stented grafts may yet prove efficacious in some settings as well. Both Drs. Hunink and Veith have contributed their experience with these two endovascular techniques.

Dr. Moore has outlined his approach to the important and controversial issue of carotid restenosis after endarterectomy, and Dr. Safi has reviewed a significant experience with the infected aortic graft, the management of which has become more controversial with the advent of in situ replacement. Dr. O'Donnell has provided an updated summary of venous reconstruction that includes an important section on preoperative physiologic evaluation, a field undergoing substantial changes. Finally, Drs. Gerhard and Creager have written a comprehensive chapter on vasospastic disorders, a chapter that may well prove to be an important primary reference.

The editorial board again hopes the reader will find in each chapter a succinct practical approach to common clinical problems encountered by clinicians caring for patients with systemic vascular disorders.

Anthony D. Whittemore, M.D.
Editor-in-Chief

Contents

Advances in the Noninvasive Diagnosis and Surgical Management of Chronic Venous Insufficiency.

PART V. Issues of Basic Science   243

Raynaud's Phenomenon: Vasopastic Disease and Current Therapy.

Mosby Document Express
   Copies of the full text of journal articles referenced in this book are available by calling Mosby Document Express, toll-free, at 1-800-55-MOSBY.
   With Mosby Document Express, you have convenient 24-hour-a-day access to literally every journal reference within this book. In fact, through Mosby Document Express, virtually any medical or scientific article can be located and delivered by FAX, overnight delivery service, international airmail, electronic transmission of bit-mapped images (via Internet), or regular mail. The average cost of a complete delivered copy of an article, including copyright clearance charges and first-class mail delivery, is $12.
   For inquiries and pricing information, please call the toll-free number shown above.

PART I

Infrainguinal Arterial Disease

Infrainguinal Arterial Reconstruction—Historical Perspective

John A. Mannick, M.D.

Surgeon-in-Chief, Harvard Medical School/Brigham and Women's Hospital, Boston, Massachusetts

W hile autogenous saphenous vein grafts had been used in a few instances beginning in the early part of the 20th century to replace popliteal aneurysms, it was not until the late 1940s when both angiography and heparin were available that treatment of occlusive disease in the arteries of the leg was begun, first by DosSantos,[1] using endarterectomy, and shortly thereafter by Kunlin,[2] using reversed saphenous vein grafts. Both these techniques were applied to occlusive lesions of the superficial femoral artery only.

After these initial reports from Europe, both endarterectomy and reverse saphenous vein grafting were tried by surgeons in the United States. The superficial femoral endarterectomy utilizing loop strippers was refined on the West Coast by Wylie[3] and Cannon[4] and their associates. Because of its simplicity, saphenous vein grafting was greeted with enthusiasm by a number of surgeons, but because the saphenous vein was difficult to work with in the hands of surgeons used to bowel anastomoses, vein grafting attempts often led to strictures at the proximal and distal anastomoses. The good results reported by Kunlin were not easily duplicated and many surgeons abandoned vein grafting in favor of arterial homografts taken from cadavers which were much easier to suture.[5] Unfortunately, homografts frequently deteriorated after a few years, with aneurysm formation, which sometimes led to graft rupture, thrombosis, and distal embolization.[6, 7] This technique for infrainguinal reconstruction was quickly abandoned and synthetic vascular prostheses were used in the femoropopliteal position instead. These grafts became available in the 1950s after the initial discovery by Voorhees, Jaretski, and Blakemore[8] that vinyon-N tubes would remain patent in the arterial system in dogs. By the late 1950s bypass grafts of knitted or woven Dacron were the choice of most surgeons since they were relatively easy to handle and had proved to be biocompatible and not subject to deterioration in the body.

However, autogenous vein grafting was kept alive by some surgeons, both in the United States and abroad. Prominent among these was Dr. Robert Linton with whom I had the pleasure of working as a surgical resident in the 1950s. Linton had traveled to Europe after Kunlin's initial reports and had watched carefully how Kunlin performed his vein grafting operations. Linton brought back to the United States the Kunlin technique of performing vein graft anastomoses which consisted of spatulating the end of the vein graft and carefully suturing it end to side to the artery with small-caliber running silk sutures started at each corner and proceeding toward the middle of the anastomosis to ensure that the anastomosis was widely patent and free of kinks. This careful anastomotic technique allowed Linton and a few other surgeons to achieve success with autogenous vein grafting while others were reporting dismal early results.

By the early 1960s it was apparent to most surgeons that femoropopliteal bypasses with fabric grafts, usually Dacron, were yielding poor long-term results, with patency rates at the 5-year interval considerably less than 50% in most instances.[9, 10] As Stanley Crawford once pointed out to me, Dacron femoropopliteal grafts would remain patent in the long term only if (1) the distal anastomosis was placed above the knee joint, (2) the popliteal artery was widely patent from that point distally, and (3) there was excellent runoff all the way to the foot. In 1962 the report of Linton and Darling[11] of a large series of autogenous saphenous vein grafts in the femoropopliteal position with cumulative 5-year patency of greater than 70% caused a marked renewal of interest in the vein graft as a conduit for infrainguinal arterial reconstruction. By this time most surgeons with experience in treating vascular disease had become sufficiently practiced in the suturing of blood vessels so that adaptation of some variant of the Kunlin technique for vein graft anastomosis was not difficult.

At about this time bypass grafting to the infrapopliteal vessels began to be attempted. It is probable that the first femoral tibial bypasses were performed by McCaughan who, in 1960, reported Dacron bypasses to several tibial arteries in patients with occlusive disease. Unfortunately, the report appeared in the *Tennessee State Medical Journal* and went unnoticed nationally. In the same year Palma[12] reported a femoral-to-posterior tibial vein graft. However, the accompanying arteriogram suggests that the distal anastomosis may have been in the infrageniculate popliteal artery. The first successful tibial vein graft was probably performed by the late Andy Dale who reported his experience with several femoral–posterior tibial vein grafts at the annual meeting of the Society for Vascular Surgery in 1962. This experience was subsequently published in 1963.[13]

In 1960 I had brought Linton's technique of reverse saphenous vein grafting to the department of Dr. David Hume at the Medical College of Virginia. Hume and I performed a series of vein grafts for limb salvage beginning that year. We had begun to use femoral-tibial reverse saphenous vein grafts to treat some of these patients in 1961, and believed that we were the first to use this technique. We were therefore surprised by Dale's report in 1962. However, it does seem likely that we performed the first femoral–anterior tibial vein graft, which we reported to the Society for Vascular Surgery in 1963.[14] It was not until more than 15 years later that femoral-tibial arterial reconstructions achieved widespread acceptance; however, several groups had begun to utilize this technique in an increasing numbers of cases. By 1968 Garrett and his associates[15] at Houston were able to report a series of 56 tibial artery bypasses with reversed autogenous saphenous vein which had increased to a series of 91 cases by the following year.

It soon became apparent that tibial vein grafts did not succeed as often as femoropopliteal grafts. The 5-year cumulative patency of reconstructions to the tibial arteries was 50% or less as compared with cumulative patency of 70% or more when autogenous grafts were placed into the popliteal artery.[16, 17] This led me and my associates to suggest in 1975 that bypass grafts to an isolated popliteal artery segment with distal outflow only through collateral vessels might be preferable to tibial artery vein grafting in patients without extensive ischemic tissue loss in the foot. While papers are still being published proposing this idea,[18] most surgeons probably no longer prefer isolated segment popliteal bypasses to tibial artery vein grafts since results with tibial vein grafting improved considerably during the late 1980s.

The 1960s also saw a fading of interest in femoropopliteal endarterectomy as a treatment of infrainguinal occlusive disease. The inferior performance of endarterectomy as compared with reversed saphenous vein grafting was clearly demonstrated in the report of Darling and Linton in 1972.[19] However, proponents of short-segmental endarterectomy of the superficial femoral artery, usually performed under direct vision and with the use of patch graft angioplasty,[20] have continued to achieve good results with this technique up to the present time.

Because of widespread disillusionment with Dacron prostheses in the infrainguinal position and because of lack of suitable autogenous saphenous vein in a substantial minority of patients requiring infrainguinal arterial reconstruction, surgeons again began searching for better artificial conduits for use in bypass grafting. Several such conduits appeared in the late 1960s and early 1970s. The bovine arterial heterograft[21] was quickly abandoned because of its tendency to degenerate. The Dacron-covered human umbilical vein graft[22] still remains in use though difficult handling characteristics, late aneurysmal degeneration,[23] and long-term patency inferior to autogenous saphenous vein have prevented widespread acceptance.

The prosthesis most commonly used for infrainguinal bypass at the present time is made from expanded polytetrafluoroethylene (PTFE).[24] This graft material currently has its champions who recommend preferential use of PTFE grafts in femoropopliteal reconstruction in order to preserve the greater saphenous vein for later use after failure of the PTFE graft.[25] Most reports,[26, 27] however, suggest that the patency of PTFE grafts with the distal anastomosis in the infrageniculate popliteal artery or in the tibial vessels is discouragingly low at the 5-year interval. Whether or not the addition of autogenous vein cuffs[28] or patches[29] at the distal anastomosis will yield improved long-term patency remains to be determined. As was the case for Dacron bypass grafts, it seems clear that PTFE grafts in the hands of most surgeons will have a satisfactory 5-year patency only when the distal anastomosis is placed above the level of the knee joint with excellent runoff through the distal popliteal and tibial vessels. Indeed, there has been no adequate demonstration up to the present that PTFE femoropopliteal bypasses have performed better than Dacron bypasses.

Perhaps the outstanding development in infrainguinal arterial reconstruction in the 1980s was the improvement in the long-term success of femorotibial reconstructions with autogenous vein. This progress, I believe, was set in motion by the report of Leather, Karmody, and their associates[30] from Albany in the late 1970s delineating their experience with new techniques of in situ vein grafting. They used miniaturized instruments for precise lysis of the valves, thus allowing in situ vein grafting to be performed expeditiously and without significant damage to the vein wall. In situ grafting had been carried out by some groups throughout the 1960s, notably by Karl Victor Hall[31] who precisely placed incisions in his in situ grafts over the obstructing valves and excised the valves under direct vision. Prior attempts at valve interruption through intraluminal stripping devices had yielded inferior results to reversed vein grafts as delineated in the report of Barner et al. in 1969.[32] However, the techniques propounded by Leather and his associates made in situ grafting a feasible technique for most vascular surgeons. Though it is still not proven that in situ grafts to the distal tibial arteries have greater success than meticulously performed reversed vein grafts in the same position,[33] the in situ technique, in my opinion, has at least made distal tibial grafting easier and less time-consuming.

Other substantial technical advances in vein grafting over the past decade, in addition to the instrumentation developed by Leather and his associates, have been the use of fine, durable, and nonreactive polypropylene sutures, the use of loupe magnification, and more gentle and physiologic treatment of the vein graft's endothelium. A combination of these techniques and the accumulation of clinical experience has allowed a number of groups[33–35] to report continuous patencies (achieved by repair of 5%–15% of patent vein grafts with localized stenoses) which approach or surpass 80% at 5 years for femorotibial vein grafts and surpass 85% patency for femoropopliteal vein grafts. Along with these technical improvements in saphenous vein grafting has come the realization that the lesser saphenous vein and arm veins are also appropriate conduits when the greater saphenous veins are diseased or missing from prior use.

These improvements appear to have had a truly dramatic impact on limb salvage. For patients operated on for critical ischemia, the 5-year limb salvage now is 85% or better,[33–35] whereas a decade or so ago it was probably no greater than 60%. With the use of the duplex scanner to search preoperatively for adequate venous conduits, it is now possible to offer autogenous tissue reconstruction with vein grafts, either in situ or reversed, coupled in some instances with short endarterectomies, in 95% of patients requiring infrainguinal arterial reconstruction. Whether newer prostheses or endothelial lining of currently extant prosthetic grafts will yield results in infrapopliteal reconstruction equal to vein grafts remains a hope for the future. However, at present, the vast majority of patients can undergo durable autogenous tissue reconstruction in the infrainguinal area with the expectation of long-term limb viability.

REFERENCES

1. Dos Santos JC: Sur la desobstruction des thromboses artérielle anciennes. *Mem Acad Chir* 1944; 73:409–411.

2. Kunlin JL: Le traitement de l'artérite oblitérante par le greffe veineuse. *Arch Mal Coeur* 1949; 42:371–374.
3. Wylie EJ: Thromboendarterectomy for arteriosclerotic thrombosis of major arteries. *Surgery* 1952; 32:275–292.
4. Cannon JA, Barker WF, Kawakami IG: Femoral popliteal endarterectomy in the treatment of obliterative atherosclerotic disease. *Surgery* 1958; 43:76–93.
5. Meeker IA, Gross RE: Sterilization of frozen arterial grafts by high voltage cathode-ray irradiation. *Surgery* 1951; 29:19–28.
6. DeWeese JA, Woods WD, Dale WA: Failure of homografts as arterial replacements. *Surgery* 1959; 46:565.
7. Szilagyi DE, McDonald RT, Smith RF, et al: Biologic fate of human arterial homografts. *Arch Surg* 1957; 75:506.
8. Voorhees AB, Jaretzski A III, Blakemore AH: The use of tubes constructed from vinyon "N" cloth in bridging arterial defects: A preliminary report. *Am Surg* 1952; 135:332.
9. Edwards WS: Late occlusion of femoral and popliteal fabric arterial grafts. *Surg Gynecol Obstet* 1960; 10:714.
10. Dale WA, Mavor GE: Peripheral vascular grafts: Experimental comparison of autogenous veins, homologous arteries and synthetic tubes. *Br J Surg* 1959; 46:305.
11. Linton RR, Darling RC: Autogenous saphenous vein bypass grafts in femoropopliteal obliterative arterial disease. *Surgery* 1962; 51:62.
12. Palma EC: Treatment of arteritis of the lower limbs by autogenous grafts. *Minerva Cardioangiol Eur* 1960; 8:36.
13. Dale WA: Grafting small arteries. *Arch Surg* 1963; 86:36.
14. Mannick JA, Hume DM: Salvage of extremities by vein grafts in far-advanced peripheral vascular disease. *Surgery* 1964; 55:154–164.
15. Garrett HE, Kotch PI, Green J Jr, et al: Distal tibial artery bypass with autogenous vein grafts, analysis of 56 cases. *Surgery* 1968; 68:90.
16. Davis RC, Davies WT, Mannick JA: Bypass vein grafts in patients with distal popliteal artery occlusion. *Am J Surg* 1975; 129:421–425.
17. Reichle FA, Martinson MW, Rankin KP: Infrapopliteal arterial reconstruction in the severely ischemic lower extremity. *Ann Surg* 1980; 191:59–65.
18. Drake S, Lamont P, Chant A, et al: Femoro-popliteal versus femoro-distal bypass grafting for limb salvage in patients with an "isolated" popliteal segment. *Eur J Vasc Surg* 1989; 3:203–207.
19. Darling RC, Linton RR: Durability of femoropopliteal reconstructions, endarterectomy versus vein bypass grafts. *Am J Surg* 1972; 123:472–479.
20. Inahara T, Scott CM: Endarterectomy for segmental occlusive disease of the superficial femoral artery. *Arch Surg* 1981; 116:1547–1553.
21. Rosenberg D, Glass B, Rosenberg N, et al: Experiments with modified bovine carotid arteries in arterial surgery. *Surgery* 1970; 68:1064.
22. Dardik H, Ibrahim IM, Sprayregen S, et al: Clinical experience with modified human umbilical cord vein for arterial bypass. *Surgery* 1976; 79:618–624.
23. Miyata T, Tada Y, Takagi A, et al: A clinicopathologic study of aneruysm formation of glutareldehyde-tanned human umbilical vein grafts. *J Vasc Surg* 1989; 10:605–611.
24. Haimov H, Giron F, Jacobson JH: The expanded polytetrafluoroethylene grafts: Three years' experience with 362 grafts. *Arch Surg* 1979; 114:673.
25. Quinones-Baldrich WJ, Busuttil RW, Baker JD, et al: Is the preferential use of polytetrafluoroethylene grafts for femoropopliteal bypass justified? *J Vasc Surg* 1988; 8:219–228.
26. Veith FJ, Gupta SK, Ascer E, et al: Six year prospective multicenter randomized comparison of autologous saphenous vein and expanded polytetraflu-

oroethylene grafts in infrainguinal arterial reconstructions. *J Vasc Surg* 1986; 3:104–114.

27. Whittemore AD, Kent C, Donaldson MC, et al: What is the proper role of poly-tetrafluoroethylene grafts in infra-inguinal reconstruction. *J Vasc Surg* 1989; 10:299–305.

28. Miller JH, Foreman RK, Ferguson L, et al: Interposition vein cuff for anastomosis of prosthesis to small artery. *Aust N Z J Surg* 1984; 54:283–285.

29. Tyrrell MR, Chester JF, Vipond MN, et al: Experimental evidence to support the use of interposition vein collars/patches in distal PTFE anastomoses. *Eur J Vasc Surg* 1990; 4:95–101.

30. Leather RP, Powers SR, Karmody AM: A reappraisal of the in situ saphenous vein arterial bypass: Its use in limb salvage. *Surgery* 1979; 86:453–460.

31. Hall KV: The great saphenous vein used "in situ" as an arterial shunt after extirpation of vein valves. *Surgery* 1962; 51:492–495.

32. Barner NB, Judd D, Kaiser GC, et al: Late failure of arterialized in situ saphenous veins. *Arch Surg* 1969; 99:781.

33. Taylor LM, Edwards JM, Porter JM: Present status of reversed vein bypass grafting: Five year results of a modern series. *J Vasc Surg* 1990; 11:193–206.

34. Bandyk DF, Schmitt DD, Seabrook GR, et al: Monitoring functional patency of in situ saphenous vein bypasses: The impact of a surveillance protocol and elective revision. *J Vasc Surg* 1989; 9:286–296.

35. Donaldson MC, Mannick JA, Whittemore AD: Femoral-distal bypass with in situ greater saphenous vein. Long-term results using the Mills valvulotome. *Ann Surg* 1991; 213:457–465.

The In Situ Saphenous Vein Bypass: a 15-Year Experience

Robert P. Leather, M.D.

Professor of Surgery, Department of Vascular Surgery, Albany Medical College, Albany, New York

Benjamin B. Chang, M.D.

Assistant Professor of Surgery, Department of Vascular Surgery, Albany Medical College, Albany, New York

R. Clement Darling III, M.D.

Assistant Professor of Surgery, Department of Surgery, Albany Medical College, Albany, New York

Dhiraj M. Shah, M.D.

Professor of Surgery, Department of Vascular Surgery, Albany Medical College, Albany, New York

HISTORY

An in situ arterial bypass using the greater saphenous vein was first performed in 1959 by Rob and Kenyon at the suggestion of Karl Victor Hall, a visiting vascular fellow from Oslo, Norway. The saphenous vein was left in situ and the valves disrupted by an internal varicose vein stripper, thus rendering them incompetent. Although arterial flow was achieved at the distal end of the vein, the patency of this bypass was short-lived using the *valve fracture* technique. Although quickly abandoned by Rob and Kenyon, it was tried extensively in North America. The paper that had the greatest impact on this procedure was published by Barner and co-workers in 1969,[1] who compared their results with in situ bypass using the Rob fracture technique with those achieved with excised reversed vein grafts. The authors found a very high incidence of early failure and late stenosis in the in situ bypasses and concluded that the procedure was inferior to standard reversed vein bypass. Their paper, primarily because it reflected the experience at large with this technique, profoundly influenced the thinking of those interested in infrainguinal bypass and was largely responsible for bringing the concept of in situ bypass into disrepute and forestalling its further evaluation in North America. Thus, after the initial wave of enthusiasm in the early 1960s, in situ saphenous vein arterial bypass by the early valve fracture technique was almost universally abandoned because of venous endothelial injuries and poor results. Although the technique was at fault, it was abandoned without much effort to investigate the reasons for its failure.

Karl Victor Hall independently developed another method of performing an in situ bypass by excising the valve leaflets via a transverse venotomy in each valve sinus. This *valve excision* technique was reported in a series of 252 bypasses[2, 3] with acceptable results, but was ignored, perhaps because it was perceived to be too complex, tedious, time-consuming, and technically demanding. Thus, in the decade between its abandonment in 1969 and its resurrection by us in 1979,[4] there were only five surgical groups with any interest and experience in this technique.

With the advent of wider successful application of reversed saphenous vein bypass grafts to the tibial arteries, we returned in 1972 to the use of the saphenous vein in situ using the valve excision technique of Hall. In the course of struggling with this method and in spite of using ×3.5 operating loupes, visualization of the valve leaflets through the transverse venotomies proved to be difficult and taxing, because the leaflets are thin, flimsy, and transparent. When a leaflet was picked up with the scissor blades used to excise it, it was inevitably cut down the middle, which bisected it and rendered the valve incompetent. Thus, serendipitously, the technique of valve incision was discovered and its effectiveness rapidly became apparent.

INSTRUMENT EVOLUTION

Valve incision was originally achieved by use of scissors introduced through the open proximal end of the vein and, in more remote valve locations, by transverse venotomy at the valve site.[5] Subsequently, appropriate side branches proximal to the valve site were used in combination with specially designed narrow-shanked scissors to allow consistent and safe valve incision without injury to the vein (Fig 1).

Subsequently, the modification and adaptation of the valvulotome described by Mills eased the problem of gaining instrument access to valve sites by allowing valve incision from below (Fig 2). The valvulotome continues to be used by many groups in the open technique for the entire procedure with excellent results. However, in spite of this and the use of two operative teams, an inordinate amount of time was spent in the preparation of the thigh segment of the saphenous vein when left in situ. This portion of the vein is largest in diameter and usually not significantly tapered.

In an effort to combine the ease of instrumentation, thus expediting the procedure by minimizing the need for surgical exposure of the entire vein in the thigh and maintaining the proven increased operability, vein use, and patency rate of the method of valve incision, a precision injection-molded polystyrene intraluminal valve cutter was developed (Fig 3). This instrument achieves safe, consistent serial valve incision without mandatory exposure of each valve site. Making the instrument detachable allows its introduction *and* retrieval through the large proximal end of the saphenous vein. In addition, the cutter should only be used in the thigh portion of the vein where it can float freely in the larger vein, thereby minimizing the potential for endothelial injury. To provide both the functionally closed valve cusps for the blades to engage and a fluid medium for flotation of the valve cutter, a pressurized fluid column produced by a pneumatic transfusion cuff set at a safe pressure of 200 to

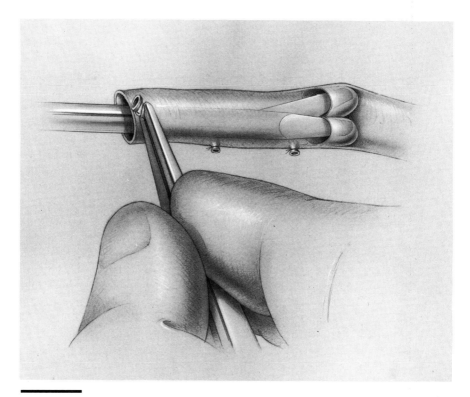

FIGURE 1.

Specially designed narrow-shank scissors with blunt tip for proximal valve incision.

300 mm Hg over a compliant plastic bag containing a dextran solution is delivered to a catheter attached directly to the cutter. This intraluminal valve cutter should be differentiated from others which are introduced and retrieved through the distal collapsed end of the vein with potential for venous injury reflected in 15% to 20% 30-day failure rates in veins less than 4 mm outer diameter (OD).[6]

Thus, all three types of instruments may be used in preparing the saphenous vein for an in situ bypass conduit. The scissors or antegrade valvulotome (Fig 4) may be introduced through the open proximal end of the vein to cut the valves down to the medial accessory branch. The valve cutter then incises valves in the mid- and distal thigh portion of the saphenous vein and the retrograde valvulotome lyses the remaining valves from the knee to the point of distal transection of the vein for anastomosis.

The evolution of instruments and constraints on their use to achieve valve incision were guided by an overriding concern for minimizing the potential for endothelial injury while producing an incompetent valve. Our data show that in the evolution of these in situ instruments[7] the patency was unchanged.

The use of preoperative venous anatomic assessment either by venography or duplex ultrasonography is not only advisable but mandatory, particularly if a valve cutter is to be used safely. A duplex ultrasonographic venous map provides the relevant information for the careful planning and execution of this procedure. Attempts to define anatomic variations at the time of surgery may result in excessive dissection, increasing the potential not only of injury to the vein but also of wound complications.

As more surgeons became involved in performing the in situ bypass, many introduced their own ideas of technique and instrumentation to simplify the procedure, but unfortunately at the expense of either patency or utilization of smaller veins.[6, 8]

These instruments (Hall, Cartier, LeMaitre, Bush, etc.) all utilize a cylindrical disruptor or cutter introduced through the distal divided end of the greater saphenous vein. Injury to the endothelial monolayer is produced primarily by the passage of these instruments retrograde along the wall of the distal, smaller end of the saphenous vein without the aid of distending intraluminal pressure. In addition, the frequency of missed valves is higher because of the increased likelihood of a valve leaflet being placed against the sinus wall.[9] Thus, results with these instruments, are satisfactory only in a high-flow situation (i.e., femoropopliteal) with larger (≥4 OD) veins. When applied to smaller veins, particularly when going to more distal tibial or pedal arteries, the importance of this degree of injury increases. In these distal bypasses, with their inherently lower flow volumes and velocities, these instruments exhibit an unacceptably high 30-day failure rate.

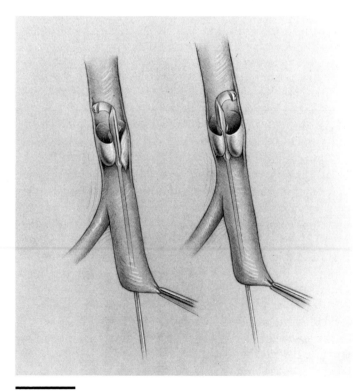

FIGURE 2.
Modified Mills retrograde valvulotome incises each valve cusp separately.

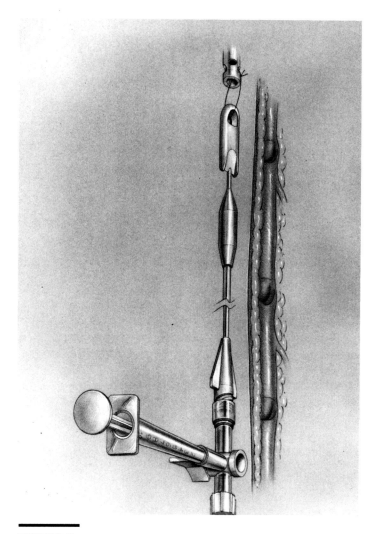

FIGURE 3.

Leather's injection-molded intraluminal valve cutter allows incision of both valve cusps at the same time. It can be used in the larger thigh portion of the saphenous vein without exposing the vein.

Therefore, although the use of these other techniques is simplistic and seductive, their inherent limitations make their applications hazardous, especially with smaller veins and more distal outflow tracts.

TECHNICAL PRINCIPLES

Technically, the crucial issue in using the greater saphenous vein in situ, and the primary reason for its excision and reversal for femoral-to-distal arterial bypass, is to remove the valvular obstruction to arterial flow and to control potential arteriovenous (AV) fistulas. All other considerations aside, leaving the saphenous vein in situ appears to be the most reliable method of achieving endothelial and vein wall preservation, provided the valves can be rendered incompetent without injury to the vein. In addi-

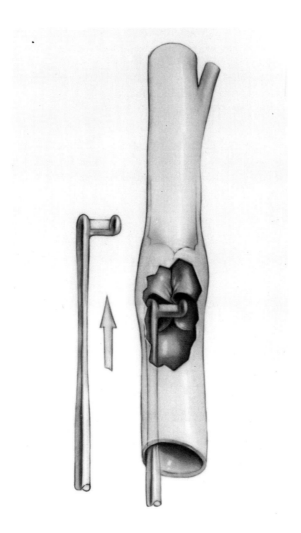

FIGURE 4.

Antegrade valvulotome, used also for proximal valve incisions.

tion, leaving the vein in situ requires both the interruption of those venous side branches, which may become AV fistulas when the vein is arterialized, and the minimal mobilization of its ends for construction of the proximal and distal anastomoses. The objective is to accomplish the vein preparation and anastomoses with a minimum of operative manipulation of the vein and especially of the endothelial surface, with particular avoidance of circumferential shear over a long segment. The simplest, most expedient, and least traumatic method of rendering the bicuspid venous valve incompetent is to cut the leaflets in the major axes, thus bisecting them. This is the essence of the valve incision technique.

A clear concept of venous valve function is important to better understand the problems encountered with valve lysis. The normal closing mechanism in a symmetric venous valve is initiated by tension along the leading edge of the valve leaflet caused by expansion of the valve sinus due to distention. This brings the edge of the leaflet toward the center of the lumen forcing it into the closed competent position. In any segment of vein where the valve is mechanically opened from below by passage of any instrument through it, the potential exists for a valve leaflet to be pushed against the wall and to remain temporarily adherent to it in the open position. This is most likely to occur in asymmetric valves, so that the valve may remain open for an indefinite period. The subsequent closure of a valve leaflet, either spontaneous or induced, by manipulation, e.g., by palpation of the pulse in the area, results in partial or even complete obstruction of arterial flow. Therefore, before the distal anastomosis is performed, deliberate attempts should be made to precipitate closure of any incompletely lysed valves by the following maneuver. With the distal vein open and free flow observed, or high flow via a fistula distally, a sponge is rolled along the in situ conduit from top to bottom or the vein is tapped gently. When the cutter is used, the most frequent location of a missed valve is in the junctional segment immediately distal to the point of the lowest cutter travel and the level of exposure of the vein. This segment should be checked routinely with the valvulotome for competency of the valve. An undiminished pulse can be transmitted through even an intact valve in a static hydraulic column.

The simple method of assessing flow from the distal divided end of the saphenous vein before construction of the distal anastomosis is very reliable in detecting any proximal hemodynamically significant lesions. If there is steady, undiminished pulsatile flow, it is unlikely that an obstructive lesion is present proximally.

Most branches of the saphenous vein drain the superficial subcutaneous tissue and their orifices are generally guarded by a competent valve, thus preventing flow away from the arterialized saphenous vein. Only valveless branches immediately become AV fistulas. However, these cutaneous branches are usually small and generally undergo spontaneous thrombosis postoperatively. This thrombosis is signaled by the development of a superficial phlebitis, the extent of which is determined by the size of the iatrogenic AV malformation. Although occasionally a large area of induration results, it is sterile and self-limiting and invariably resolves within a few days. Even if such superficial veins remain patent, the loss of distal arterial flow is generally small and does not threaten the continued patency of a bypass. As a rule, only branches with sufficient flow to visualize the deep venous system with radiopaque dye on the completion angiogram or with high flow by Doppler ultrasound need be ligated.

The effects of AV fistulas on in situ saphenous vein bypass hemodynamics and patency has been of great concern to some, even to the point of regarding these as a frequent cause of in situ bypass occlusion. On the other hand, there are opposing opinions, that AV fistulas help keep the bypass patent. From the onset more than 15 years ago, it has been our practice to ligate only large fistulas that are hemodynamically significant. Most of the residual subcutaneous iatrogenic AV malformations undergo spontaneous thrombosis. We have studied more than 600 such bypasses longitudinally using duplex ultrasonic scanning to assess overall hemodynamic function. The results indicate a steady reduction in fistula flow with no overall effect on distal perfusion (Fig 5). There is a small group of patients in whom high fistula flow is poorly tolerated, usually those

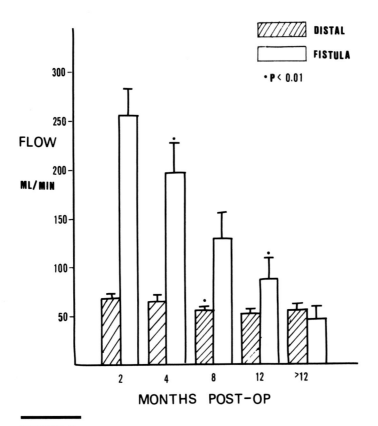

FIGURE 5.
Changes in fistula flow and distal bypass flow during the first 12 months after in situ bypass. Fistula has little effect on distal bypass flow.

with limited inflow capacity due to proximal stenosis or a small vein (<3 mm OD). In most patients, however, the flow capacity of the in situ conduit far exceeds the volume demanded by a fistula, thus allowing adequate, undiminished distal perfusion.

The allegation that fistulas are a potential cause of occlusive bypass failure has not proved true in our experience. The probable cause of failure in this setting is endothelial injury in the distal vein, the portion of the in situ conduit proximal to the fistula remaining patent because of flow to the fistula. For these reasons, we regard residual fistulas as, at most, an annoyance to the patient and the surgeon, but not as a crucial determinant of thrombosis of the bypass.

SURGICAL TECHNIQUE

After preparation and sterile draping of the entire extremity, warm (37° C) papaverine solution (60 mg/500 mL Plasmolyze or normal saline solution) is injected percutaneously into the subcutaneous tissue adjacent to the saphenous vein along its course below the knee. This is aided by duplex mapping of the vein. The proximal saphenous vein, which lies immediately deep to membranous superficial fascia, is then exposed, and papaverine solution is infiltrated into the surrounding tissue to minimize spasm (Fig 6).

Although the common femoral artery has been considered the proper site for proximal anastomosis of all distal bypasses, there is evidence that use of the unobstructed superficial femoral artery or the profunda femoris artery in the limb salvage patient population is equally satisfactory. Furthermore, technical circumstances such as a previous surgical scar or exposure of the common femoral artery or its encasement with circumferential calcification make either the deep femoral (profunda femoris) or the superficial femoral artery a valid alternative inflow source. In spite of its less accessible anatomic location, the deep femoral artery is usually less invested with thick or calcified plaque than either the common or superficial femoral artery and, therefore, frequently provides the most satisfactory site for proximal anastomosis.

The proximal operative field is best approached from the medial aspect by incision of the subcutaneous tissue immediately lateral to the saphenous vein down to the underlying investing myofascia. Dissection laterally in this fusion plane to the superficial femoral artery is bloodless. The fascia is incised over the superficial femoral artery and, if it is occluded, a segment of 3 to 5 cm can be excised, thus facilitating exposure of the deep femoral artery. If patent, a plane is developed between the femoral vein and the superficial femoral artery. The lateral circumflex femoral vein is often divided and the proximal deep femoral artery lies immediately deep to it.

The most satisfactory site of proximal anastomosis having been determined, the length of the proximal saphenous vein required to reach it

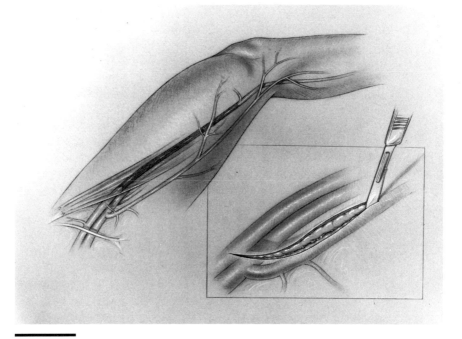

FIGURE 6.

The position of the greater saphenous vein and the proximal incision.

is known. If the common femoral artery is to be used as the inflow source, a complete dissection of the saphenous bulb and secure ligation of its branches are carried out. If additional length is required to facilitate anastomosis to the common femoral artery, a portion of the anterior aspect of the common femoral vein is removed in continuity with the saphenous bulb. The vein is closed using 6–0 nonabsorbable (Prolene) suture.

The valve leaflets at the saphenofemoral junction (first valve) are excised, removing only the transparent portion, leaving the usually prominent insertion ridge intact. The second valve, usually present 3 to 5 cm distal to the first, can be incised easily with a retrograde valvulotome through a side branch distal to the valve before the vein is divided, or alternatively cut either with scissors or an antegrade valvulotome through the open end of the vein after division, as is the valve immediately distal to the medial accessory branch. These valves are identified by gently distending the vein through its open end with dextran solution and are cut with special scissors while the valve is held in the functionally closed position by fluid trapped between the open end of the saphenous vein and the valve with the thumb and index finger around the shank of the scissors.

The plane of closure of the valve cusps is invariably parallel to the skin. This dictates the orientation of all instruments with relation to the valve cusps.

If a valve cutter cannot be used, the location of the next valve site is determined by advancing a 6F soft catheter, the infusion running through it under 200-mm Hg pressure, until it impacts in the valve sinus. This location is marked on the skin and the proximal anastomosis is carried out. The saphenous vein is thus initially arterialized. The rest of the vein is exposed and the valves are incised using the retrograde valvulotome via a branch of sufficient length distal to the valve (open method).

If the cutter is to be used, a 3- to 5-cm incision is made 5 mm posterior to the position of the main saphenous vein below the knee which has been marked preoperatively on the skin. Identifying a predetermined branch and using it to gain access to the lumen of the saphenous vein is done without disturbing the saphenous vein itself. A no. 3 Fogarty catheter is introduced into the saphenous vein through this side branch and passed proximally with the leg straightened to exit through the open end of the vein. The catheter is then divided at an acute angle at the 20- or 30-cm mark, whichever is closer to the open end of the vein. The intraluminal valve cutter (2 or 3 mm in diameter) is screwed onto the catheter and a 6F or 8F catheter is then secured to the cutter with a loop of fine suture.

The leading cylinder of the cutter is drawn into the vein, providing a partial obturator obstruction to venous flow while permitting visualization of the cutting blade and minimal resistance in torque, thus allowing precise orientation of the cutting edges at 90 degrees to the plane of closure of the valves, i.e., to the plane of the overlying skin surface. The catheter-cutter assembly is then drawn slowly distally while the dextran solution (500 mL of dextran 70 containing 1,000 units of heparin and 120 mg of papaverine) is introduced through the catheter at 200 to 300-mm Hg pressure with a pressure seal provided by a 1-mm Silastic vessel loop

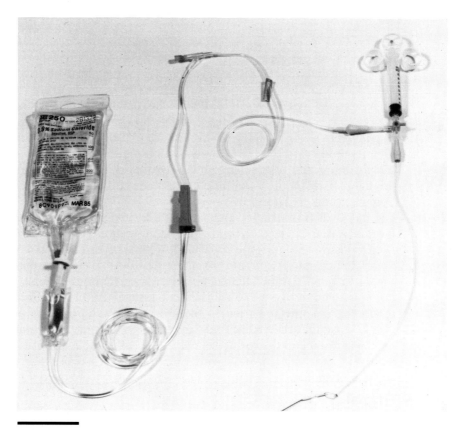

FIGURE 7.

The vein is distended and the valve cusps are rendered closed by the dextran-heparin-papaverine solution introduced from a plastic bag via a soft catheter.

secured by a small hemostat around the most proximal end of the saphenous vein (Fig 7). This pressurized fluid column snaps each successive valve to the closed position so that the cusps are efficiently engaged by the blades of the cutter. A slight but definite resistance is felt as the cutter encounters each valve and cuts the leaflets. Greater resistance than this should be managed by turning the cutter through 45 degrees and making another attempt at advancement. If this does not produce the desired result, the cutter should be withdrawn, dismounted, and the area of impaction exposed directly. The amount of allowable resistance can be learned only by experience.

The cutter is advanced to a predetermined safe distance, generally to the knee joint level, and is then withdrawn to the femoral exposure. It may be desirable to pass the cutter twice at a slightly different orientation. The cutter is dismounted and the catheter removed from the saphenous vein. Proximal anastomosis of the saphenous vein to the selected inflow artery is performed end to side using 6–0 or 7–0 Prolene suture with a continuous parachute technique; the pulsatile impulse thus provided makes the location of the next competent valve, usually below the knee, readily apparent.

The remaining valves are incised by a retrograde valvulotome introduced through a side branch or the distal end of the vein. In passing the valvulotome intraluminally to and from a valve site, it is important that any pressure on the vein wall resulting from its curving path be exerted on the shaft of the instrument rather than on the projecting blade tip. This lessens the likelihood of the blade becoming lodged in the side branch and lacerating the vein wall. This instrument is so designed that it engages a leaflet, centers itself, and cuts the leaflet in its longitudinal axis. It is then readvanced, carefully rotated through 180 degrees, and withdrawn, thus engaging the remaining leaflet. However, before the cutting force is applied to the tip of the valvulotome, it should be maneuvered toward the center of the vein lumen by depression of the vein itself, allowing division of the remaining leaflet without the risk of entering a side branch, which is invariably present, close to all valve sinuses. The anterior valve cusp is usually incised first. One set of valves should be incised at a time to make it completely incompetent.

Unobstructed pulsatile arterial flow is thus brought to the desired level. Before transection and mobilization of the distal vein, exposure of the anticipated outflow anastomotic site is carried out. This is desirable not only to minimize the warm ischemia time of the endothelium but also to assess the appropriate length required, always allowing an additional 1 to 2 cm so that the manipulated and thus traumatized terminal portion can be excised and discarded. The distal anastomosis is completed using a 70 or 80 Prolene continuous suture with parachute technique in an end-to-side manner.

After completion of the distal anastomosis, flow in the bypass as well as the outflow vessel is confirmed and a quantitative appraisal is made by the use of the sterile Doppler ultrasonic probe. A completion angiogram is then performed with radiopaque reference markers (19-gauge needles in their plastic containers attached to the skin by sterile adhesive strips, a radiologic strip marker, or skin clips) to correlate the roentgenographic position of the fistulas with the surface anatomy. With increasing experience with quantitative Doppler analysis, the on-table angiogram is done less frequently in our institution when there is any question.

RESULTS

Among more than 2,000 patients in whom the ipsilateral greater saphenous vein was present requiring a distal arterial reconstruction for limb preservation, an in situ bypass was attempted in more than 95%. Of these, less than 6% could not undergo reconstruction by the in situ technique in toto. However, half of these operations were successfully completed with segments of autogenous vein grafts (a partial in situ bypass). Life table analysis of secondary patency of bypasses for all patients is shown in Table 1. The results of popliteal in situ bypasses are shown in Table 2 and tibial bypasses in Table 3. Patient demographics are shown in Table 4. Most bypasses were done for limb salvage (Table 5). A majority of bypasses were carried down to an infrapopliteal artery (Table 6).

Early detection of stenoses and correction of defects with in situ conduits before occlusion occurs can be achieved by a comprehensive surveillance program. Our patients are seen and examined every 3 to 4

TABLE 1.
Total in Situ Bypasses — Secondary Patency

Interval (Mo)	Bypasses at Risk	Occlusions	Interval Patency	Cumulative Patency
1−1	1,853	72	0.958	0.958
2−12	1,512	66	0.947	0.907
13−24	913	26	0.967	0.877
25−36	638	13	0.976	0.856
37−48	431	16	0.958	0.820
49−60	309	6	0.977	0.801
61−72	213	5	0.973	0.780
73−84	148	4	0.968	0.755
85−96	98	1	0.988	0.745
97−108	66	2	0.964	0.719
109−120	44	2	0.944	0.679

months up to the second year, and every 6 months thereafter. Each examination includes pulse volume recordings and segmental pressures and audible Doppler assessment along the course of the bypass. Direct visualization of the conduit and estimates of volume flow by duplex ultrasonic scanning, both at rest and after reactive hyperemia induced by 3 minutes of tourniquet occlusion, have been used for evaluation.

Among 1,853 in situ conduits constructed, 110 stenotic lesions developed in 88 patients. More than 70% of these occurred within the first 12 months (82/110). Thirty-seven occurred in the distal mobilized segment; 34 in the proximal mobilized segment, and 39 in the midportion of the bypass conduit. Stenotic lesions tend to occur with increased frequency in smaller veins, 45 (10%) occurring in 470 veins of 3.0 mm or

TABLE 2.
Popliteal in Situ Bypasses — Secondary Patency

Interval (Mo)	Bypasses at Risk	Occlusions	Interval Patency	Cumulative Patency
0−1	577	24	0.956	0.956
2−12	490	19	0.954	0.912
13−24	318	9	0.968	0.883
25−36	244	2	0.990	0.875
37−48	167	8	0.947	0.829
49−60	129	3	0.973	0.806
61−72	87	3	0.959	0.773
73−84	57	2	0.961	0.743
85−96	43	0	1.000	0.743
97−108	31	2	0.929	0.690
109−120	23	0	1.000	0.690

TABLE 3.
Tibial in Situ Bypasses—Secondary Patency

Interval (Mo)	Bypasses at Risk	Occlusions	Interval Patency	Cumulative Patency
0–1	1276	48	0.959	0.959
2–12	1022	47	0.944	0.905
13–24	595	17	0.966	0.874
25–36	394	11	0.967	0.846
37–48	264	8	0.965	0.816
49–60	180	3	0.981	0.800
61–72	126	2	0.982	0.785
73–84	91	2	0.973	0.764
85–96	55	1	0.978	0.747
97–108	35	0	1.000	0.747
109–120	21	2	0.889	0.664

less as compared with 45 (3%) in 1,338 veins of 3.5 mm or larger. All of these stenoses were treated operatively by vein patch angioplasty and all but five remained patent beyond 30 days. There were 97 (5%) residual AV fistulas that required ligation under local anesthesia 3 days to 54 months after the initial procedure. There were 85 occlusions within 30 days (immediate patency rate, 96%) and 69 deaths in the same period (operative mortality, 3.7%).

DISCUSSION

Femoral-to-infrapopliteal bypasses using greater saphenous vein in situ (long bypasses) have shown excellent results in long-term follow-up. For such bypasses there is general agreement that autogenous vein is the best conduit. Although there are some reports of acceptable patency using excised greater or lesser saphenous vein in the infrainguinal positions,, many of these bypasses were short and were done for lesser indications.[6, 9] We strongly believe that for long distal bypasses the in situ technique attributes its potential benefit by a tapering conduit, physiologic

TABLE 4.
Demographics of Patients Undergoing in Situ
Bypasses (n = 1,853)

Males 1,190 (64%)
Females 663 (36%)
Diabetic patients 963 (52%)
Smokers 702 (38%)
Average age = 68 yr (range, 12–99 yr)

TABLE 5.
Indications for in Situ Bypass

Indication	n
Claudication	93
Microembolism	30
Gangrene	159
Nonhealing ulcer	185
Rest pain	576
Gangrene with rest pain	342
Ulcer with rest pain	401
Blunt trauma	6
Penetrating trauma	15
Operative trauma	4
Aneurysm	39
Invasive foot infection	3
Total	1,853

preservation of venous endothelium and wall, and minimal trauma to the vein.

Furthermore, while there is controversy regarding the technique of in situ bypass, in our opinion it is immaterial what technique is used as long as certain principles of this operation are adhered to. The valves of the vein must be made incompetent with a minimum of trauma, and circumferential injury to the vein should be avoided.[10] A minimal amount of vein should be mobilized before arterialization, and hemodynamically significant fistulas should be ligated. Any technique which avoids these injurious processes should be successful in performing in situ arterial bypasses.

TABLE 6.
In Situ Bypasses—Sites of Distal Anastomosis (All Indications)

Above-knee popliteal	48
Below-knee popliteal	529
Tibioperoneal trunk	53
Proximal anterior tibial	40
Midanterior tibial	146
Distal anterior tibial	98
Dorsalis pedis	124
Proximal posterior tibial	241
Distal posterior tibial	106
Proximal peroneal	373
Distal peroneal	95

In situ bypasses require careful preparation. Merely retaining the saphenous vein in situ does not substitute for sustained care, patience, and attention to detail as well as consistent, meticulous surgical technique aided by optical magnification. Before attempting to adopt this technique, a surgeon should see it performed by an experienced operating team. In addition, familiarity with the use and feel of all instruments should be gained, perhaps ex vivo on discarded valve-bearing vein segments.

In conclusion, in situ saphenous vein arterial bypass has provided excellent results in long-term follow-up in spite of long bypasses, compromised outflow tracts, and various patient risk factors.

REFERENCES

1. Barner HB, Judd DR, Kaiser GC, et al: Late failure of arteriologic "in situ" saphenous vein. *Arch Surg* 1969; 99:781.
2. Hall KV: The greater saphenous vein used "in-situ" as an arterial shunt after vein valve extirpation. *Acta Chir Scand* 1964; 128:245–257.
3. Hall KV, Rostad H: In situ vein bypass in the treatment of femoro-popliteal atherosclerotic disease: A ten year study. *Am J Surg* 1978; 136:158.
4. Leather RP, Powers SR, Karmody AM: A reappraisal of the "in-situ" saphenous vein arterial bypass. *Surgery* 1979; 86:453–460.
5. Leather RP, Corson JD, Karmody AM: Instrumental evolution of the valve incision method of "in-situ" saphenous vein bypass. *J Vasc Surg* 1984; 1:113–123.
6. Moody AP, Edwards PR, Harris PL: In situ versus reversed femoropopliteal vein grafts: Long-term follow-up of a prospective, randomized trail. *Br J Surg* 1992; 79:750–752.
7. Leather RP, Shah DM, Chang BB, et al: Resurrection of the in situ saphenous vein bypass: 1000 cases later. *Ann Surg* 1988; 208:435.
8. Gruss JD, Bartels D, Vargas H, et al: Arterial reconstruction for distal disease of the lower extremities by the in-situ vein graft technique. *J Cardiovasc Surg* 1982; 23:231–234.
9. Harris PL, How TV, Jones DR: Propsective randomized clinical trial to compare in situ and reversed saphenous vein grafts for femoropopliteal bypass. *Br J Surg* 1987; 74:252–255.
10. Parent FN III, Gandhi R, Wheeler JR, et al: Angioscopic evaluation of valvular disruption during in situ saphenous vein bypass. *Ann Vasc Surg*, 1994; 8:24–30.

Infrapopliteal Short Vein Graft Bypass

Kurt R. Wengerter, M.D.

Assistant Professor of Surgery, Albert Einstein College of Medicine, Montefiore Medical Center, Bronx, New York

Ross T. Lyon, M.D.

Assistant Professor of Surgery, Jack D. Weiler Hospital of the Albert Einstein College of Medicine, Bronx, New York

Frank J. Veith, M.D.

Professor of Surgery, Albert Einstein College of Medicine, Chief of Vascular Surgery, Montefiore Medical Center, Bronx, New York

T he common femoral artery is the chosen site for graft origin in the majority of limbs requiring bypass to the infrapopliteal arteries for limb-threatening lower extremity ischemia. The large percentage of patients with occlusive disease of the superficial femoral and popliteal arteries makes this the appropriate choice. As a result, long segments of vein, 50 to 95 cm in length, are frequently needed for these bypass procedures. However, when disease of the femoral and popliteal vessels is minimal or absent, an alternative exists. A shorter bypass graft to a distal vessel can be performed, with inflow from the *popliteal* or *tibial* vessel. Benefits of a short bypass graft include the ability to be more selective of the segment of vein used, and the ability to perform a vein graft bypass when autogenous vein is limited. The primary concern about these grafts, however, has been the risk of disease progression of the inflow tract. Development of a significant stenosis or occlusion of the femoral, popliteal, and in some cases the tibial arteries, can cause graft failure. If the frequency and rate of disease progression in the inflow arteries surpasses the rate and frequency of disease occurring in the length of vein graft needed to bypass these arteries, then the short vein graft bypass would be at a distinct disadvantage.

HISTORIC PERSPECTIVE

Since the first report describing the lower extremity vein graft bypass some 45 years ago, the preferred site of origin for these bypass grafts has traditionally been the common femoral artery. This vessel is not only the most proximal vessel in the leg and typically easy to access, it is also relatively free of disease, especially on its anterior aspect. Indeed, the high frequency of disease in the superficial femoral artery has made use of the common femoral as the site of graft origin necessary in most cases. Since

Advances in Vascular Surgery, vol 2
© 1994, Mosby–Year Book, Inc.

early lower extremity bypass procedures were performed to bypass superficial femoral artery occlusive disease, the use of a more distal inflow site was usually not an issue. In addition, when a sufficient length of vein was not available, or if the vein was of poor quality, a readily available alternative existed: Dacron, and later, polytetrafluoroethylene, served as prosthetic graft materials. While results with these prosthetic grafts for femoropopliteal bypass were generally not quite as good as vein, acceptable patency and limb salvage were achieved,[1-3] especially at the above-knee position. As the distal limits of revascularization were later extended beyond the popliteal artery, and longer vein grafts were required, the availability of vein became a more significant limiting factor. Prosthetic graft material was not an attractive alternative for routine use in bypass grafts to distal vessels when sufficient vein was not available. Autogenous vein was strongly preferred because of significantly better patency.[1] Thus, alternative approaches were needed to help meet the increasing requirements for vein to revascularize more distal vessels.

A number of ways exist to extend the use of the vein, especially when a limited amount of acceptable vein is available. Commonly, alternative vein sources are utilized when the amount of greater saphenous vein is limited. These include the lesser saphenous, cephalic, or basilic veins. Over 20 years ago, Linton and Wilde[4] described techniques for the management of a small-diameter proximal segment of reversed vein graft, which limits the amount of adequate-size vein available. One approach involved patching the proximal superficial femoral artery with an elongated anastomosis, in effect patching a segment of the superficial femoral artery. Another technique described placement of a vein patch on the artery, with the proximal anastomosis of the bypass placed at the lower end of the patch. Both techniques resulted in a shorter bypass graft by the use of a form of patch angioplasty, with the graft being shortened by the length of the patch. They represent an early approach to shortening the bypass graft to accommodate a lack of sufficient good-quality vein.

In cases where alternative, more distal inflow sites are available, it is often possible to place a shorter bypass graft, thereby using the *minimal* amount of vein necessary for the bypass. This is possible only when vessels distal to the common femoral artery remain patent. One of the earliest techniques for placing a short bypass graft was use of the profunda femoris artery as the inflow site. This was reported as early as 1964,[5] and a number of studies later appeared in the 1970s[6-8] confirming the usefulness of this inflow site. In these reports, the primary indication for placement of the graft origin in the profunda was the avoidance of a scarred or infected groin. Many of these grafts were placed below an aortobifemoral bypass graft and were considered a useful alternative to anastomosis to the limb of the aortobifemoral graft, since the approach to the profunda did not require dissection through the prior wound, or exposure of the graft, with the associated risk of infection. One group,[7] however, reported that in a third of their cases the shorter bypass was necessitated by a limited amount of available vein. They concluded that this technique had the added benefit of reducing the length of vein needed. We have also found the profunda femoris artery useful for bypass graft inflow for similar reasons.[9] Our results with the use of the mid- and distal segments of the profunda femoris artery for the proximal anastomosis in bypasses to the popliteal as well as distal arteries demonstrated that even the more distal portions of this vessel could be used successfully. In addition, the bypass grafts we reported were performed not only for secondary procedures but also for primary procedures when the length of available vein was limited.

As strides were made in the performance of more distal bypass procedures primarily for the limb salvage objective, surgical techniques and expertise in handling these smaller vessels in the ankle and foot improved. As a result, in the late 1970s and early 1980s, more and more *distal* bypass procedures were performed to treat occlusive disease of the infrapopliteal vessels. Bypasses to ankle and pedal arteries became common, and grafts 85 to 95 cm in length were routinely used. In turn, this allowed a greater number of diabetic patients with distal disease to be treated. In these patients, the superficial femoral, popliteal, and even proximal portions of the tibial and peroneal vessels were frequently patent, while extensive occlusive disease of the tibial arteries produced the limb-threatening lesions. Thus, a more distal site of origin for the bypass graft, with unobstructed inflow, was possible. In many cases the use of more distal vessels for graft origin was out of necessity: limited availability of autologous vein, previous surgical scarring, the presence of infection, or severe obesity prevented the use of the common femoral, and in some cases even the superficial femoral arteries. The ability to use a shorter bypass made the use of autogenous vein feasible in these cases.

Our initial success with superficial femoral artery inflow sites, as well as the need to treat patients with secondary bypass grafts and more limited sources of vein, led to the use of the popliteal vessels for graft inflow. In 1981, we reported results demonstrating a satisfactory outcome with inflow from arteries distal to the common femoral.[10] It became apparent that the use of shorter vein grafts also allowed a greater degree of selection of the segment of vein to be used, and obviated the need to use diseased or small-diameter portions of available vein which could lower patency rates.[11–12] An added advantage was the avoidance of wounds in the groin and thigh in many cases, as well as an overall reduction in the length of the vein harvest wounds required.

Others have also found the superficial femoral and popliteal arteries to be valuable inflow sites. In 1986, Cantelmo et al.[13] reported 32 arterial reconstructive procedures performed between 1976 and 1984 in which a vessel below the common femoral artery was used for inflow. Selection for these cases was based on the absence of a hemodynamically significant superficial femoral or popliteal artery lesion above the level of the proximal anastomosis, and the finding of a palpable popliteal pulse. In 16 procedures the distal superficial femoral or proximal popliteal artery was used, and in another 16 the distal popliteal was used. The distal anastomosis was at the infrapopliteal level in all cases. The authors reported 79% graft patency at 3 years, and a limb salvage rate of 82%. They found that the site of origin of the proximal anastomosis did not affect graft patency, and in only one case was progression of disease in the inflow vessels found to place patency of the bypass graft at risk.[13] In 1983 Schuler et al.[14] also reported an experience with the use of bypass grafts originating from the distal superficial femoral and popliteal arteries. A follow-up study by this group in 1988[15] reported long-term results with 49 bypasses from the superficial femoral in 12% and the popliteal artery in 88% of cases. In 80% of cases the distal anastomosis was to a distal tibial vessel. They found a 1-year graft patency of 83%, and a 5-year patency of 41%, while the limb salvage rate was 69% at 6 years. These early reports were later confirmed by data from our group[16] and others.[17] All demonstrated the utility of arterial reconstructions originating below the common femoral artery.

Our favorable experience with inflow from the popliteal artery led us to use even more distal vessels for inflow, and we began to utilize infrapopliteal vessels as inflow in selected cases.[18] In 1982, the report by Danza[19] was the first documentation of the use of infrapopliteal vessels for the origin of distal bypass procedures. Our initial experience, reported in 1985,[18] demonstrated that this procedure was feasible and useful. In the 14 cases reported, we found graft patency to be 70% at 3 years, and an amputation (below the knee) was needed in only one case. These early reports, as well as our most recent data,[20] have established that these very short tibial-distal grafts provide good graft patency and limb salvage, and support the conclusions of the popliteal-distal studies that the outcome with short vein grafts was at least comparable to long distal grafts.

PREOPERATIVE ASSESSMENT

The patient with tibial occlusive disease and limb-threatening ischemia is initially considered as a candidate for a popliteal–distal artery bypass on the basis of a palpable popliteal pulse. The presence of a strong popliteal pulse indicates a significant stenosis of the inflow vessels is not likely. This must be confirmed by an arteriogram, since significant stenoses and occlusions can be found proximal to a pulse when the collateral circulation is good, especially in the presence of poor outflow due to the tibial occlusions. The arteriogram is performed to completely evaluate vessels providing inflow to the graft, including the infrarenal aorta, the iliac arteries, the common and superficial femoral arteries, the popliteal artery, and the proximal tibial vessels. Special attention must be placed on evaluating the proximal superficial femoral artery. At its origin there is frequently overlap on the arteriogram with the deep femoral artery. A stenosis at this point can easily be missed if special views are not obtained to visualize the origin of these two vessels separately. This is achieved by taking an oblique image of the groin, to "open up" the bifurcation of the common femoral artery.[21]

Of course, the tibial and pedal vessels also must be seen well to determine the appropriate site for the distal anastomosis. With proper attention placed on the details of performing the arteriogram, including the optimal rate and volume of contrast injection, as well as the timing of the images after injection, good visualization of the tibial and pedal arteries can routinely be obtained.[21] As a result, we have not had to rely on intraoperative prebypass arteriography for visualization of the distal vessels.

Once the arteriogram is performed, it usually becomes clear whether a short vein graft bypass can be performed. If there is no significant stenosis of the inflow vessels, we would preferentially perform a popliteal—distal artery bypass. If a tibial vessel is also patent proximally in the calf, and the vein available for the bypass is severely limited, then a tibial artery—tibial artery bypass should be performed. Another reason for moving the proximal anastomosis to the tibial artery is the presence of scarring or infection in the popliteal region making access to the popliteal artery difficult or unsafe. In general, if sufficient vein is available, the popliteal artery below the knee is preferred since this vessel is easily approached, it is larger, and the anastomosis is technically easier than one to a smaller tibial vessel.

PROXIMAL STENOSIS

The decision to utilize the short popliteal-distal bypass becomes more difficult when there is disease present in the femoral or popliteal vessels. One must then determine the significance of these stenoses on the basis of the arteriogram. Pressure cannot be reliably measured during the arteriogram since the catheter would have to traverse the stenosis and falsely elevate the reading. Thus, visual assessment of the stenosis with estimation of the degree of luminal narrowing must be used to determine its significance. The presence of a mild stenosis, or even several mild stenoses in the common femoral or superficial femoral arteries, has not been found to reduce graft patency in this group of bypass grafts. Rosenbloom et al.[21] found that a stenosis of 20% or less did not decrease graft patency in their review of 49 bypasses originating from the distal superficial femoral and popliteal arteries. Our review[15] of 153 nonsequential popliteal—distal artery bypass grafts also demonstrated that placement of the bypass below some degree of stenosis was acceptable. In fact, placement of the graft below a stenosis of up to 35% diameter narrowing was not found to decrease graft patency. In 56 procedures where the proximal superficial femoral or popliteal artery had a stenosis of up to 20%, graft patency was found to be similar to patency in a group of 20 grafts placed below a 21% to 35% stenosis. Placement of the graft below an untreated stenosis of greater than 35% does decrease patency, and we found the 2-year primary patency of 18 grafts placed below a stenosis of 36% to 50% was only 53% ($P = .25$).[15]

The relatively safe use of an inflow vessel distal to a stenosis in the thigh is consistent with the findings of Walsh et al.[22] who studied the natural history of superficial femoral stenoses with both arteriography and duplex ultrasonography. In the 45 arteries that were analyzed, the mean stenosis progression rate was only 4.5% per year. Of those that ultimately went on to occlusion of the superficial femoral artery, the mean rate of progression was 12% per year, with the maximum rate at 30% per year. This would suggest that follow-up of the graft and the inflow tract with duplex ultrasonography performed at standard intervals would be able to detect progression to a critical stenosis. Of note, diabetes mellitus, highly prevalent in those patients undergoing short vein graft distal bypasses, was not associated with an increased rate of progression.

ANGIOPLASTY

If a significant stenotic lesion of the iliac vessels is found proximal to an intended lower extremity bypass, usually an angioplasty of that vessel is performed. If the lesion is not severe, a pressure measurement is taken above and below the stenosis. If a gradient of more than 10 to 15 mm Hg is found, angioplasty is indicated. Pressures are also measured after the angioplasty is performed. If a gradient greater than 15 to 20 mm Hg persists after angioplasty, or if the stenosis is recurrent, a Palmaz intraluminal stent (Johnson & Johnson) is usually placed.

Whether a distal bypass graft is to be performed or not, a stenosis of the superficial femoral or popliteal artery can be successfully treated with angioplasty, especially if the lesion is short and nonocclusive. If the initial failure rate, which can range from 10% to 50%, is excluded, the 1-year patency of the superficial femoral and popliteal arteries is about 80%, and the 3-year patency is approximately 60%, with the best results occurring in short (<3 cm) nonocclusive lesions.[23–25] We have treated patients with ischemia and gangrene or rest pain with angioplasty of the superficial femoral or popliteal arteries, even if there was evidence of multilevel disease. In cases where the gangrene is limited, or when there are very discrete chronic ulcerations, we have found this approach to be useful, especially when the amount of vein is known to be limited, or the patient is a poor risk for surgery.

The results of the angioplasty must be monitored closely, and if the segmental pressures and pulse volume amplitude do not increase sufficiently, more invasive treatments, such as bypass, are performed. If angioplasty is successful and calf pressures and pulse amplitudes increase but ankle or foot measurements do not increase substantially, the ischemic lesions are not likely to heal, and a bypass procedure must be considered. In this circumstance, a short vein graft bypass from the popliteal artery distal to the angioplasty site can be performed. We have reviewed our own experience with the placement of a short vein graft bypass below angioplasty of the superficial femoral or popliteal artery in 19 cases.[15] The degree of luminal narrowing ranged from 24% to 85%, and all lesions were reportedly less than 3 cm in length. None of the vessels treated by angioplasty were occluded. In 9 of these cases the patient underwent bypass surgery within 10 days of the angioplasty, for a mean of 5.7 days of observation after the angioplasty. In the remaining 10 cases a longer period of observation or delay occurred, from 2 weeks to 7 months, or an average of 2.4 months. In the latter group, the longer period of delay was due to observation of the ischemic lesions for healing as a result of the angioplasty alone. When healing did not occur, the bypass procedure was performed. We believe this period of observation has allowed us to select out angioplasty failures. Indeed, this is an important concern since reportedly 73% of angioplasty failures occur in the first month.[26] With this selection process, the resulting patency rate of those short vein graft bypass grafts placed below angioplasty-treated superficial femoral and popliteal artery stenoses was similar to grafts placed without proximal stenotic lesions.[15] An added benefit of the placement of the graft below an angioplasty may be the increased runoff through the treated vessel which may have a protective effect on patency of the angioplasty site. Jeans et al.[26] have shown that the best angioplasty results occur when there is adequate runoff; when there are no patent calf vessels to provide outflow from the popliteal artery below the angioplasty, a much lower patency rate is seen.[26] Since the short vein graft bypass typically increases flow through the superficial femoral and popliteal arteries, it may also increase angioplasty patency.

INTRAOPERATIVE ASSESSMENT

If the pulse at the proximal anastomsis site of the short vein graft distal bypass intraoperatively is noted to be weak either *prior to* or *after* the performance of the bypass graft, a pressure measurement at the proximal anastomosis must be carried out. This involves puncture of the vessel at the hood of the anastomosis with insertion of a "butterfly" needle. The catheter is connected to the anesthesiologist's pressure transducer and the pressure is measured after calibration of the setup. This measurement is compared to the "systemic" pressure measurement, which usually is monitored via a radial artery line. If a pressure gradient of more than 10 to 12 mm Hg is measured between the site of the proximal anastomosis and the radial artery, further investigation for the cause should be performed. In most cases the cause of the gradient can be deduced from the preoperative arteriogram. Usually a stenotic lesion will be present. If the cause is not evident, and the gradient is sufficiently high to warrant immediate therapy, then a pressure measurement at the common femoral artery level should be obtained. This is performed either by passing a catheter proximally from the popliteal anastomosis under fluoroscopic control, or by transcutaneous puncture of the femoral artery.

If the gradient is localized to the superficial femoropopliteal artery segment, then the decision must be made whether this is to be treated. Essentially three options exist. First, an inflow procedure from the common femoral artery to the distal graft could be performed, either with vein or prosthetic graft material. This converts the bypass into a sequential graft. This option is preferred when the gradient is high, although proper preoperative assessment reduces the likelihood of this event. The second option would be to perform an intraoperative angioplasty. This works when the occlusive lesion is short. To perform intraoperative angioplasty, adequate visualization of the lesion is necessary, and fluoroscopy must be used. Alternatively, duplex scan evaluation utilizing an ultrasound angioplasty catheter localization system (Echocath, New Brunswick, N.J.) of the angioplasty catheter can be used, although intraoperative experience is limited.[27] Typically, the lesion can be dilated with a Tegwire (Boston Scientific, Boston) angioplasty catheter. This is a relatively short angioplasty catheter which includes the guidewire on its tip, thus simplifying the procedure. A completion arteriogram of the angioplasty-treated vessel is usually performed to confirm restoration of the lumen. The third alternative would be to not treat the stenosis, but to observe or to perform a percutaneous angioplasty postoperatively. Ideally, this should be used only when the gradient is relatively mild (<20 mm Hg). If observation or delayed angioplasty is chosen, usually for reasons of inexperience with angioplasty, lack of appropriate equipment, or the intra-operative condition of the patient, postoperative anticoagulation should be considered, especially when the gradient is greater than 20 mm Hg.

If the gradient is localized to vessels proximal to the femoral artery, the options are similar: bypass, intraoperative angioplasty, or observation with possible postoperative percutaneous angioplasty.[28] The unexpected need for an inflow bypass to treat a gradient should be rare since the pre-operative assessment should thoroughly evaluate and aggressively treat lesions in the iliac arteries. Intraoperative or postoperative angioplasty or stent placement remains the most attractive choice if a significant iliac stenosis is present. It should be noted that on occasion we have found a gradient between the femoral artery and the radial artery which was *not* associated with an iliac lesion. In this circumstance, passage of a cath-eter from the femoral artery proximally into the aorta will allow more ac-curate determination of the pressure gradient across the iliac arteries. Thus, a falsely elevated radial artery catheter reading may be responsible for a gradient found when the radial artery is used for measurement of systemic pressure and compared to pressure in the femoral artery.

GRAFT MATERIAL

As with other distal arterial bypass grafts, ipsilateral greater saphenous vein is the graft material of choice for short vein graft infrapopliteal re-constructions. Ideally, the vein segment should be harvested from the lower leg (calf) to incorporate the arterial exposure incisions, thus mini-mizing the total length of the incisions. An important advantage of the short vein graft bypass is that the surgeon may be more selective in choos-ing the portion of vein to be used for the graft. If only 30 to 40 cm of vein are needed, one can be selective with the segment taken from the 80- or 90-cm total length of greater saphenous vein available. Segments of the vein containing calcification, thickened walls, or fibrotic stenoses are known to increase the risk of failure[12] and the ability to *completely* ex-clude these areas helps to maximize graft patency. Segments in which the vein is small can also be excluded, since a vein diameter of 3.0 mm or less is likely to reduce hemodynamic efficiency of the graft, and has been shown to be associated with decreased reversed vein graft patency.[11]

When a sufficient length of ipsilateral greater saphenous vein is not available, the contralateral greater saphenous, lesser saphenous, cephalic, or basilic vein can be used for the bypass. The short length required for the graft reduces the need to harvest, and then splice together, multiple segments of vein. This is especially true when a tibial-tibial bypass is per-formed. These procedures usually require less than 20 cm of vein graft, a length which often can be obtained from one of the sources listed above, even when most veins have been used for multiple previous procedures. Thus, when the amount of vein available is very limited, the ability to perform a short vein graft bypass can permit the use of vein where it oth-erwise would not be possible. Conversely, if this is the first procedure performed, the use of a short vein graft conserves vein and leaves more for possible subsequent ipsilateral or contralateral procedures.

The in situ graft bypass is not a practical technique for the short vein graft bypass, and has not been adopted by many groups performing this procedure. The in situ approach requires 8 to 10 cm of mobilization of the proximal and distal ends of the graft to allow transposition onto the arteries at both ends. Sufficient mobilization is necessary to avoid twisting and acute angulation at the anastomoses. The popliteal-to-distal artery short vein grafts, however, average only 33 cm in length. If 16 cm is mobilized (8 cm from each end), about one half of the graft would be removed from its bed, and only one half would remain "in situ." In our experience frequently even more graft must be mobilized at each end. Since an important advantage of the in situ vein graft is believed to be the maintenance of vasa vasorum, this supposed advantage would be lost. In addition, the size match advantage of the in situ graft does not occur in most of these cases. The greater saphenous vein is usually *smallest* around the knee and proximal calf, where it is used for the proximal anastomosis into the popliteal-to-distal graft, while it is *larger* near the ankle and foot, close to the distal anastomosis. There has been only one series reporting use of the in situ technique for the popliteal-to-distal bypass,[29] and this primarily reported on the use of the lesser saphenous vein.

MONTEFIORE EXPERIENCE

We have reviewed and reported our experience at Montefiore Medical Center and the hospital of the Albert Einstein College of Medicine with the use of short infrapopliteal bypass grafts.[10, 15, 17, 19] Over a 12-year period, we have performed nearly 200 popliteal-to-distal and tibial-to-distal artery bypasses, all for limb-threatening ischemia. Indications included gangrene or nonhealing ulcers in 180 procedures, or 92%. Only 15 procedures (8%) were performed for severe rest pain or acute ischemia, and none for claudication. The patients were somewhat younger than those undergoing long-segment vein graft bypass. The average age was 66 years, compared with 74 years for those receiving long-segment vein bypass.[30] The patients undergoing the tibial-tibial bypass were the youngest, an average of 60 years of age.

POPLITEAL-TO-DISTAL BYPASS

One-hundred fifty-three popliteal-to-distal artery bypasses were reviewed.[15] Only nonsequential graft procedures were included, and the graft length ranged from 6 to 54 cm, with an average of 33 cm (Fig 1). The primary graft patency for this group was 71% at 1 year, 65% at 2 years, and 55% at 5 years (Fig 2). The 30-day operative mortality was 3.9%, and an additional 8.5% of patients were determined to have had a postoperative myocardial infarction. At 1 year after the procedure, the life table patient survival was 73%, which dropped to 53% by 5 years. A viable limb resulted after 77% of the procedures at 1 year, and a limb salvage rate of 73% was found at 5 years (see Fig 2). Factors which affected graft patency and limb salvage included outflow and vein graft diameter. When the bypass was performed to a compromised outflow tract which did not have straight-line flow (not via collaterals) to the foot, or was not associated with a patent pedal arch, the primary graft patency rate at 2 years was 54% (n = 19). However, when the outflow tract was not compromised, the primary graft patency at 2 years was significantly better,

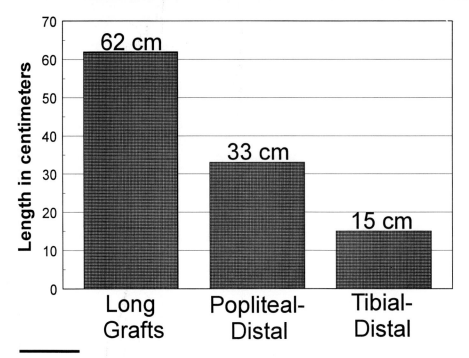

FIGURE 1.

Average vein graft length by type of bypass. The long graft group consisted of 125 vein graft bypasses from the common femoral and proximal superficial femoral arteries. (Data from Wengerter KR, Veith FJ, Gupta SK, et al: *J Vasc Surg* 1991; 13:189–199.)

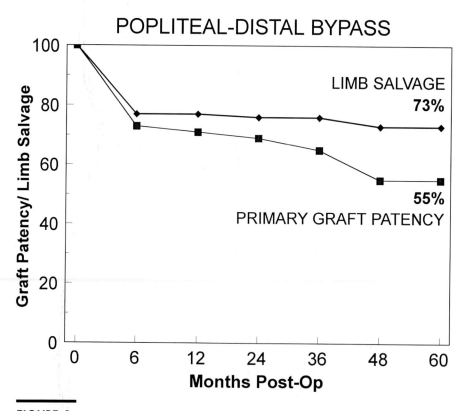

FIGURE 2.

Results of 153 popliteal–distal artery bypasses: primary life table graft patency and limb salvage.

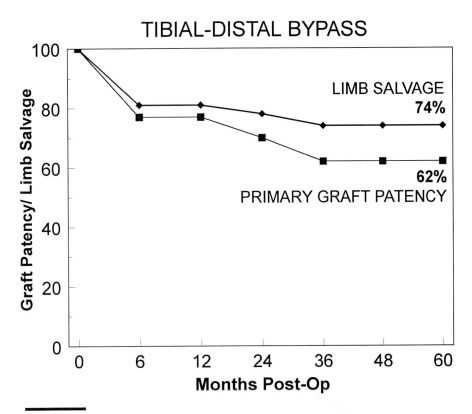

FIGURE 3.

Results of 42 tibial–distal artery bypasses: primary life table graft patency and limb salvage.

72% ($P < .05$). Limb salvage was also affected, and was significantly better (82% vs. 61% at 3 years, $P < .005$) when the outflow tract was good.[15]

TIBIAL-TO-DISTAL BYPASS

Forty-two bypasses to either tibial (20) or pedal (22) arteries from tibial vessels were evaluated.[19] These included 32 nonsequential procedures, and 10 sequential grafts in which a bypass to the popliteal or tibial artery was performed before the tibial–distal artery graft. These grafts were on average 15 cm in length, and ranged from 8 to 33 cm (see Fig 1). Primary graft patency was 76% at 1 year, and 65% at 5 years(Fig 3). Patient survival was 95% at 1 year and 55% at 5 years, and the limb salvage rate was 81% at 1 year and 73% at 5 years (see Fig 3).[19]

WOUND INFECTION

Short vein graft bypass procedures should be expected to have a lower wound infection rate than longer bypass graft procedures based on two features of these grafts. First, the procedure usually does not involve an incision in the groin, and thus avoids the area most commonly associated with infection in lower extremity revascularizations. Groin wound infections occur in approximately 2% of bypass procedures in the legs, and are responsible for the greatest number of exposed and infected bypass grafts.[31] The difficulty in keeping this area clean (especially in the obese patient with an overlying pannus), the close proximity to the perineum, the frequent movements in the tissues associated with the hip joint and the large number of lymphatics crossing the area that are frequently disrupted by the surgery, are all suspected as reasons for an increased infection rate. Since short distal vein grafts avoid this area completely, they have a great advantage in reducing wound breakdown and infection. A second reason these grafts should have a lower infection rate is the shorter length of vein harvest wound. On average, these grafts are about 41 cm longer. This translates into a shorter length vein harvest wound, and less wound means less chance for infection.

Of the 195 short vein graft distal bypass procedures we have reviewed, the infection rate was found to be 6% overall for serious wound breakdown and infection. These wounds correspond to Johnson classification class 3 and 4 wound infections,[32] where class 3 includes those wounds with separation of the skin edges, while class 4 wounds involve exposure of the graft. For comparison, the rate of serious wound complication for long bypass grafts reported in the Montefiore randomized series comparing in situ and reversed grafts[30] was reviewed. The grafts in that study were from the common femoral or proximal superficial femoral arteries only, and the average vein graft length was 62 cm, as noted. There were a total of 24 cases of class 3 and 4 wound complications for the group of 125 long vein grafts reported in that study, for a rate of 19%. This difference in the serious wound complication rate was statistically lower in the short vein graft group ($P < .001$) by chi-square analysis.

DIABETES MELLITUS

Patients who are candidates for short vein bypass of tibial arterial lesions are predominantly diabetic. This well-known "pattern of disease" for atherosclerosis in the lower extremities of those with diabetes mellitus includes heavy involvement, frequently with occlusions, of the calf arteries.[33] In addition, there usually is sparing of disease in more proximal vessels, especially when other factors, such as a history of smoking or advanced age, are not present. Thus, in the nonsmoking diabetic patient, the femoral vessels are frequently free of disease, and the iliac arteries are almost always free of significant disease. This provides the setting for the short vein graft bypass: tibial arterial occlusive disease with minimal disease in the vessels proximal to the tibial arteries.

Studies reporting large numbers of short vein graft infrapopliteal bypasses have uniformly noted a high percentage of diabetic patients in the population undergoing this procedure. Sidaway et al.[34] reported 74% of patients receiving superficial femoral or popliteal–distal artery bypasses were diabetic. Likewise, Cantelmo et al.[13] found a history of diabetes mellitus in 77% of their short vein graft group. In our reviews of short vein graft distal bypasses, 87% of patients undergoing popliteal–distal artery bypass were diabetic,[15] and 90% of those receiving a distal–distal artery bypass were diabetic.[19] In comparison, only 62% of patients were diabetic in our review of 125 long bypasses, which included grafts that extended from the common or proximal superficial femoral arteries to in-

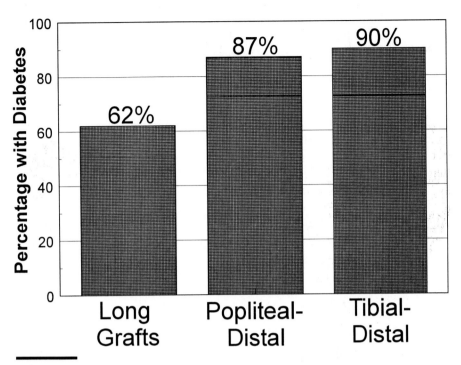

FIGURE 4.

Percentage of distal artery bypass graft patients with diabetes mellitus by type of graft. The long graft group consisted of 125 vein graft bypasses from the common femoral and proximal superficial femoral arteries. (Data from Wengerter KR, Veith FJ, Gupta SK, et al: *J Vasc Surg* 1991; 13:189–199.)

frapopliteal arteries[30] (Fig 4). The difference in the percentage of diabetic patients in these two groups was statistically significant by chi-square analysis ($P < .001$). While graft patency has not clearly been shown to be adversely affected by the presence of diabetes mellitus in limbs with similar severities of disease,[35, 36] limb salvage does appear to be more difficult. This may be due to problems with resolving infection in these patients, and a higher incidence of renal failure which is associated with a greater number of amputations despite a patent graft.[37]

SUMMARY

The short infrapopliteal vein graft bypass is a useful alternative to a long bypass graft when the superficial femoral and popliteal arteries are relatively free of disease. Durability of the procedure is confirmed by graft patency and limb salvage rates that are similar to or better than long vein grafts, and the complication rate is low. Even when a stenosis of the inflow vessels exists, short vein graft bypass results are good if a successful angioplasty can be performed, or if the stenosis is mild (<35%). The use of the popliteal-to-distal and tibial-to-tibial vein graft bypass is an important approach to maximizing vein graft utilization since it conserves vein and can allow performance of an autogenous vein graft bypass when there is a shortage of usable vein.

REFERENCES

1. Veith FJ, Gupta SK, Ascer E, et al: Six year prospective multicenter randomized comparison of autologous saphenous vein and expanded polytetrafluoroethylene grafts in infrainguinal arterial reconstructions. *J Vasc Surg* 1986; 3:104–114.

2. Abbott WM, Darling RC Jr: Comparison of PTFE and Dacron grafts for femoropopliteal bypass: Do we need a randomized prospective study?, in Veith FJ (ed): *Current Critical Problems in Vascular Surgery*, vol 5. St Louis, Quality Medical Publishing, 1993, pp 56–61.

3. Rosenthal D, Evans D, McKinsey J, et al: Prosthetic above-knee femoropopliteal bypass for intermittent claudication. *J Cardiovasc Surg* 1990; 31:462–468.

4. Linton RR, Wilde WL: Modifications in the technique for femoropopliteal saphenous vein bypass autografts. *Surgery* 1970; 67:234–242.

5. Farley JJ, Kiser JC, Hitchcock CR: Profunda femoris-popliteal shunt. *Ann Surg* 1964; 160:23–25.

6. Bole P, Andronaco JT, Purdy R, et al: The use of profunda femoris–popliteal bypass to compensate for short autogenous vein graft: A report of two cases. *J Cardiovasc Surg* 1973; 14:329–332.

7. Stabile BE, Wilson SE: The profunda femoris–popliteal artery bypass. *Arch Surg* 1977; 112:913–918.

8. Hershey FB, Auer AL: Extended surgical approach to the profunda femoris artery. *Surg Gynecol Obstet* 1974; 138:88–90.

9. Nunez AA, Veith FJ, Collier P, et al: Direct approaches to the distal portions of the deep femoral artery for limb salvage bypasses. *J Vasc Surg* 1988; 8:576–581.

10. Veith FJ, Gupta SK, Samson RH, et al: Superficial femoral and popliteal artery as inflow sites for distal bypasses. *Surgery* 1981; 90:980–989.

11. Wengerter KR, Veith FJ, Gupta SK, et al: Influence of vein size (diameter) on infrapopliteal reversed vein graft patency. *J Vasc Surg* 1990; 11:525–531.

12. Panetta TF, Marin ML, Veith FJ, et al: Unsuspected pre-existing saphenous vein disease: An unrecognized cause of vein bypass failure. *J Vasc Surg* 1992; 15:102–112.

13. Cantelmo NL, Snow R, Menzoian JO, et al: Successful vein bypass in patients with an ischemic limb and a palpable popliteal pulse. *Arch Surg* 1986; 121:217–220.

14. Schuler JJ, Flanigan DP, Williams LR, et al: Early experience with popliteal to infrapopliteal bypass for limb salvage. *Arch Surg* 1983; 118:472–476.

15. Wengerter KR, Yang PM, Veith FJ, et al: A twelve-year experience with the popliteal-to-distal artery bypass: The significance and management of proximal disease. *J Vasc Surg* 1992; 15:143–151.

16. Marks J, King TA, Baele H, et al: Popliteal-to-distal bypass for limb threatening ischemia. *J Vasc Surg* 1992; 15:755–760.

17. Veith FJ, Ascer E, Gupta SK, et al: Tibiotibial vein bypass grafts: A new operation for limb salvage. *J Vasc Surg* 1985; 2:552–557.

18. Danza R: The use of bypass grafts for obstructive lesions of tibial and peroneal arteries. *J Cardiovasc Surg* 1982; 23:59–64.

19. Lyon RT, Veith FJ, Marsan BU, et al: Eleven-year experience with tibio-tibial bypass: An unusual but effective solution to distal tibial artery occlusive disease and limited autologous vein. *J Vasc Surg*, 1994; 220:61–69.

20. Sprayregen S: Principles of angiography, in Haimovici H (ed): *Vascular Surgery Principles and Techniques*. New York, McGraw Hill, 1976, pp 39–66.

21. Rosenbloom MS, Walsh JJ, Schuler JJ, et al: Long term results of infragenicu-

lar bypasses with autogenous vein originating from the digtal superficial femoral and popliteal arteries. *J Vasc Surg* 1988; 7:691–696.

22. Walsh DB, Gilbertson JJ, Zwolak RM, et al: The natural history of superficial femoral artery stenoses. *J Vasc Surg* 1991; 14:299–304.

23. Capek P, McLean GK, Berkowitz HD: Femoropopliteal angioplasty. Factors influencing long-term success. *Circulation* 1991; 83(suppl I):I-70–I-80.

24. Gallino A, Mahler F, Probst P, et al: Percutaneous transluminal angioplasty of the arteries of the lower limbs: A 5 year follow-up. *Circulation* 1984; 70:619–623.

25. Johnston KW, Rae M, Hogg-Johnston SA, et al: 5-year results of a prospective study of percutaneous transluminal angioplasty. *Ann Surg* 1987; 206:403–413.

26. Jeans WD, Armstrong S, Cole SE, et al: Fate of patients undergoing transluminal angioplasty for lower-limb ischemia. *Radiology* 1990; 177:559–564.

27. Brenner BJ, Cluley SR, Hollier LH, et al: Ultrasound-guided balloon angioplasty: What is its role?, Veith FJ (ed): *Current Critical Problems in Vascular Surgery*, vol 5. St Louis, Quality Meducal Publishing, 1993, pp 217–220.

28. Gupta SK, Kram HB, Veith FJ, et al: Significance and management of inflow gradients unexpectedly generated after femorofemoral or femorodistal bypasses, in Veith FJ (ed): *Current Critical Problems in Vascular Surgery*, vol. 5. St Louis, Quality Medical Publishing, 1993, pp 138–142.

29. Shandall AA, Leather RP, Corson JD, et al: Use of the short saphenous vein in situ for popliteal-to-distal artery bypass. *Am J Surg 1987*; 154:240–244.

30. Wengerter KR, Veith FJ, Gupta SK, et al: Prospective randomized multicenter comparison of in situ and reversed vein infrapopliteal bypasses. *J Vasc Surg* 1991; 13:189–199.

31. McIntyre KE Jr: Wound complications following vascular reconstruction, in Berhard VM, Towne JB (eds): *Complications in Vascular Surgery*. St Louis, Quality Medical Publishing, 1991, pp 291–300.

32. Johnson JA, Cogbill TH, Strutt PJ, et al: Wound complications after infrainguinal bypass. *Arch Surg* 1988; 123:859–862.

33. Haimovici H: Arteriographic patterns of atherosclerotic occlusive disease of the lower extremity, in Haimovici H (ed): *Vascular Surgery Principles and Techniques*. New York, McGraw-Hill, 1976, pp 240–263.

34. Sidaway AN, Menzoian JO, Cantelmo NL, et al: Effect of inflow and outflow sites on the results of tibioperoneal vein grafts. *Am J Surg* 1986; 152:211–214.

35. Bernhard VM. Bypass to the popliteal and infrapopliteal arteries, in Rutherford RB (ed): *Vascular Surgery*, ed 3. Philadelphia, WB Saunders, 1989, pp 692–704.

36. Stemmer EA: Influence of diabetes mellitus on the patterns and complications of vascular occlusive disease, in Moore WS (ed): *Vascular Surgery. A Comprehensive Review*. Philadelphia, WB Saunders, 1991, pp 390–402.

37. Sanchez LA, Goldsmith RN, Rivers SP, et al: Limb salvage surgery in end-stage renal disease: Is it worthwhile? *J Cardiovasc Surg* 1992; 33:344–348.

Distal Reconstructions to the Dorsal Pedis Artery in Diabetic Patients

Frank B. Pomposelli, Jr., M.D.

Assistant Professor of Surgery, Harvard Medical School; Vascular Surgeon, New England Deaconess Hospital, Boston, Massachusetts

Frank W. LoGerfo, M.D.

Professor of Surgery, Harvard Medical School; Chief, Division of Vascular Surgery, Department of Surgery, New England Deaconess Hospital, Boston, Massachusetts

F oot problems are the most common cause of hospitalization for patients with diabetes mellitus with about 20% receiving in-hospital care during their lifetime and accounting for an annual health care cost of approximately $1 billion.[1] The primary pathologic mechanisms of ischemia and neuropathy set the stage for pressure necrosis, ulceration, infection, and gangrene.[2] When significant ischemia is present, successful salvage of the limb requires the prompt restoration of maximum arterial flow to the foot. Correction of ischemia through arterial reconstruction, however, has been hampered by a misconception that there is an untreatable occlusive lesion at the arteriolar level. This idea originated from a study by Goldenberg and associates[3] who performed soft tissue microscopic evaluation of amputated limb specimens from diabetic patients. They described observing a PAS (periodic acid-Schiff)-positive material occluding the arterioles and labeled this process "arteriolosclerosis." A subsequent prospective study[4] of amputation specimens from diabetic and nondiabetic patients, however, demonstrated no histologic evidence of an arteriolar occlusive lesion associated with diabetes. Other anatomic[5] and physiologic studies[6, 7] have failed to demonstrate evidence of a small artery or arteriolar occlusive lesion in these patients.

Rejection of the small vessel disease theory is critically important since if such an occlusive lesion were present in the microcirculation, arterial reconstruction would not be effective in achieving healing. In fact, the most compelling evidence against the existence of small vessel disease may be the observation that the results of lower extremity bypass grafting in diabetic patients equal or exceed those achieved in nondiabetic patients.[8]

As in nondiabetic patients the cause of lower extremity ischemia is atherosclerotic occlusion. When atherosclerosis occurs in diabetes, the histologic picture is no different from that in nondiabetic patients. Its incidence, however, appears to be much higher in diabetic patients[9] as is the incidence of claudication.[10] The most important characteristic of atherosclerosis and diabetes is a difference in the pattern of occlusive disease. While atherosclerosis in nondiabetic patients most often involves the aortoiliac segment or superficial femoral arteries, Strandness et al.[4] and Conrad[5] both demonstrated in prospective studies that occlusive disease in diabetic patients tends to involve the infrageniculate, or so-called tibial arteries. Moreover, they also demonstrated that in spite of extensive infracrural occlusions the foot arteries are often spared, which has been confirmed by a recent angiographic study.[11]

The refinements in the technique of distal bypass that have occurred over the past decade have made arterial reconstruction to the small arteries of the distal leg and foot technically feasible,[12] with results comparable to more proximal reconstructions.[13, 14] Because imaging the distal arteries of the leg and foot is now relatively simple, we have been influenced in our own practice to attempt, whenever possible, to bypass to the best vessel in continuity with the pedal circulation in preference to isolated popliteal or tibial segments. When severe tibial occlusive disease is seen on the preoperative arteriogram, the best vessel to restore a palpable foot pulse is often found to be the dorsalis pedis artery. We initially began performing pedal bypass in patients with no other available option for a limb-salvaging arterial bypass. Early results were encouraging enough that we expanded our indications and standardized our tech-

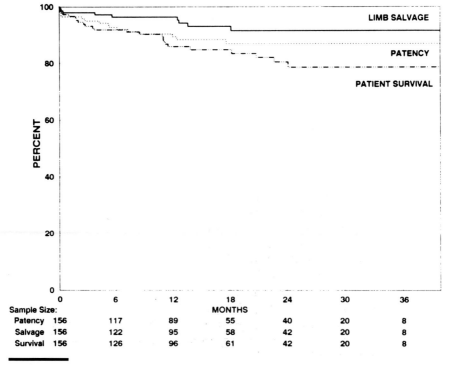

FIGURE 1.

Cumulative limb salvage patency and patient survival in 156 dorsalis pedis bypasses. (From Pomposelli FB, Jepsen SJ, Gibbons GW, et al: *Arch Surg* 1991; 126:724–729. Used by permission.)

nique.[15] In our most recent follow-up of 156 dorsalis pedis vein bypass grafts, graft patency and limb salvage are 87.1% and 91.6% respectively at 3 years' follow-up[16] (Fig 1). As with all distal arterial reconstructions, success with dorsalis pedis artery bypass is dependent upon both proper patient selection and excellent surgical technique.

PATIENT SELECTION CRITERIA

The complexity and technical difficulty of these procedures are such that they should be reserved for patients with truly limb-threatening ischemia. Table 1 lists the clinical criteria and surgical indications in 367 consecutive patients undergoing this procedure at the New England Deaconess Hospital between October 1985 and October 1992. These procedures constituted 19.2% of the 2,099 lower extremity bypasses performed during that time period and approximately 25% of the lower extremity procedures performed on diabetic patients at our institution in the last 3 years. Nearly all of these procedures were performed for limb-threatening indications. It should be noted that claudication alone is not an appropriate indication for pedal bypass, and, in fact, may not be improved, especially if there are occlusive tibial lesions present that prevent retrograde flow from the dorsalis pedis artery to the vascular bed supplying the calf muscles.

Infection is a common complication accompanying ischemic foot lesions in diabetic patients, occurring in approximately 50% at the time of presentation. Prompt control of active spreading infection is the important first step in treatment of these patients. Because of the polymicrobial nature of these infections, all patients presenting with infection should be started on broad-spectrum intravenous antibiotics. Patients with deep space infection or abscess should undergo prompt incision and drainage with debridement or open partial forefoot amputation, as required. The need to control sepsis may delay revascularization for several days, but should not lead to further progression of foot necrosis, provided that arterial reconstruction is done promptly once active spreading infection and cellulitis have resolved. The decision to perform arteriography and vascular reconstruction should be made during this waiting period, which is usually no longer than 5 to 7 days. Further delays while waiting for healing by secondary intention or mistakenly thinking further necrosis is solely due to infection may lead to loss of opportunity to salvage the foot.

In evaluating ischemia, the most important finding on physical examination other than the presenting ischemic lesion is the absence of a palpable foot pulse. It is important to remember that it is not uncommon for many diabetic patients to have a strongly palpable popliteal pulse in the presence of advanced foot ischemia if the atherosclerotic occlusions are confined to the tibial or peroneal arteries.[17] It is erroneous to consider such patients "unreconstructible" without the benefit of an arteriogram encompassing the foot circulation. Several studies[18, 19] have confirmed the frequency of this finding in diabetic patients with foot ischemia and the high likelihood of limb salvage with arterial reconstruction. In our reported experience,[16] greater than 50% of patients undergoing dor-

TABLE 1.

Clinical Criteria and Indications for Pedal Bypass in 367 Consecutive Patients Treated From 1985 to 1992 at the New England Deaconess Hospital

	No. of Patients (%)
Demographics	
Male	253 (69)
Female	114 (31)
Mean age	58 yr
Risk factors*	
Diabetes	350 (96)
Prior MI	115 (29)
Angina	88 (22)
Prior CABG	43 (11)
Hypertension	219 (54)
Smoking	194 (48)
Dialysis	21 (5.0)
Indications	
Ulcer	290 (72)
Gangrene	47 (12)
Rest pain	25 (6.0)
Failed foot amputation	13 (3.0)
Failed bypass graft	13 (3.0)
Popliteal aneurysm	1.0 (0.25)
Associated infection	222 (55)

*MI = myocardial infarction; CABG = coronary artery bypass grafting.

salis pedis bypass had a palpable popliteal pulse present at the time of initial presentation.

Doppler ankle pressures are of limited value in these patients. The mean ankle-brachial ratio in patients with open foot lesions in our noninvasive vascular laboratory was unexpectedly high (0.67). Artifactual elevation of the ankle systolic pressures is well recognized[20] and probably due to calcification of the tunica media (Mönckeberg's sclerosis). Pulse volume tracings, however, which are unaffected by medial calcinosis, are usually markedly abnormal at the forefoot level in most, but not all patients. These findings underscore the importance of not overly relying on noninvasive criteria in determining the severity of ischemia in patients with diabetes mellitus. Generally, the absence of a palpable foot pulse in the clinical setting of an ischemic foot ulcer or ischemic rest pain is all that is required in deciding to perform an arteriogram.

ARTERIOGRAPHY

Ultimately the decision of when to perform a dorsalis-pedis bypass is based on a carefully performed femoral arteriogram. Because of the propensity for diabetic patients to have occlusive lesions in the tibial arteries, it is essential that arteriograms not be terminated at the midtibial level, as is commonly done in nondiabetic patients, but that they incorporate the complete infrapopliteal circulation, including the foot vessels. Visualizing the infrapopliteal vessels in diabetic patients can be difficult due to the extensive nature of their occlusive disease. Fears about inducing renal failure from the multiple contrast injections required to image the infrapopliteal vessels are sometimes used as excuses for limiting these studies. In our experience, however, this has rarely been a problem in those patients with normal renal function, and when it does occur almost never requires dialysis for management. Intravenous hydration of the patient prior to arteriography should be a routine which greatly reduces the risk of contrast-induced renal failure.

Lower extremity arteriography in diabetic patients has been simplified by the development of intraarterial digital subtraction angiography[21, 22] which has become our preferred method for imaging the lower extremity circulation. Although the smaller, computer-generated digital subtraction images have somewhat inferior resolution when compared with standard contrast arteriography, the image quality has generally been adequate and is improving as the technology evolves (Fig 2). Visualization of the foot vessels is also possible by a skilled angiographer with conventional arteriography, although it is likely to require a greater volume of contrast agent. Regardless of the method of arteriography used, anteroposterior and lateral foot views must be included with the infrapopliteal

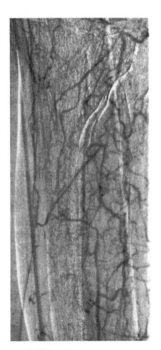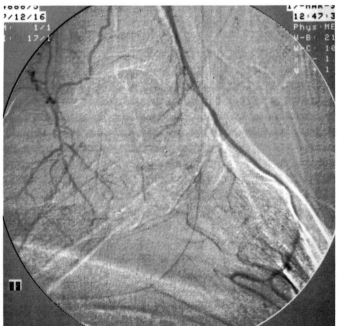

FIGURE 2.

Intraarterial digital subtraction arteriogram of the infrapopliteal vessels *(left panel)* and pedal vessels *(right panel)*. The dorsalis pedis artery is widely patent and connects to a patent distal arch. The posterior tibial and plantar vessels are occluded.

portion of the arteriogram in order to have as complete a picture as possible of the location of all significant stenoses and occlusion. The pattern of occlusive disease may suggest several possible options for arterial reconstruction, and it is important not to exclude the dorsalis pedis artery, which is often a better option for outflow than a more diseased proximal vessel.

TECHNICAL CONSIDERATIONS

When planning a pedal bypass, the individual pattern of occlusive disease may present the vascular surgeon with several different bypass options. Isolated popliteal artery segments[23] visualized proximal to a patent dorsalis pedis artery are potentially available as outflow sites that are technically easier to bypass than pedal vessels and require a shorter conduit. When the superficial femoral artery is patent, inflow can be taken from either the common femoral artery, the time-honored approach,[24] or more distally, usually the popliteal artery.[19] Although the superiority of autogenous vein in infrapopliteal reconstructions is now firmly established,[25] there is little consensus among vascular surgeons as to which method of preparing the conduit is best, with in situ grafts,[26] reversed vein grafts[27] and translocated nonreversed grafts,[28] all having specific advantages and disadvantages.

It is our strong opinion that the only appropriate conduit for pedal bypass is autogenous vein. However, beyond this principle we believe that a flexible approach toward reconstructing pedal bypasses is most appropriate. Using all of the described techniques has been advantageous in specific circumstances to shorten the length of the procedure, decrease its complexity, and avoid the creation of potentially troublesome wounds without a detrimental effect on results. The following is an outline of our approach.

OUTFLOW CONSIDERATIONS: WHEN TO CHOOSE THE DORSALIS PEDIS ARTERY

Limb salvage in diabetic patients with foot ischemia and tissue loss is most likely when a successful bypass results in the return of a palpable foot pulse. In the past, achieving this endpoint was often compromised because arteriograms rarely included the complete distal circulation, missing areas of significant occlusive disease in the infrapopliteal vessels. Moreover, even when tibial occlusive disease was recognized, bypasses distal to the popliteal artery were infrequently performed because technical difficulties were encountered which often resulted in early graft thrombosis. When a superficial femoral artery occlusion was present but the popliteal artery was patent, i.e., isolated, segment, a technically easier femoropopliteal bypass was often performed in the hope that collateral circulation would be sufficient to improve foot perfusion. Following successful femoropopliteal bypass, if primary healing did not occur, a limb-sparing partial foot amputation was tried, and, if unsuccessful, converted to a below-knee amputation.

The improved results with distal arterial reconstructive surgery and arteriography in the past decade have made these compromises unneces-

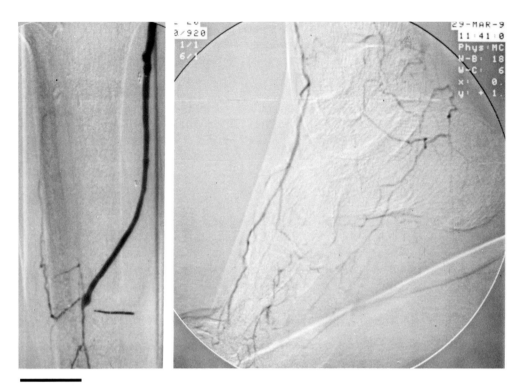

FIGURE 3.

Arteriogram in a patient whose ischemic foot ulcer failed to heal after a successful femoroperoneal in situ bypass. The graft is patent, but the distal peroneal artery does not have open branches to the foot. The dorsalis pedis artery is also
patent. The patient underwent a second procedure from the distal end of his previously placed vein graft to the dorsalis pedis artery.

sary. With a complete imaging of the lower extremity circulation, it is
usually possible to choose an outflow artery that will restore a palpable
foot pulse. This has been our goal, especially when tissue loss is present.
If a more proximal bypass to the popliteal, anterior tibial, or posterior
tibial arteries cannot achieve this goal owing to distal obstruction, we
preferentially bypass to the foot itself when the dorsalis pedis artery is
patent. Although the modern results with peroneal artery bypass have
generally been excellent,[29, 30] there are occasional instances where a successful peroneal bypass does not result in adequate restoration of arterial
flow to the foot to achieve healing (Fig 3). Moreover, the location of the
peroneal artery can make its exposure and fashioning the anastomosis
more difficult than with the more superficial and readily accessible dorsalis pedis artery, especially in obese patients or when dealing with calcified arteries. However, dorsalis pedis bypass is unnecessary when a
more proximal bypass will restore foot pulses and should not be done
when there is inadequate conduit to reach the foot, when the dorsal foot
is infected, or when the dorsalis pedis artery appears on the arteriogram
to be occluded or severely diseased.

INFLOW CONSIDERATIONS

The time-honored approach in infrainguinal arterial reconstruction has
been to always take inflow from the common femoral artery in order to

avoid late graft failure from disease progression in the superficial femoral artery. In diabetic patients, however, the superficial femoral artery is frequently spared of significant atherosclerosis, which is a potential advantage in performing a dorsalis pedis bypass. By taking inflow from a more distal location, usually the popliteal artery, a shorter vein graft is required and avoids the need for dissection in the groin and thigh, which are common locations for wound complications in these patients. Several studies[17–19] have reported excellent long-term patency with popliteal-based inflow procedures showing that concerns about the progression of disease in the superficial femoral artery are unfounded. We routinely take inflow from the distal superficial femoral or popliteal artery provided that the artery is free of significant disease more proximally, which we define as no stenosis greater than 30% of the transverse diameter or no pressure gradient across any lesion present proximal to the site of the proximal anastomosis. Sixty percent of our patients undergoing pedal arterial reconstruction have had their grafts based on inflow sites distal to the common femoral artery, with no apparent decrease in patency noted in follow-up of 36 months.[16]

PREPARATION OF THE VEIN GRAFT

For many years, the reversed saphenous vein graft had been the mainstay of infrainguinal arterial reconstruction. However, in recent years, the in situ[26] method has become popular since Leather et al.[31] devised a simple and atraumatic method for cutting the valves. Reports of improved vein use and long-term patency rates with the in situ graft have led some authors to suggest that it possesses some biologic advantages over reversed vein grafts. However, strong evidence supporting this is lacking.[32] As pointed out by Taylor et al.,[33] not only are the modern results with reversed vein grafts, including the rate of vein utilization, equivalent to those of the in situ method but as many as 20% of patients requiring distal bypass may have absent or incomplete saphenous veins making an in situ bypass impossible.

In constructing a dorsalis pedis bypass, several practical considerations make all current preparation techniques useful including removing the vein but still cutting the valves (translocated nonreversed vein graft).[28] One such consideration is the size discrepancy between the saphenous vein and the inflow and outflow arteries which is most pronounced when constructing a pedal bypass from the common femoral artery. Using an in situ graft minimizes the size mismatch and results in the most technically satisfactory anastomosis, both proximally, at the femoral artery, and distally, in the foot. Moreover, the in situ method has proved to be less laborious and time-consuming than removing and reversing the whole saphenous vein simply to overcome the valves. Cutting the valves with the vein left in situ is far quicker and has been facilitated in recent years in our practice by the use of angioscopy.[34]

One disadvantage of using the in situ technique is the need for exposing the foot extension of the saphenous vein in order to have adequate length of conduit to reach the dorsalis pedis artery. This necessitates the creation of a second foot incision parallel to the one required to expose the dorsalis pedis artery. The skin bridge between these two incisions will occasionally become ischemic if there is extensive tension from wound closure, particularly when there is significant foot edema or if the graft is tunneled under the skin bridge. One way to avoid the problem entirely is by using a shorter translocated vein graft based on a more distal inflow site. With this technique, the second foot incision can be avoided by obtaining the extra length of vein required to reach the dorsalis pedis artery from the proximal portion of the exposed vein. As previously described, use of a distal inflow site also avoids the need to expose the proximal saphenous vein in the groin or upper thigh, which can result in significant wound morbidity, particularly in obese patients. Using the vein nonreversed may also be advantageous to optimize size matchup between the vein graft and artery. In circumstances where the caliber of the saphenous vein is larger at the ankle than at the knee, we use the vein reversed for the same reasons. The types of vein grafts used and the inflow sites chosen in our series are depicted in Table 2.

The advantage of the flexible approach to pedal bypass is that the surgeon can fashion the procedure to the patient's individual anatomy based on practical considerations rather than theoretical concerns. There does not appear to be any disadvantage in terms of graft durability with this approach. In follow-up extending out to 3 years, cumulative patency rates have been comparable for in situ and translocated vein grafts and pedal bypasses with common femoral or popliteal artery inflow.[15]

TABLE 2.
Inflow Source and Conduit Configuration in 384 Pedal Bypasses Performed From 1985 to 1992.*

	n (%)	
Inflow source		
Common femoral	129	34
Distal SFA/Pop†	231	60
Tibial artery	5	1
Previously placed graft	19	5
Total	384	100
Conduit		
In situ	148	39
Reversed	110	29
Nonreversed	68	18
Arm	27	7
Composite vein	31	8
Total	384	100

*All procedures were performed with autogenous vein
†SFA/Pop = superior femoral artery or popliteal artery.

DORSALIS PEDIS BYPASS AND FOOT INFECTION

Foot infection, which frequently accompanies ischemic tissue loss in diabetic patients,[35] is often multimicrobial and can spread rapidly causing extensive soft tissue destruction. Abscess and osteomyelitis are not uncommon and may be accompanied by severe systemic toxicity. Patients requiring a pedal bypass in this situation are a source of particular concern because the distal anastomosis is placed in such close proximity to the infection. In one recent report where pedal bypass was only modestly successful as a limb salvage procedure, difficulty with postoperative infection was a principle problem.[36] In our own experience, approximately 10% of our patients undergoing pedal bypass have had postoperative wound infections requiring further debridement and drainage.[37] These have resulted in one death and two major amputations due to graft infec-

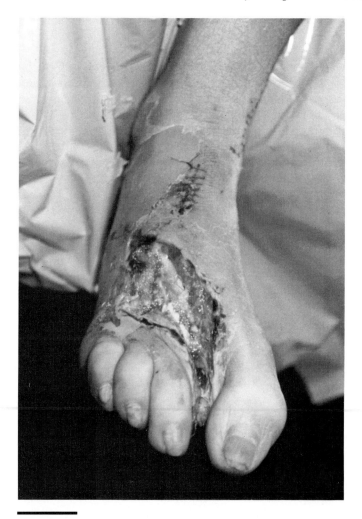

FIGURE 4.

This patient presented with an ischemic second toe which became infected and required an open toe amputation and debridement of the distal dorsal foot. Following control of the infection, a bypass to the dorsalis pedis artery was performed followed by a split-thickness skin graft several days later.

tion. Nonetheless, pedal bypass has been safely performed in the majority of patients with foot infection, provided the infection is properly treated first.

In treating combined ischemia and infection, the cornerstone of therapy is rapid control of active, spreading infection. Signs of control of active infection include resolution of cellulitis, lymphangitis, edema, and crepitus, coupled with loss of fever, leukocytosis, and return of glycemic control. When a surgical debridement or partial forefoot amputation is required to control infection, it should be done promptly and before entertaining any thoughts of arteriography or vascular surgery. Once the active infection has been controlled and localized, pedal bypass can be safely performed provided the dissection of the dorsalis pedis artery and the location of the distal anastomosis do not encroach upon open wounds and cellulitis has resolved, especially in areas of any proposed surgical incisions (Fig 4). As stated previously, further delay may result in progression of ischemic necrosis and loss of the opportunity to salvage the foot. The complexities and high costs of managing these patients is evident in the study by Tannenbaum et al.[37] reviewing experiences with pedal bypass in 56 patients presenting with significant infection. Control of sepsis necessitated debridement or open amputation in 25 cases and delayed bypass by a average of 10.7 days. Following successful bypass, 7 (12.5%) patients developed serious wound infections, including one that resulted in death. Postbypass foot procedures were needed in 36 cases to achieve healing, and total hospital stay averaged 29.8 days. In addition, 20 patients had a total of 35 readmissions for related foot problems which delayed ultimate healing by an average of 5.5 months. In spite of these difficulties, graft patency and limb salvage rates were 91.8% and 97.8%, respectively, at 36 months.

SURGICAL CONSIDERATIONS

Previous studies have demonstrated the high incidence of significant coronary artery disease in diabetic patients with peripheral vascular disease.[38] Many of these patients do not experience the typical symptoms and signs of coronary ischemia in spite of the presence of advanced coronary artery disease.[39] The urgent nature of the limb-threatening ischemia may make the time delay for a complete cardiac evaluation and correction of significant coronary artery disease impossible if limb salvage is to be achieved. For these reasons, patients undergoing dorsalis pedis artery bypass in our institution routinely have pulmonary arterial catheters and radial arterial lines placed prior to general endotracheal, epidural, or spinal anesthesia. Pulmonary arterial pressures and cardiac index are frequently monitored to avoid fluid overload and hypoxemia, can lead to congestive heart failure and myocardial infarction. Intravenous nitroglycerin and loop diuretics are used liberally to reduce filling pressures when ventricular performance is adversely affected. Following surgery, all patients are kept in a monitored setting with pulmonary arterial catheters in place for approximately 2 or 3 days until resuscitative intravenous fluid in the "third space" has been mobilized and dry body weight has been achieved. Although costly and difficult, we believe that this approach is responsible for the comparatively low number of perioperative deaths (1.8%) and myocardial infarctions (5.4%) in our series.

The dorsalis pedis artery is exposed as the first step in the surgical procedure. A longitudinal incision is made 1 cm distal to an imaginary transverse line between the distal ends of the malleoli, and 1 cm lateral to the extensor hallucis longis tendon. The artery is found beneath a dense fascial layer, the inferior extensor retinaculum. A sterile, continuous-wave Doppler probe has proved to be helpful in localizing the artery. The dorsalis pedis artery gives off its lateral tarsal branch proximally and bifurcates into the deep plantar and first dorsal metatarsal arteries distally. Usually the segment between these branches is where the anastomosis is placed. If this segment is found to be diseased or heavily calcified, alternative sites can be chosen distally or proximally, or in some cases one of the branch vessels, particularly the lateral tarsal artery, can be used if it is large enough. Occasionally, finding the appropriate site for the distal anastomosis may require exposing the artery more distally or proximally. As a result, we prefer to always expose it through a longitudinal incision and have not used a transverse incision as suggested by Weaver and Yellin.[40]

Once the artery has been exposed, attention is directed toward harvesting the vein. Generally, it is best to start at the ankle and work proximally, exposing only as much vein as needed depending on the level of inflow chosen. When the common femoral artery is the inflow site, obtaining adequate vein length requires exposure of the complete saphenous vein including its extension onto the foot, the medial marginal branch. As previously described, this results in a second incision on the dorsal foot running parallel to the arterial incision with a fairly narrow intervening bridge of skin and subcutaneous tissue between them. This skin bridge is a potential area of troublesome wound problems resulting from skin necrosis when it becomes devitalized from undermining by excessive dissection or tunneling the vein graft through it, which should be avoided (Fig 5). When possible, a shorter translocated vein graft arising from a distal inflow site should be used and the extra length of vein needed to reach the foot should be harvested from the proximal end of the vein (Fig 6). Translocated vein grafts can be used either reversed or nonreversed depending on which gives the best size match between the vein graft and artery. This is particularly true of arm vein grafts which often have great differences in diameter between their proximal and distal ends. In recent years, we have been using the angioscope in preparation of vein grafts. Angioscopically directed valve cutting has proved less traumatic than "blind" cutting, especially in thin-walled arm veins.[35] Angioscopy has also proved useful in discovering areas in vein grafts of stricture from old trauma and sites of recanalization from previous thrombosis, which are common due to venipuncture and which are not always apparent by visual inspection of the vein's exterior surface. If not excised, these lesions become areas of intimal hyperplasia that may result in late graft failure.[41]

Occasionally, when no outflow vessel is visible on the arteriogram, and amputation appears to be otherwise inevitable, dorsalis pedis bypass may still be possible if an audible Doppler signal is heard on the dorsal

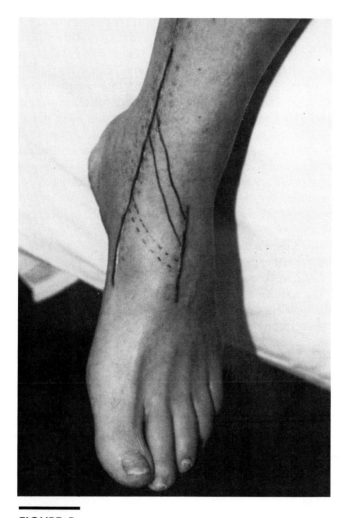

FIGURE 5.

Tunneling a femoral–dorsalis pedis in situ bypass. This photograph was taken 6 months after surgery. The *solid vertical lines* mark the incisions for harvesting the saphenous vein and exposing the dorsalis pedis artery. The *transverse lines* mark the actual location of the graft. The *dotted lines* depict the incorrect position for tunneling the graft through the skin bridge between the two incisions (see text).

foot over the usual location of the artery. The artery is located with a sterile Doppler probe and then exposed by making an incision directly over the Doppler signal. Often the source of the Doppler signal is a small collateral vessel and the procedure is terminated. If the artery is present, suitability for bypass must be determined before proceeding. The patient is given heparin, and the artery is opened longitudinally. If backbleeding is encountered, a small coronary dilator is inserted to both gauge the luminal diameter and determine if the artery is patent for any distance. Generally the artery must have a lumen diameter of at least 1 mm and reasonable outflow to be acceptable. Outflow is then assessed by inserting a small angiocatheter (22 gauge) and gently injecting heparinized balanced salt solution. If flow meets very little resistance, we continue the procedure. High resistance or inability to inject means inadequate outflow, and the procedure is abandoned. These maneuvers have proved more reliable than on-table arteriography of the dorsalis pedis artery which has proved to be difficult both to perform and to interpret. "Blind" exploration of the dorsalis pedis artery, however is becoming a less frequent procedure in our more recent practice. In our early series, this was performed in 11.5% of extremities. More recently, however, these cases only make up 7.2% of our total series and 5.7% of our last 300 cases. We attribute this to improved resolution of our current generation of digital subtraction angiography equipment and the increasing experience and expertise of our angiographers in imaging foot arteries. Nevertheless, there are sill occasional patients in whom foot amputation is imminent due to ischemia when blind exploration of the dorsalis pedis artery may uncover an outflow vessel suitable for bypass.

Several other technical points that can mean the difference between success or failure deserve emphasis. Patience, meticulous technique, and attention to detail are essential. Excellent lighting, with a headlight if necessary, and magnification improve technical proficiency with such small arteries. Fine instruments and sutures, usually 6−0 and 7−0 polypropylene on cardiovascular cutting needles, alleviate the difficulties in performing anastomoses on calcified arteries. We avoid clamping or fracturing[42] heavily calcified arteries by using intraluminal coronary occluders for hemostatic control. The importance of not tunneling the graft through the skin bridge has already been emphasized. A corollary is that fine plas-

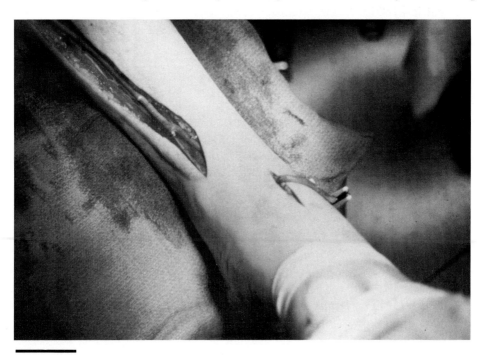

FIGURE 6.
Using a translocated vein graft avoids the need for a second foot incision by obtaining the extra length of vein needed to reach the foot from the proximal end of the vein. This approach is preferred when the popliteal artery is used for inflow.

tic surgical closures should be used for all foot and distal leg wounds. We avoid the use of skin staples in these areas, which can cause excessive wound tension and necrosis, especially with the inevitable foot swelling that occurs after bypass. Elevation of the foot or elastic bandages over the foot and lower leg are helpful in controlling edema and reducing skin tension.

When infected ulcers or wounds are present, adhesive plastic drapes are used to isolate them from the surgical wound. A sterile surgical glove placed over the toes and distal forefoot is an effective surgical barrier that does not obstruct access to the dorsal foot. Foot incisions must not encroach on areas of infection or gangrene.

SUMMARY

Improvements in angiography and in the technique and results of distal arterial reconstruction have made extreme distal bypass to the foot vessels a safe and effective treatment for limb-threatening ischemia. This has proved especially important for patients with diabetes mellitus who are most likely to require these procedures owing to the predilection for atherosclerotic occlusions to involve the crural arteries but spare the foot vessels. We are now performing pedal bypasses in approximately 25% of our diabetic patients undergoing lower extremity revascularization. Our increased use of this procedure can be partly attributed to a more liberal application of lower extremity revascularization in our diabetic patients, but is also due to the selection of the dorsalis pedis artery in preference to more proximal vessels, as previously outlined. Our decision to bypass to the dorsalis pedis artery is principally determined by our desire to restore palpable foot pulses in all patients with tissue loss or gangrene, which serves to both maximize arterial blood flow in the foot and avoid the potential need for a secondary vascular reconstruction if a bypass into a more proximal isolated segment does not result in foot healing. Since the results of pedal reconstruction are comparable to or better than those of contemporary series of tibioperoneal artery bypass grafts,[29, 30, 43–45] this approach seems justified.

The most unattractive aspect of pedal bypass grafting is its very distal location necessitating a lengthy conduit and long procedure. Being flexible with regard to inflow and vein technique, however, can simplify the surgical procedure, decrease operating time, and avoid potentially troublesome wound problems without adversely affecting results.

The presence of foot infection complicates the management of these patients owing to the frequent need for prebypass debridement or open toe or ray amputation, or both, to control active sepsis. Ultimately, foot healing is often delayed and may require additional procedures following successful bypass grafting. It is somewhat surprising that limb salvage has been more successful in these patients than in patients without infection.

We have been encouraged to note that our aggressive management of ischemia with incorporation of the dorsalis pedis bypass into our vascular surgical armamentarium has led to a decline in all levels of amputation[46] (Fig 7) and also in the lengths of stay and cost of hos-

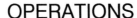

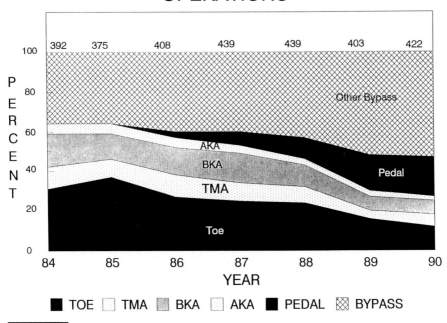

FIGURE 7.

The impact of arterial reconstruction on limb amputations at the New England Deaconess Hospital over a 7-year period. The decline in the incidence of both major and minor amputations has closely corresponded with the increasing use of pedal arterial reconstructions. AKA = above-knee amputation; BKA = below-knee amputation; TMA = transmetatarsal amputations. (From LoGerfo FW, Gibbons GW, Pomposelli FB, et al: *Arch Surg* 1992; 127:617–621. Used by permission.)

pitalization[47] of patients with ischemic, diabetic foot problems. Increasing use of the dorsalis pedis bypass has been the most important advance enabling us to improve outcome for these patients. Our results further show that the presence of diabetes should in no way diminish the vascular surgeon's expectation for successful limb salvage. A carefully planned approach including prompt control of infection, expert arteriography and a well-constructed arterial reconstruction affords a likelihood of successful limb salvage that should equal or exceed that in nondiabetic patients.

REFERENCES

1. Grunfeld C: Diabetic foot ulcers: Etiology, treatment and prevention. *Adv Intern Med* 1991; 37:103–132.
2. Levin ME: The diabetic foot: Pathophysiology, evaluation and treatment, in Levin ME, O'Neal LW (eds): *The Diabetic Foot*, ed 4. St Louis, Mosby–Year Book, 1987, pp 1–50.
3. Goldenberg SG, Alex M, Joshi RA, et al: Nonatheromatous peripheral vascular disease of the lower extremity in diabetes mellitus. *Diabetes* 1959; 8:261–273.
4. Strandness DE Jr, Priest RE, Gibbons GE: Combined clinical and pathologic

study of diabetic and nondiabetic peripheral arterial disease. *Diabetes* 1964; 13:366–372.

5. Conrad MC: Large and small artery occlusion in diabetics and nondiabetics with severe vascular disease. *Circulation* 1967; 36:83—91.

6. Barner HB, Kaiser GC, Willman VL: Blood flow in the diabetic leg. *Circulation* 1971; 43:391–394.

7. Irwin ST, Gilmore J, McGrann S, et al: Blood flow in diabetics with foot lesions due to "small vessel disease." *Br J Surg* 1988; 75:1201–1206.

8. Rosenblatt MS, Quist WC, Sidawy AN, et al: Lower extremity vein graft reconstruction: Results in diabetic and non-diabetic patients. *Surg Gynecol Obstet* 1889; 171:331–335.

9. Beach KW, Bedford GR, Bergelin RO, et al: Progression of lower-extremity arterial occlusive disease in type II diabetes mellitus. *Diabetes Care* 1988; 11:464–472.

10. Brand FN, Abbott RD, Kannel WB: Diabetes, intermittent claudication and risk of cardiovascular events; The Framingham Study. *Diabetes* 1989; 38:504–509.

11. Menzoian JO, LaMorte WW, Paniszyn CC, et al: Symptomatology and anatomic patterns of peripheral vascular disease: Differing impact of smoking and diabetes. *Ann Vasc Surg* 1989; 3:224–228.

12. Baird RJ, Tatassaura H, Miyagishima R: Saphenous vein bypass grafts to the arteries of the ankle and foot. *Ann Surg* 1979; 172:1059–1063.

13. Buchbinder D, Pasch AR, Rollins DL, et al: Results of arterial reconstruction of the foot. *Arch Surg* 1986; 121:673–677.

14. Andros G, Harris RW, Salles-Cunha SX, et al: Bypass grafts to the ankle and foot. *J Vasc Surg* 1988; 7:785–794.

15. Pomposelli FB, Jepsen SJ, Gibbons GW, et al: Efficacy of the dorsalis pedis bypass for limb salvage in diabetic patients: Short-term observations. *J Vasc Surg* 1990; 11:745–752.

16. Pomposelli FB, Jepsen SJ, Gibbons GW, et al: A flexible approach to infrapopliteal vein grafts in patients with diabetes mellitus. *Arch Surg* 1991; 126:724–729.

17. Cantelmo NL, Snow JR, Menzoian JO, et al: Successful vein bypass in patients with an ischemic limb and a palpable popliteal pulse. *Arch Surg* 1986; 121:217–220.

18. Schuler JJ, Flanigan P, William LR, et al: Early experience with popliteal to infrapopliteal bypass for limb salvage. *Arch Srug* 1983; 118:472–476.

19. Veith FJ, Gupta SK, Samson RH, et al: Superficial femoral and popliteal arteries as inflow sites for distal bypasses. *Surgery* 1981; 90:980–990.

20. Sumner DS: Noninvasive assessment of peripheral arterial occlusive disease, in Rutherford RB (ed): *Vascular Surgery*, ed 3. Philadelphia, WB Saunders, 1989, pp 61–111.

21. Turnipseed WD, Detmer DE, Berkoff HA, et al: Intra-arterial digital angiography: A new diagnostic method for determining limb salvage candidates. *Surgery* 1982; 93:322–327.

22. Blakeman BM, Littooy FN, Baker WH: Intra-arterial digital subtraction angiography as a method to study peripheral vascular disease. *J Vasc Surg* 1986; 4:168–173.

23. Mannick JA, Jackson BT, Coffman JD: Success of bypass vein grafts in patients with isolated popliteal artery segments. *Surgery* 1967; 61:17–25.

24. Noon GP, Diethrich EB, Richardson WP, et al: Distal tibial bypass: Analysis of 91 cases. *Arch Surg* 1983; 99:770–775.

25. Veith FJ, Gupta SK, Ascer E, et al: Six year comparison of autologous saphe-

nous vein and expanded polytetrafluoroethylene grafts in infrainguinal arterial reconstructions. *J Vasc Surg* 1986; 3:104–114.

26. Leather RP, Powers SR, Karmody AM: A reappraisal of the in situ saphenous vein arterial bypass: Its use in limb salvage. *Surgery* 1979; 86:453–461.

27. Taylor LM, Phinney ES, Porter JM: Present status of reversed vein bypass for lower extremity revascularization. *J Vasc Surg* 1986; 3:288–297.

28. Thompson RW, Mannick JA, Whittemore AD: Arterial reconstruction at diverse sites using nonreversed saphenous vein. *Ann Surg* 1987; 205:747–751.

29. Corson JD, Karmody AM, Shah DM, et al: In situ vein bypasses to distal tibial and limited outflow tracts for limb salvage. *Surgery* 1984; 96:756–763.

30. Plecha EJ, Seabrook GR, Bandyk DF, et al: Determinants of successful peroneal artery bypass. *J Vasc Surg* 1993; 17:97–106.

31. Leather RP, Shah CM, Corson JD, et al: Instrumental evolution of the valve incision method of in situ saphenous vein bypass. *J Vasc Surg* 1984; 1:113–123.

32. Cambria RP, Megerman J, Brewster DC, et al: The evolution of morphologic and biomechanical changes in reversed and in situ vein grafts. *Ann Surg* 1987; 202:50–155.

33. Taylor LM, Edwards JM, Porter JM: Present status of reversed vein bypass grafting: Five year results of a modern series. *J Vasc Surg* 1990; 11:193–205.

34. Miller A, Stonebridge PA, Tsoukas AI, et al: Angioscopically directed valvulotomy: A new valvulotome and technique. *J Vasc Surg* 1991; 13:813–821.

35. Gibbons GW: The diabetic foot: Amputations and drainage of infection. *J Vasc Surg* 1987; 5:800—802.

36. Harington EB, Harrington ME, Schanzer H, et al: The dorsalis pedal bypass—moderate success in difficult situation. *J Vasc Surg* 1992; 15:409–416.

37. Tannenbaum GA, Pomposelli FB, Marcaccio EJ, et al: Safety of vein bypass grafting to the dorsal pedal artery in diabetic patients with foot infections. *J Vasc Surg* 1992; 15:982–988.

38. Kannel WB, McGee DL: Diabetes and cardiovascular disease. The Framingham Study. *JAMA* 1979; 241:2035–2038.

39. Nesto RW, Watson FS, Kowalchuk GJ, et al: Silent myocardial ischemia and infarction in diabetics with peripheral vascular disease: Assessment by dipyridamole thallium-201 scintigraphy. *Am Heart J* 1990; 120:1073–1077.

40. Weaver FA, Yellin AE: Efficacy of the dorsal pedal bypass for limb salvage in diabetic paients: Short-term observations (letter). *J Vasc Surg* 1991; 13:565.

41. Stonebridge PA, Miller A, Tsoukas AI, et al: Angioscopy of arm-vein infrainguinal bypass grafts. *Ann Vasc Surg* 1991; 5:170–175.

42. Ascer EA, Veith FJ, Gupta SK: Infrapopliteal bypasses to heavily calcified rock-like arteries. *Am J Surg* 1986; 152:220–223.

43. Evans WE, Bernard VW: Tibial artery bypass for limb salvage. *Arch Surg* 1970; 100:477–481.

44. Leather RP: In situ saphenous vein arterial bypass to the tibial arteries. *J Vasc Surg* 1984; 1:912–913.

45. O'Mara CS, Kilgore TL Jr, McMullan MH, et al: Distal bypass for limb salvage in very elderly patients. *Am J Surg* 1987; 53:66–69.

46. LoGerfo FW, Gibbons GW, Pomposelli FB, et al: Trends in the care of the diabetic foot: Expanded role of arterial reconstruction. *Arch Surg* 1992; 127:617–621.

47. Gibbons GW, Marcaccio EJ, Burgess AM, et al: Improved quality of diabetic foot care, 1984 vs. 1990. *Arch Surg* 1993; 128:1–6.

Tourniquet Control for Distal Bypass

Willis H. Wagner, M.D.
Clinical Assistant Professor of Surgery, University of Southern California
School of Medicine; Chief, Division of Vascular Surgery, Cedars-Sinai Medical
Center, Los Angeles, California

David V. Cossman, M.D.
Medical Director, Vascular Laboratory; Attending, Division of Vascular Surgery,
Cedars-Sinai Medical Center, Los Angeles, California

Richard L. Treiman, M.D.
Clinical Professor of Surgery, University of Southern California School of
Medicine; Senior Attending, Division of Vascular Surgery, Cedars-Sinai Medical
Center, Los Angeles, California

T ibial and pedal artery reconstruction has increased significantly over
the last decade. Improved diabetic management has reduced microvascular complications that limit longevity. Nevertheless, the incidence
of macrovascular disease has not abated.[1, 2] With the graying of the population we have witnessed an increase in symptomatic tibial vessel occlusive disease in both diabetic and nondiabetic patients. Primary amputations are rarely performed as current limb salvage rates with autogenous
infrainguinal procedures exceed 85%.[3, 4] These factors have made distal
bypasses the most common arterial reconstructive procedures performed
in our practice.

TABLE 1.
Complications of Vascular Occlusive Devices*

Early complications
  Embolization
  Acute thrombosis
  Mural dissection
Late complications
  Late thrombosis
  Accelerated local atherosclerosis
  Fibroproliferative intimal stenosis
  Pseudoaneurysm

*From Bunt TJ, Manship L, Moore W: *J Vasc Surg* 1985;
  2:495. Used by permission.

While optimal utilization of autogenous vein is responsible for a large measure of the improved results with distal bypasses, other technical elements have contributed. Atraumatic manipulation of the vein minimizes endothelial damage and may reduce graft thrombosis.[5, 6] Routine loupe magnification and headlight illumination have substantially improved the ability to construct error-free small vessel anastomoses. Despite an emphasis on atraumatic technique, little progress has been made in eliminating the injury induced by vascular clamps (Table 1). Standard means of arterial isolation require circumferential dissection, artery and vein manipulation, and apposition of frequently rigid, calcified vessel walls. Each of these steps has the potential for injury which may cause early or late graft occlusion.

IATROGENIC INJURY

VASCULAR CLAMPS

Henson and Rob,[7] in 1956, were the first investigators to show histologic evidence of arterial wall damage caused by vascular clamps. Ultrastructural injury to the intima and media by arterial clamps has been demonstrated consistently in subsequent studies.[8-12] Atherosclerotic arteries are particularly susceptible to clamp injury, unrelated to the thickness of the intima at the site of clamp placement.[13-15] The spectrum of damage ranges from endothelial cell disruption detected by electron microscopy (Fig 1) to gross arterial wall fracture. Clamp-related intimal injury can cause early failure of an arterial reconstruction and is easily missed by completion arteriography.[15]

Vascular clamps induce physiologic alterations as well as structural damage. Endothelial cell injury caused by application of a clamp is associated with a significant reduction in local fibrinolytic activity.[16] In animal models local arterial and venous fibrinolytic activity does not return to normal until 3 weeks after the trauma (Fig 2). Since the human endothelial cell turnover rate is considerably slower than in most species, this recovery period may be prolonged in the clinical setting. Arterial wall vasomotor dysfunction has also been correlated with structural injury detected by electron microscopy. Standard metal clamps disturb both endothelial cell-mediated relaxation and the response of smooth muscle cells to nitroprusside.[17]

ALTERNATIVE OCCLUDING DEVICES

Modification of standard metal clamps has reduced arterial injury. Soft jaw insets incorporated into the Fogarty clamp significantly reduce, but do not eliminate, the damage caused by DeBakey, Potts, or Satinsky clamps.[8, 10, 11, 17] Unfortunately, the bulky nature of the Fogarty clamps makes them difficult to use in occluding tibial arteries.

Electron microscopic studies of Silastic vessel loop damage have produced contradictory data. This variation is related to the spectrum of pressure which can be generated by elastic loops. If applied at the minimum pressure necessary to occlude a compliant artery, loops cause minimal or no endothelial injury relative to other occlusive devices tested.[10-12]

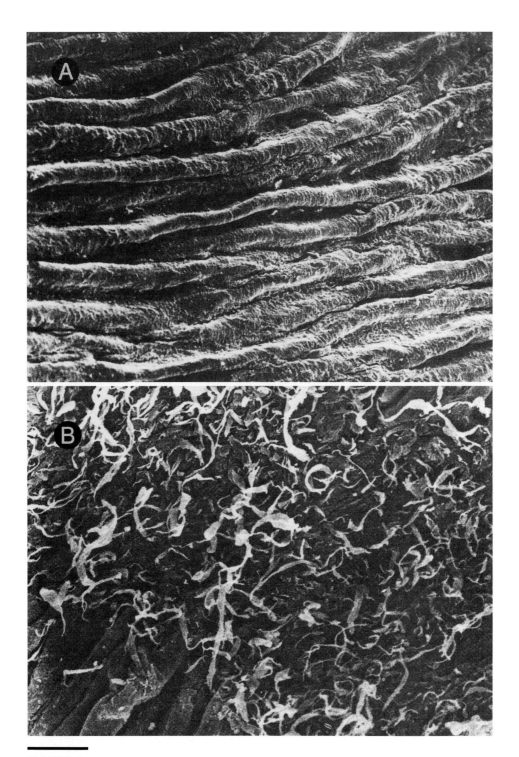

FIGURE 1.

Scanning electron photomicrographs of canine artery showing normal, control intimal surface **(A)** and extensive intimal stripping with disruption of endothelial elements throughout area of clamp application **(B).** (From Moore WM, Bunt TJ, Hermann GD, et al: *J Vasc Surg* 1988; 8:422–427. Used by permission.)

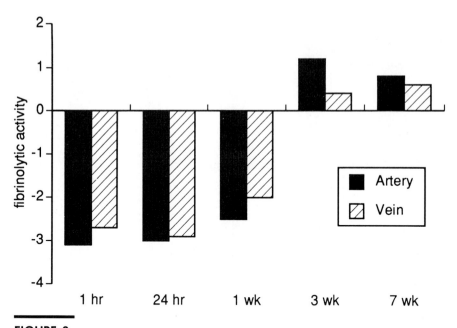

FIGURE 2.

Fibrinolytic activity in clamped segment of arteries and veins compared to controls. (From Risberg B, Bylock A: *Acta Chir Scand* 1981; 147:25–32. Used by permission.)

However, if the tension on the loops is increased, the degree of injury approaches that found with a clamp.[17, 18] Clinically, the minimal occlusive vessel loop tension may be difficult to predict without first opening the artery. Although vessel loops are relatively atraumatic on normal arteries, the frequently calcified, atherosclerotic tibial vessels cannot be occluded using atraumatic tensions.

Intraarterial balloons have been used to prevent clamp injury. As with most occluding devices, the energy transmitted to the vessel wall is variable and difficult to assess in the operating room. At low pressures (300 mm Hg) balloons cause minimal intimal injury. At intermediate to high pressures (700–1200 mm Hg), delayed intimal thickening as well as gross intimal and medial disruption occurs.[19] Balloon catheters are useful in controlling calcified large-caliber arteries; however, they are cumbersome and unsuited for small arteries below the knee.

Bulb-tipped intraluminal occluders are a less obtrusive modification of the balloon technique.[20, 21] These internal occluders are composed of silicone bulbs at either end of a flexible shaft attached to a pull-tab (Fig 3). The bulbs are of equal size on either end and are available with internal diameters (IDs) ranging from 1.0 to 3.0 mm in 0.25-mm increments (Biovascular, St. Paul, Minn). Like intraluminal balloons, use of these devices does not require circumferential vessel dissection. Before our adoption of the tourniquet technique of arterial control, we often used intraluminal occluders. While they are less traumatic than metal clamps, they fall short of the ideal occlusive device. In order to prevent bleeding from arterial side branches, collaterals must be dissected and controlled or the distal anastomosis placed in an arterial segment without branches. The

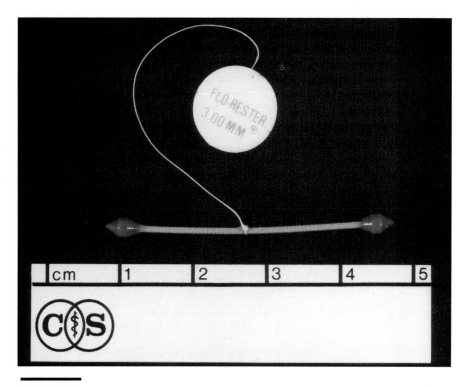

FIGURE 3.

Intraluminal occluder with silicone tips connected to a pull-tab.

latter is not always possible because distal reconstructions usually must be performed within the narrow confines of available artery, irrespective of the presence of side branches. The surgeon must be careful to avoid placing sutures through the occluder's bulbs as they have a consistency similar to the arterial wall. Inconsistency in the diameter of the perianastomotic artery may require a different-sized bulb for adequate control of both the proximal and distal lumina. Simultaneous use of two different-sized occluders is awkward and limits visualization of the anastomosis. Intraarterial positioning of the occluders can cause intimal injury or plaque dissection. Despite these limitations, we continue to use the intraluminal occluders in the rare instance that tourniquet control is not adequate.

CLINICAL SIGNIFICANCE

Experimental evidence that clamp injury causes late stenosis is equivocal. Dobrin et al.[22] found no evidence of stenosis or alteration of arterial distensibility 6 months after clamp trauma using a nonatherosclerotic canine model. In contrast, DePalma and colleagues[23] used a similar model but induced hypercholesterolemia in the experimental group. At 13 months, the hyperlipemic dogs had significant atheroma at areas of clamp injury, compared with no atheroma in the group taking a regular diet. Expression of clamp injury appears to be attenuated by individual risk factors.

The significance of histologic or physiologic clamp injury in the clinical setting is likewise uncertain. In 1981, Whittemore et al.[24] noted that an isolated juxta-anastomotic arterial stenosis, presumably due to clamp injury, was occasionally the cause of graft failure. Over the subsequent decade, duplex scan surveillance of infrainguinal reconstructions has provided substantial insight into the cause of intermediate and late graft failures. The most frequently identified lesions are intrinsic graft stenoses.[25-27] Focal, distal arterial stenoses attributable to an occluding device are inconsistently noted. During a 6-year study of over 300 consecutive reversed vein grafts, Mills[28] identified only one such lesion. In contrast, color-flow duplex surveillance of our last 100 patients having infrapopliteal bypass, prior to conversion to the tourniquet technique, identified two stenoses and two occlusions immediately distal to the tibial anasto-

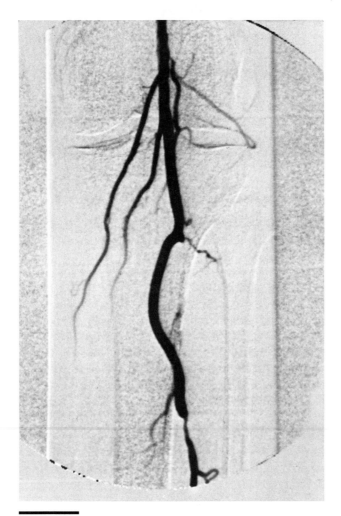

FIGURE 4.

Perianastomotic stenosis 1 year after popliteal-peroneal reversed saphenous vein bypass. Vessel loops were used to control the peroneal artery during the initial operation after the intraluminal occluder did not provide adequate hemostasis. (From Wagner WH, Treiman RL, Cossman DV, et al: *J Vasc Surg* 1993; 18:637–647. Used by permission.)

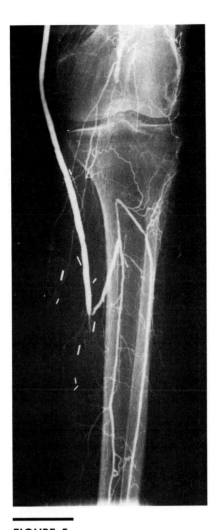

FIGURE 5.

Distal occlusion and proximal stenosis of previously normal posterior tibial artery 7 months following arm vein bypass due to severe myointimal hyperplasia. Artery was initially controlled with vessel loops.

mosis. Two of the lesions were repaired using tourniquet control in symptomatic patients (Figs 4 and 5). The remaining two grafts are still patent with only retrograde runoff. Since mid-1991, when we adopted tourniquet control as the routine, we have not identified any distal juxta-anastomotic stenoses by duplex surveillance.

TOURNIQUET CONTROL

HISTORY

Use of the tourniquet dates back to ancient Roman times, although it consisted of only a simple constricting band.[29]. In the 16th century, Ambrose Paré recommended using a tourniquet device to perform amputations.[30] Several modifications were introduced during the 17th century to tighten the band and provide more effective hemostasis. Early in the 18th century, Petit, who coined the word *tourniquet* from the French *tourner*, to turn, invented a screw modification of the technique.[30] In 1904, Harvey Cushing described the pneumatic tourniquet that could be rapidly inflated with a bicycle pump. He advocated use of this instrument to minimize bleeding during craniotomy and to provide a bloodless field for "cocaine operations" on the hand.[31]

Exsanguination of the limb before application of the tourniquet is an essential step in providing a dry field. In the 1860s, Lister routinely elevated the limb before securing the tourniquet.[32] Credit for the use of an elastic material wrapped tightly around the limb is generally given to Johann Friedrich August von Esmarch. However, the original material used by Esmarch was a rubber tube the thickness of a finger which was used as a tourniquet after the limb had been compressed by bandages. The elastic wrap, which approximates what is currently referred to as an "Esmarch bandage," was designed by von Langenbeck, as a modification of the equipment used by Esmarch.[29]

VASCULAR SURGICAL APPLICATIONS

In 1888, Rudolph Matas was the first to use a tourniquet for an arterial operation.[33] After an unsuccessful attempt to control a brachial artery pseudoaneurysm with a proximal compressing device, an Esmarch bandage applied above the aneurysm allowed Matas to perform the first endoaneurysmorrhaphy. The concept of tourniquet control for vascular reconstruction lay dormant for nearly a century. In 1979, Scheinin and Lindfors[34] described the repair of four popliteal artery aneurysms with proximal pneumatic tourniquet occlusion. During the same year, Bernhard et al.[35] presented a series of 40 popliteal and tibial artery operations using the tourniquet. They found the technique safe and it simplified the construction of the distal anastomosis. Despite these early encouraging series, vascular surgeons have been reluctant to use the tourniquet fearing irreversible aggravation of limb ischemia, thrombosis of collateral vessels, bleeding from occult venous injury, and inability to compress calcified, diabetic arteries.[36] While Bernhard and his prior collaborators at the Medical College of Wisconsin continue to use tourniquet control,[37] only recently have other vascular surgeons reported further experience with this technique. In 1991, Myers[38] described 35 infrageniculate bypasses (20 popliteal, 15 tibial) performed with thigh tourniquet control. There were no complications associated with the tourniquet except the inability to control inflow in one patient with a heavily calcified, patent superficial femoral artery (SFA). In a subsequent report, Collier[39] described his experience with 93 popliteal and tibial artery reconstructions using tourniquet control. There were no operative complications and duplex surveillance up to 18 months after surgery showed no evidence of distal juxta-anastomotic arterial stenosis.

Shindo and colleagues[40] used a modification of the tourniquet technique to perform 49 infrapopliteal artery bypasses. They used an Esmarch bandage to both exsanguinate the limb and create a bloodless field. Use of the Esmarch bandage alone to compress the thigh is not recommended due to inability to control the applied pressure. However, the authors did not identify any complications with this technique and attributed their admirable 5-year primary patency rate of 82% to the atraumatic exposure and control of the distal artery.[40]

In 1991, we first used the thigh tourniquet for inflow occlusion on a patient with a diffusely calcified, rock-hard tibial artery that could not be controlled with vessel loops or clamps. Improved visualization of the distal anastomosis, free of blood or occluding devices, and the requirement for minimal circumferential and longitudinal dissection of the artery, encouraged us to expand the application of tourniquet occlusion to all tibial artery reconstructions. In 1993, we reported our initial experience with 88 tibial and pedal artery procedures.[41] This has been expanded by an additional 75 infrapopliteal operations.

PREOPERATIVE EVALUATION

One concern that has limited application of the tourniquet technique is the potential inability to control inflow through noncompliant thigh vessels. We have not found it necessary to establish femoral artery compressibility preoperatively. The goal of preoperative noninvasive vascular testing of patients with nonhealing foot lesions or rest pain is to determine the severity and the anatomic level of the occlusive disease. A combination of the ankle-brachial index and tibial artery waveform analysis indicates the degree of pedal ischemia. Until 1988, limited localization of atherosclerotic lesions was provided by sequential blood pressure cuff measurements. Color-flow duplex scanning now provides much more accurate localization of the infrainguinal disease.[42] Therefore, we have abandoned cuff pressure measurements except at the ankle.

Arterial calcification seen on plain radiographs of the thigh has been suggested as a contraindication to using the tourniquet in orthopedic procedures.[29, 43, 44] Preoperative assessment of ankle Doppler flow with thigh cuff compression has theoretical appeal in predicting tourniquet failures. In practice, although many of our patients are diabetic with calcified distal vessels, the femoral artery in the area encompassed by the tourniquet is usually occluded or spared of significant calcification. Collateral arteries in the thigh are virtually always compressible despite severe medial calcinosis of larger vessels. We found that noncompliance of the tibial arteries at the ankle did not correlate with failure of tourniquet occlusion.[41]

Patients with patent, rigid femoral arteries are at greatest risk for incomplete hemostasis with the thigh tourniquet. This has occurred once during the 309 reported cases.[34, 35, 38–41] Since our initial experience, the tourniquet has failed to provide an adequately bloodless field in two additional patients, both with patent, calcified SFAs. Hemostasis was achieved without difficulty using conventional occlusive devices. Presumably, these few tourniquet failures could have been predicted by preoperative assessment with a thigh cuff. However, the incidence of incomplete hemostasis is sufficiently low (1%) that it does not warrant changing our vascular laboratory protocol.

TECHNIQUE

Femoral Inflow

The technique of tourniquet control is equally applicable to reversed or in situ vein bypassing. The proximal artery is prepared for anastomosis in standard fashion. The vein is then either removed from its bed for reversed bypassing or left in situ. Standard approaches to the tibial arteries are used. The most common target vessel has been the peroneal artery (Fig 6). The dissection for the distal anastomoses is significantly limited. After identifying the target vessel, no further dissection of the tibial artery or veins is performed if a sufficient length of artery wall is available for anastomosis. Crossing veins are divided only as required to gain access to one wall of the least diseased portion of the artery. Dissection of the tibial artery resembles that used for coronary arteries in the bloodless field afforded by extracorporeal circulation.

The patient is systemically anticoagulated in preparation for the anastomoses. The proximal anastomosis is performed first to allow assessment of the flow through the vein and to prevent rotation of the graft. The end of the graft is occluded with a clip and the distended vein is allowed to seek its proper orientation. All vein grafts are placed subcutaneously to

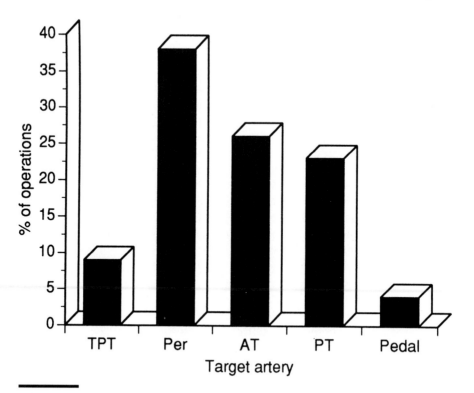

FIGURE 6.

Site of distal reconstruction of 88 tibial or pedal arteries. *TPT* = tibioperoneal trunk; *Per* = peroneal artery; *AT* = anterior tibial artery, *PT* = posterior tibial artery, *Pedal* = dorsalis pedis or plantar artery. (From Wagner WH, Treiman RL, Cossman DV, et al: *J Vasc Surg* 1993; 18:637–647. Used by permission.)

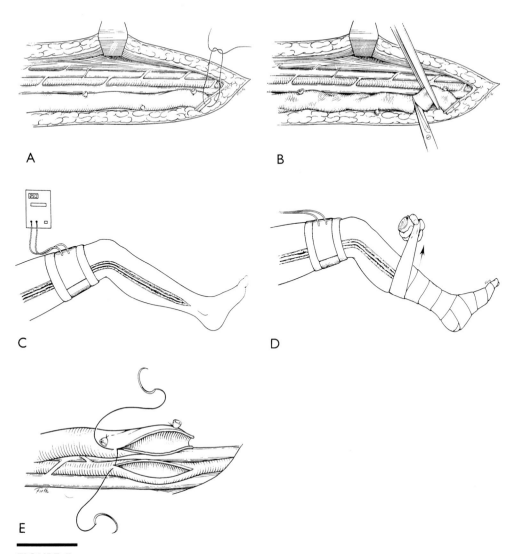

FIGURE 7.
Technique specific to tourniquet control After proximal anastomosis, the distended vein is secured to the distal wound **(A)**. The vein is emptied **(B)** and the tourniquet is placed in the thigh **(C)**. An Esmarch bandage exsanguinates the leg **(D)** and the tourniquet is inflated. The distal anastomosis is performed in standard fashion without dissecting veins or arterial branches **(E)**. (See text for details.)

facilitate postoperative duplex surveillance and revision. After extension of the leg, the end of the vein graft is placed in the distal wound and fixed to the subcutaneous tissue or muscle with a clip or suture (Fig 7,A). It is important to carefully determine the appropriate vein length and secure the graft at this point. Subsequent application of the Esmarch bandage can cause rotation of the vein and inflation of the tourniquet restricts vein movement by fixation in the thigh. A spring-loaded Fogarty bulldog clamp is placed on the proximal graft and blood is drained from the vein by incising it distally (Fig 7,B). The vein must be emptied prior to compression by both the Esmarch bandage and the tourniquet, as endothelial damage and graft rupture can occur from generation of high intraluminal pressures.

A sterile towel is wrapped around the distal thigh to pad the skin. We do not use cotton cast padding as it sheds into the underlying vein harvest wounds. A 12- to 18-cm-wide tourniquet is placed over the towel and connected to an automatic pressure inflator (Fig, 7,C). A curved cuff is more efficient than a straight cuff in transmitting pressure to the deep soft tissue.[45] The inflating device must have a feedback loop that allows constant maintenance of the set pressure. The leg is elevated and the Esmarch bandage is applied from the toes to the tourniquet (Fig, 7D). We have individualized the tourniquet pressure based on the circumference of the thigh, the degree of arterial calcification, and the systolic blood pressure. The most common pressure used in 250 mm Hg (Fig 8). We have attempted to be conservative with the pressure, as neuromuscular complications are related to the maximal transmitted pressure and the duration of inflation.

An arteriotomy is made that is approximately two to three times the diameter of the graft (Fig 7,E). After opening the artery there is occasionally a trickle of residual blood in the lumen. Squeezing the calf will usually evacuate this blood and create a dry field. The vein is cut to the appropriate length and the distal anastomosis is performed in running fashion. Over the last 3 years we have used a 7-0 nonabsorbable (Prolene)

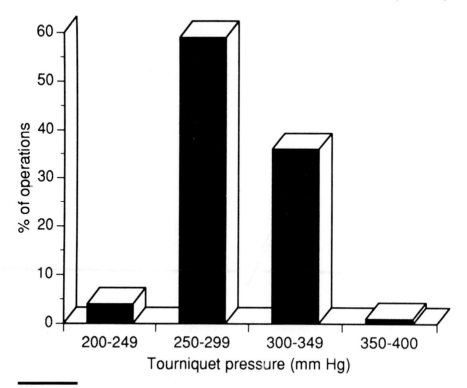

FIGURE 8.

Tourniquet pressures used during 88 infrapopliteal reconstructions. (From Wagner WH, Treiman RL, Cossman DV, et al: *J Vasc Surg* 1993; 18:637–647. Used by permission.)

suture on a BV-175 needle (Ethicon, Somerville, N.J.). This smaller needle allows more precise suture placement and, paradoxically, more easily penetrates calcified arteries than standard, larger needles.

After completion of the distal anastomosis the tourniquet is deflated and a duplex scan is obtained. Tourniquet times have been under 1 hour in all cases. Most single anastomoses can be performed with tourniquet times of 15 to 25 minutes. The visualization of the distal anastomosis with tourniquet control is so superior to the field encumbered by clamps or other occluding devices that we now selectively obtain completion arteriograms. If a palpable pulse or normal Doppler flow is present and if the completion duplex scan is normal, an arteriogram is usually not performed.

Popliteal or Tibial Inflow

When both anastomoses are below the tourniquet there are minor modifications of the procedure. Unlike preparation for anastomosis to the femoral arteries, the wall of the inflow artery is dissected as little as necessary to place the graft. When both anastomoses are below the tourniquet and a reversed vein is used, the distal anastomosis is created first. Since there is no arterial inflow, this allows manual distention of the vein through the proximal graft. After the distal anastomosis is completed a Fogarty bulldog is temporarily applied to the distal vein and the graft is distended with heparinized saline to assess orientation and length. The bulldog is then released and the proximal anastomosis to either the popliteal or the proximal tibial artery is performed. Disruption of the valves with the in situ technique allows distention of the vein in either direction. Therefore, the sequence of the anastomoses is not important.

RISKS OF TOURNIQUET CONTROL

Aside from incomplete hemostasis in less than 1% of patients, the only reported complication attributed to tourniquet control for infrapopliteal artery bypass is a single case of muscle necrosis. Bernhard et al.[35] reported superficial myonecrosis of the medial head of the gastrocnemius muscle. Omission of heparin anticoagulation during the period of tourniquet ischemia was believed to have caused local stasis and thrombosis. The muscle was debrided and the patient was discharged ambulating with a patent graft.

Although the risk of tourniquet control for arterial reconstruction appears minimal, local and systemic complications have been reported with orthopedic procedures (Table 2). Chronic limb ischemia or arterial calcification have been considered contraindications to the use of a tourniquet for orthopedic reconstructions.[29, 30] Therefore, most clinical and experimental investigation of the risks of tourniquet compression is limited to limbs without arterial occlusive disease. Chronic diabetic microvascular and atherosclerotic macrovascular insufficiency may attenuate or exacerbate these risks to an unknown degree. Although most of the complications that have been reported in orthopedic patients occurred with tourniquet times and pressures less than we have used, it is possible that our

TABLE 2.

Potential Risks of Tourniquet Control

Inadequate hemostasis
Neurologic
  Numbness
  Paresis
  Paralysis
Muscle injury
Skin damage
Metabolic
  Acidosis
  Hyperkalemia
  ↑ Oxygen consumption
  ↑ Carbon dioxide production
  Oxygen free radical production
Sickle cell crisis
Edema
Pulmonary embolism
↑ Fibrinolytic activity
Sepsis
Vein trauma
Deep vein thrombosis
Arterial injury
  Atheroembolism
  Intimal injury
  Thrombosis
  Inflow graft occlusion

patients are at heightened risk. Conversely, systemic anticoagulation used during bypass surgery may lessen the adverse effects of tourniquet inflation.

NEUROLOGIC

The primary complication of tourniquet occlusion is neuromuscular injury, predominantly in the area under the tourniquet. A posttourniquet syndrome consisting of stiffness, pallor, edema, weakness, and subjective numbness has been characterized in orthopedic patients.[45, 46] These findings are largely reversible within a week but the edema may persist for months. Many of these symptoms are indistinguishable from those seen in patients after infrainguinal bypass using conventional occlusive techniques. We have had two patients with transient neurologic symptoms following use of the tourniquet: one had subjective numbness of the toes for several days; the other had transient footdrop after bypass to the anterior tibial artery. In neither case could the cause of the patient's symptoms be unequivocally attributed to use of the tourniquet.

Objective evaluation of postmeniscectomy patients after use of the tourniquet showed a 72% incidence of electromyographic (EMG) abnormalities.[47] The incidence of EMG changes is directly related to the duration of tourniquet inflation and the applied pressures. Despite these EMG findings, clinically detectable deficits were mild and occurred with tourniquet times greater than 1 hour.[48] A similar study of patients having infrainguinal arterial reconstruction would be complicated by the high incidence of preexisting nerve dysfunction. Hunter and associates[49] found abnormal nerve conduction studies in up to 78% of patients with chronic lower extremity ischemia.

In 1954, Moldaver[50] described a more severe syndrome of tourniquet paralysis characterized by loss of touch, motor, pressure, vibration, and position senses with preservation of temperature sensation, pain, and sympathetic fibers. The incidence of clinically significant lower extremity nerve palsy related to use of a tourniquet was estimated at 1 in 13,000 in a 1974 report.[51] All cases occurred with use of an Esmarch bandage alone as the sole compressive device, a practice known to cause variable, excessive pressures. Advances in pneumatic tourniquet design currently allow greater control over the applied pressure. To minimize the risk of nerve injury, the lowest possible occlusive pressure is desired. Nomograms based on thigh circumference in patients without arterial disease

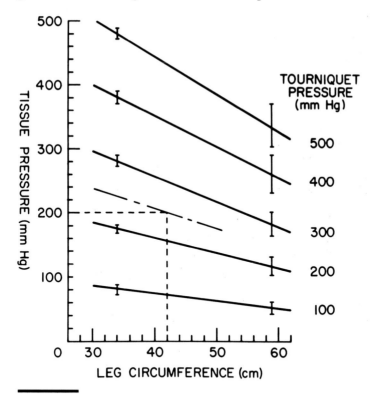

FIGURE 9.

Nomogram relating tourniquet pressure to underlying tissue pressure and thigh circumference. The *sloping lines* represent the mean soft tissue pressures in thighs of different circumferences at given (constant) tourniquet pressures. Assuming compliance of the femoral artery, the tourniquet pressure that will overcome individual systolic blood pressure is estimated using leg circumference. (From Shaw JA, Murray DG: J Bone Joint Surg [Am] 1982; 64:1150. Used by permission.)

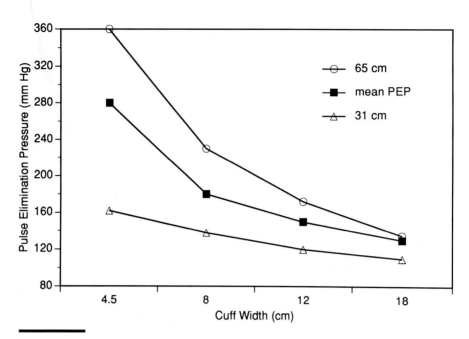

FIGURE 10.
The relationship between pulse elimination pressure *(PEP)* and cuff width. The *middle plot* represents the mean PEP for all subjects (N = 12). The *top* and *bottom curves* represent the largest and smallest thigh circumference used in this study. (From Crenshaw AG, Hargens AR, Gershuni DH, et al: *Acta Orthop Scand* 1988; 59:450. Used by permission.)

provide an estimate of the tourniquet pressure necessary to result in closure of the femoral artery[52] (Fig 9). These values are inadequate in many patients undergoing infrainguinal bypass owing to variable degrees of medial calcinosis and atherosclerosis, We have found that a pressure of 250 mm Hg is adequate in most patients. This pressure is more effectively transmitted to the deep soft tissues with a 12- or 18-cm-wide cuff than with a smaller cuff[53] (Fig 10).

The basis of the nerve disorder associated with tourniquet use has been the subject of considerable investigation.[45, 54, 55] Electrophysiologic studies suggest that the greatest nerve conduction abnormality exists at the border of the tourniquet.[56] Early anatomic findings of invagination of the nodes of Ranvier are frequently cited as evidence of mechanical deformation as the cause of clinical dysfunction.[54] However, these changes occurred only at supraphysiologic pressures of 1,000 mg Hg for 1 to 3 hours. More recent studies have concluded that the shear stress induced by the tourniquet border increases microvascular permeability and intraneural edema.[45] The resulting rise in endoneural fluid pressure impairs local tissue nutrition analogous to a muscle compartment syndrome and causes a conduction block.

MUSCULAR AND CUTANEOUS

Muscle damage, like nerve injury, occurs primarily under the tourniquet cuff and is related to pressure and duration of tourniquet inflation[45, 57]

(Fig 11). Within the range of 125- to 350-mm Hg applied pressure, there are few histologic changes in the muscle under the tourniquet after 1 to 2 hours. After 2 hours, sensitive quantitative analysis of muscle injury shows significant injury in the compressed thigh muscles.[45] Ischemia does not appear to be the sole deleterious factor, as the leg muscles distal to the tourniquet show minimal changes up to 4 hours after cuff inflation. Mechanical deformation of the underlying muscle ultrastructure appears to be a significant contributing cause of dysfunction.[58, 59] Regional hypothermia and short periods of reperfusion limit muscle damage.[46, 60, 61] However, tourniquet inflation times and pressures used in vascular surgery have generally not been associated with significant muscle injury. Routine anticoagulation during bypass surgery may prevent further injury due to microvascular thrombosis. Blisters and full-thickness skin necrosis under the tourniquet are rare occurrences. Cutaneous complications are unlikely when pressures and inflation times are minimized.

METABOLIC, HEMODYNAMIC, SYSTEMIC

Physiologic consequences of tourniquet-induced muscle ischemia result in transient systemic effects. Release of the tourniquet is associated with a rise in potassium, lactate, carbon dioxide production, oxygen uptake,

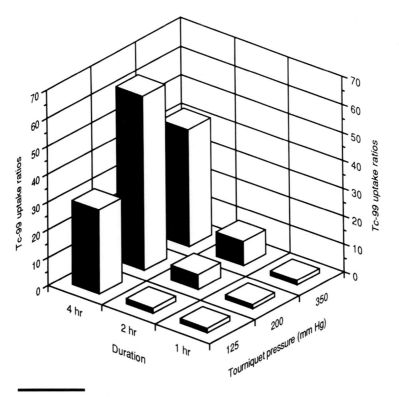

FIGURE 11.

Mean [99m]technetium pyrophosphate uptake ratios after continuous tourniquet application in rabbits (Data from Pedowitz RA: *Acta Orthop Scand Suppl* 1991; 245:1–33.)

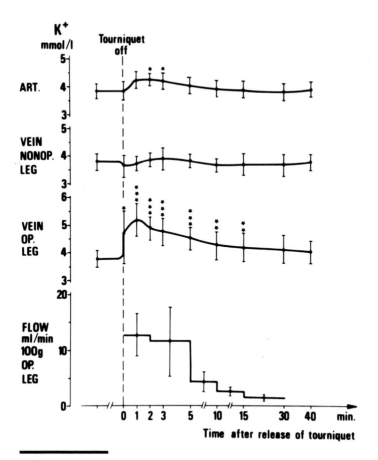

FIGURE 12.

Mean changes in arterial *(ART.)* and venous serum potassium levels and limb blood flow in the operated *(OP.)* and nonoperated *(NONOP.)* lower extremity after release of a thigh tourniquet for orthopedic reconstruction (N = 11). * = P <.05; ** = $P < .01$; *** = $P < .001$. (From Larsson J, Bergstrom J: *Acta Chir Scand* 1978; 144:68. Used by permission.)

and byproducts of oxygen-derived free radicals.[62-66] A concomitant drop in blood pressure and increase in heart rate may be due to the vasoactive effects of these metabolites or to local hemodynamic effects[63, 67] (Fig 12). The systemic effects of these metabolic and hemodynamic changes are usually mild and completely reversed within 30 minutes of tourniquet release. Although preexisting renal, pulmonary, and cardiac disease in vascular surgery patients can potentially increase the magnitude, duration, and clinical consequences of these alterations, we have not observed any adverse effects following release of the tourniquet. A potential risk of the local stasis, acidosis, and hypoxia caused by tourniquet occlusion is induction of a sickle cell crisis in a susceptible patient. Effective exsanguination of the limb with the Esmarch bandage and maintenance of optimal oxygenation and acid-base status have prevented this complication in orthopedic patients.[68]

After reperfusion, muscle blood flow increases five to ten times normal along with a significant drop in the peripheral vascular resistance of the involved limb.[67] Increased flow through the graft as a result of this reactive hyperemia may have a salutary effect on early graft patency. Conversely, reduction in vascular resistance and increase in vascular permeability associated with release of the tourniquet may exacerbate the usual postoperative limb swelling.

Ipsilateral infection of the foot or leg is considered a contraindication to compression with an Esmarch bandage in orthopedic patients.[29] Expression of bacteria into the lymphatics and the venous circulation can theoretically increase systemic and local wound infections. However, nonhealing infected or colonized foot lesions are common indications for infrainguinal bypass. We have not appreciated any unanticipated remote infectious complications following vascular reconstruction. Our wound complication rate with tourniquet control was identical to a similar group of our patients having infrainguinal bypass prior to adoption of the tourniquet.[69]

VASCULAR

Iatrogenic venous injury during tibial reconstruction has been virtually eliminated by tourniquet control. The dissection of the tibial artery is performed prior to inflation of the tourniquet and is limited to the wall where the anastomosis is to be placed. Collapse of the tibial veins after exsanguination of the limb significantly improves visualization of the anastomosis and prevents further risk of injury. Tourniquet control is particularly invaluable when reoperation in the same area of a tibial artery is required.

Systemic heparinization during vascular surgery limits the risk of deep vein thrombosis (DVT) in patients having infrainguinal reconstruction. Tourniquet occlusion may further reduce this risk. The veins are emptied and the transient ischemia induced by tourniquet control has been associated with very high levels of local fibrinolytic activity.[70] Experience with orthopedic procedures suggests that tourniquet control may decrease the rate of DVT.[71] We initially screened all patients with postoperative duplex scans, but abandoned this policy when no abnormal scans were found. There are two case reports of pulmonary emboli after applying a tourniquet in orthopedic patients with presumed acute DVT.[72, 73] Therefore, diagnosis of a recent DVT is a contraindication to tourniquet control because of the risk of extruding an inadequately adhered clot. We do not know whether a remote, prior DVT poses any significant risk.

Injury to a patent SFA under the tourniquet is a remote possibility. There have been rare reports of atheroemboli, intimal injury, and thrombosis of the SFA using the tourniquet for orthopedic reconstruction.[74, 75] Postoperative duplex surveillance of tibial bypasses originating below a patent SFA have not shown any evidence of arterial injury due to tourniquet control.[39, 41] Sequential or jump grafts to distal arteries require compression of a patent femoropopliteal bypass by the tourniquet. Graft thrombosis has been prevented by routine systemic anticoagulation and, when feasible, local irrigation of heparin within the graft.

CONCLUSION

No method of vascular isolation is without risk. However, thigh pneumatic tourniquet control appears to be the least traumatic means of arterial occlusion available for infrapopliteal bypass. Since the advent of modern coronary revascularization, cardiac surgeons have appreciated the simplicity of creating anastomoses with myocardial arrest. Tourniquet control induces a regional state of circulatory arrest that provides an unobstructed view of the artery lumen and significantly limits the required dissection.

REFERENCES

1. Haffner SM, Stern MP, Hazuda HP, et al: Cardiovascular risk factors in confirmed prediabetic individual. *JAMA* 1990; 263:2893–2898.
2. Nathan DM: Long-term complications of diabetes mellitus. *N Engl J Med* 1993; 328:1676–1685.
3. Dalman RL, Taylor LM Jr: Basic data related to infrainguinal revascularization procedures. *Ann Vasc Surg* 1990; 4:309–312.
4. Schneider JR, Walsh DB, McDaniel MD, et al: Pedal bypass versus tibial bypass with autogenous vein: A comparison of outcome and hemodynamic results. *J Vasc Surg* 1993; 17:1029–1040.
5. Adcock OT, Adcock GLD, Wheeler JR, et al: Optimal techniques for harvesting and preparation of reversed autogenous vein grafts for use as arterial substitutes: A review. *Surgery* 1984; 96:886–894.
6. Cambria RP, Megerman J, Abbott WM: Endothelial preservation in reversed and in situ autogenous vein grafts. *Ann Surg* 1985; 202:50–55.
7. Henson GF, Rob CG: A comparative study of the effects of different arterial clamps on the vessel wall. *Br J Surg* 1956; 43:561–564.
8. Harvey JG, Gough MH: A comparison of the traumatic effects of vascular clamps. *Br J Surg* 1981; 68:267–272.
9. Bunt TJ, Manship L, Moore W: Iatrogenic vascular injury during peripheral revascularization. *J Vasc Surg* 1985; 2:491–498.
10. Moore WM, Manship LL, Bunt TJ: Differential endothelial injury caused by vascular clamps and vessel loops: I. Normal vessels. *Am Surg* 1985; 51:392–400.
11. Manship LL, Moore WM, Bynoe R, et al: Differential endothelial injury caused by vascular clamps and vessel loops: II. Atherosclerotic vessels. *Am Surg* 1985; 51:401–406.
12. Moore WM Jr, Bunt TJ, Hermann GD, et al: Assessment of transmural force during application of vascular occlusive devices. *J Vasc Surg* 1988; 8:422–427.
13. Slayback JB, Bowen WW, Hinshaw DB: Intimal injury from arterial clamps. *Am J Surg* 1976; 132:183–189.
14. Guidoin R, Doyon B, Blais P, et al: Effects of traumatic manipulation on grafts, sutures, and host arteries during vascular surgery procedures. *Res Exp Med (Berl)* 1981; 179:1–21.
15. Coelho JCU, Sigel B, Flanigan DP, et al: Arteriographic and ultrasonic evaluation of vascular clamp injuries using an in vitro human experimental model. *Surg Gynecol Obstet* 1982; 155:506–512.
16. Risberg B, Bylock A: Vascular trauma induced by clamping—correlation be-

tween surface ultrastructure and fibrinolytic activity. *Acta Chir Scand* 1981; 147:25–32.

17. Barone GW, Conerly JM, Farley PC, et al: Assessing clamp-related vascular injuries by measurement of associated vascular dysfunction. *Surgery* 1989; 105:465–471.

18. Pabst TS, Flanigan DP, Buchbinder D: Reduced intimal injury to canine arteries with controlled application of vessel loops. *J Surg Res* 1989; 47:235–241.

19. McCaughan JJ, Young JM: Intra-arterial occlusion in vascular surgery, *Ann Surg* 1970; 171:695–703.

20. Edwards WH, Mulherin JL: An internal vessel occluder for distal limb bypass. *Ann Thoracic Surg* 1979; 27:472–473.

21. Griffin JB, Meng RL: Internal vessel occlusion: an improved technique for small vessel anastomosis. *J Vasc Surg* 1986; 4:616–618.

22. Dobrin PB, McGBurrin JF, McNulty JA: Chronic histologic changes after vascular clamping are not associated with altered vascular mechanics. *Ann Vasc Surg* 1992; 6:153–159.

23. DePalma RG, Chidi CC, Sternfeld WC, et al: Pathogenesis and prevention of trauma-provoked atheromas. *Surgery* 1977; 4:429–437.

24. Whittemore AD, Clowes AW, Couch NP, et al: Secondary femoropopliteal reconstruction. *Ann Surg* 1981; 193:35–42.

25. Bandyk DF, Schmitt DD, Seabrook GR, et al: Monitoring functional patency of in situ saphenous vein bypasses: The impact of a surveillance protocol and elective revision. *J Vasc Surg* 1989; 9:286–296.

26. Mills JL, Harris EJ, Taylor LM, et al: The importance of routine surveillance of distal bypass grafts with duplex scanning: A study of 379 reversed vein grafts. *J Vasc Surg* 1990; 12:379–389.

27. Donaldson MC, Mannick JA, Whittemore AD: Causes of primary graft failure after in situ saphenous vein bypass grafting. *J Vasc Surg* 1992; 15:113–120.

28. Mills JL: Mechanisms of vein graft failure: The location, distribution, and characteristics of lesions that predispose to graft failure. *Semin Vasc Surg* 1993; 6:78–91.

29. Fletcher IR, Healy TE: The arterial tourniquet. *Ann R. Coll Surg Engl* 1983; 65:409–417.

30. Mullick S: The tourniquet in operations upon the extremities. *Surg Gynecol Obstet* 1978; 146:821–826.

31. Cushing H: Pneumatic tourniquet: with special reference to their use in craniotomies. *Med News* 1904; 84:577–580.

32. Klenerman L: The tourniquet in surgery. *J Bone Joint Surg [Br]* 1962; 44:937–943.

33. Friedman SG, Friedman MS: Matas, Antyllus, and endoaneurysmorrhaphy. *Surgery* 1989; 105:761–763.

34. Scheinin TM, Lindfors O: Simplified repair of popliteal aneurysms. *J Cardiovasc Surg* 1979; 20:189–192.

35. Bernhard VM, Boren CH, Towne JB: Pneumatic tourniquet as a substitute for vascular clamps in distal bypass surgery. *Surgery* 1980; 87:709–713.

36. Mannick JA, DeWeese JA, Porter JM, et al: Infrainguinal bypass grafting techniques (symposium). *Contemp Surg* 1991; 39:39–59.

37. Towne JB: In situ saphenous vein bypass open technique. *Semin Vasc Surg* 1993; 6:166–170.

38. Myers KA: Semi-closed, ex-situ, non-reversed or reversed autogenous vein grafting. *J Cardiovasc Surg* 1991; 32:110–116.

39. Collier PE: Atraumatic vascular anastomoses using a tourniquet. *Ann Vasc Surg* 1992; 6:34–37.

40. Shindo S, Tada Y, Sato O, et al: Esmarch's bandage technique in distal by-pass surgery. *J Cardiovasc Surg* 1992; 33:609–612.
41. Wagner WH, Treiman RL, Cossman DV, et al: Tourniquet occlusion technique for tibial artery reconstruction. *J Vasc Surg* 1993; 18:637–647.
42. Cossman DV, Ellison JE, Wagner WH, et al: Comparison of dye arteriography to arterial mapping with color-flow duplex imaging in the lower extremities. *J Vasc Surg* 1989; 10:522–529.
43. Jeyaseelan S, Stevenson TM, Pfitzner J: Tourniquet failure and arterial calcification. *Anaesthesia* 1981; 36:48–50.
44. Klenerman L, Lewis JD: Incompressible vessels (letter). *Lancet* 1976; 1:811–812.
45. Pedowitz RA: Tourniquet-induced neuromuscular injury. *Acta Orthop Scand Suppl* 1991; 245:1–33.
46. Sapega AA, Heppenstall RB, Chance B, et al: Optimizing tourniquet application and release times in extremity surgery. *J Bone Joint Surg [Am]* 1985; 67:303–314.
47. Weingarden SI, Louis DL, Waylonis GW: Electromyographic changes in postmeniscectomy patients. *JAMA* 1979; 241:1248–1250.
48. Saunders KC, Louis DL, Weingarden SI, et al: Effect of tourniquet time on postoperative quadriceps function. *Clin Orthop* 1979; 143:194–199.
49. Hunter GC, Song GW, Nayak NN, et al: Peripheral nerve conduction abnormalities in lower extremity ischemia: the effects of revascularization. *J Surg Res* 1988; 45:96–103.
50. Moldaver J: Tourniquet paralysis syndrome. *Arch Surg* 1954; 68:136–144.
51. Middleton RWD, Varian JP: Tourniquet paralysis. *Aust N Z J Surg* 1974; 44:124–128.
52. Shaw JA, Murray DG: The relationship between tourniquet pressure and soft-tissue pressure in the thigh. *J Bone Joint Surg [Am]* 1982; 64:1148–1151.
53. Crenshaw AG, Hargens AR, Gershuni DH, et al: Wide tourniquet cuffs more effective at lower inflation pressures. *Acta Orthop Scand* 1988; 59:447–451.
54. Ochoa J, Fowler TJ, Gilliatt RW: Anatomical changes in peripheral nerves compressed by a pneumatic tourniquet. *J Anat* 1972; 113:433–455.
55. Nitz AJ, Matulionis DH: Ultrastructural changes in rat peripheral nerve following pneumatic tourniquet compression. *J Neurosurg* 1982; 57:660–666.
56. Pedowitz RA, Nordborg C, Rosenqvist AL, et al: Nerve function and structure beneath and distal to a pneumatic tourniquet applied to rabbit hindlimbs. *Scand J Plast Reconstr Surg Hand Surg* 1991; 25:109–120.
57. Pedowitz RA, Friden J, Thornell LE: Skeletal muscle injury induced by a pneumatic tourniquet: an enzyme- and immunohistochemical study in rabbits. *J Surg Res* 1992; 52:243–250.
58. Gersoff WK, Ruwe P, Jokl P, et al: The effect of tourniquet pressure on muscle function. *Am J Sports Med* 1989; 17:123–127.
59. Pedowitz RA, Gershuni DH, Schmidt AH, et al: Muscle injury beneath and distal to a pneumatic tourniquet: A quantitative animal study of effects of tourniquet pressure and duration. *J Hand Surg* 1991; 16A:610–621.
60. Swanson AB, Livengood LC, Sattel AB: Local hypothermia to prolong safe tourniquet time. *Clin Orthop* 1991; 262:200–208.
61. Pedowitz RA, Gershuni DH, Friden J, et al: Effects of reperfusion intervals on skeletal muscle injury beneath and distal to a pneumatic tourniquet. *J Hand Surg* 1992; 17A:245–255.
62. Haljamae H, Enger E: Human skeletal muscle energy metabolism during and after complete tourniquet ischemia. *Ann Surg* 1975; 182:9–14.

63. Larsson J, Bergstrom J: Electrolyte changes in muscle tissue and plasma in tourniquet-ischemia. *Acta Chir Scand* 1978; 144:67–73.
64. Friedl HP, Till GO, Trentz O, et al: Role of oxygen radicals in tourniquet-related ischemia-reperfusion injury of human patients. *Klin Wochenschr* 1991; 69:1109–1112.
65. Hoka S, Yoshitake J, Arakawa S, et al: VO_2 and VCO_2 following tourniquet deflation. *Anaesthesia* 1992; 47:;65–68.
66. Lee TL, Tweed WA, Singh B: Oxygen consumption and carbon dioxide elimination after release of unilateral lower limb pneumatic tourniquets. *Anesth Analg* 1992; 75:113–117.
67. Larsson J, Lewis DH: The local hemodynamic effects of operation in a bloodless field. *Eur Surg Res* 1978; 10:24–32.
68. Adu-Gyamfi Y, Sankarankutty M, Marwa S: Use of a tourniquet in patients with sickle cell disease. *Can J Anaesth* 1993; 40:24–27.
69. Wagner WH, Levin PM, Treiman RL, et al: Early results of infrainguinal arterial reconstruction with a modified biological conduit. *Ann Vasc Surg* 1992; 6:325–333.
70. Petaja J, Myllynen P, Myllyla G, et al: Fibrinolysis after application of a pneumatic tourniquet. *Acta Chir Scand* 1987; 153:647–651.
71. Kroese AJ, Stiris G: The risk of deep-vein thrombosis after operations on a bloodless lower limb. A venographic study. *Injury* 1976; 7:271–273.
72. Austin M: The Esmarch bandage and pulmonary embolism. *J Bone Joint Surg [Br]* 1963;45:384–385.
73. McGrath BJ, Hsia J, Epstein B: Massive pulmonary embolism following tourniquet deflation. *Anesthesiology* 1991; 74:618–620.
74. Williams TA, Baerg RH, Beal WS: Acute arterial occlusion secondary to the use of a pneumatic thigh tourniquet. *J Am Podiatr Med Assoc* 1986; 76:464–465.
75. DeLaurentis DA, Levitsky KA, Booth RE, et al: Arterial and ischemic aspects of total knee arthroplasty. *Am J Surg* 1992; 1:164:237–240.

Determinants of Long-Term Success After Infrainguinal Vein Bypass

Jonathan B. Towne, M.D.
Professor and Chairman, Department of Vascular Surgery/Surgery, Medical
College of Wisconsin, Milwaukee, Wisconsin

T he success of infrainguinal arterial reconstructions is influenced by changes in the anatomic and hemodynamic characteristics of the inflow artery, the outflow artery, and the bypass conduit. The two disease processes that primarily affect long-term patency are the progression of atherosclerosis and the development of fibrointimal hyperplasia. The progression of atherosclerosis in the inflow and outflow artery can result in a diameter-reducing stenosis that threatens bypass patency. The development and progression of fibrointimal hyperplasia to diameter-reducing lesions resulting in bypass failures are related to injurious effects of modifying a poor-quality venous conduit, correcting technical errors, handling the vein, and performing the anastomosis. The superior long-term patency rates in recent series of vein bypasses (i.e., in situ and reversed) have largely been attributed to improved surgical technique and increase in experience of the vascular surgeons.[1-3]

A decade ago we adopted the in situ saphenous vein bypass technique for the management of limb-threatening ischemia. Preference for this bypass technique was based on the superiority of autogenous reconstruction, the ability to use the ipsilateral saphenous vein, and the accessibility of the bypass for postoperative surveillance and revision. During the 1980s we studied the learning curve associated with initial success, the effect of technical errors on early patency, the pathophysiologic mechanisms that decrease primary patency, and the favorable impact of a surveillance protocol on elective revision on secondary patency. Our results have improved with increasing experience in performing the in situ saphenous vein bypass.[1] Commitment to the study of the in situ bypass has permitted a unique opportunity to assess the advantages and limitations of this technique as well as the determinant factors of long-term patency. We evaluated the outcome of 361 consecutive in situ saphenous vein bypasses performed during the last decade to determine the influence of operative decisions regarding the selection and management of the inflow artery, the outflow artery, and the venous conduit on long-term patency. We also evaluated the effect of reconstruction of a diseased inflow artery or modification of the conduit during the operative procedure.

Advances in Vascular Surgery, vol 2
© 1994, Mosby–Year Book, Inc.

MODIFIED VEIN

A *modified conduit* was defined as the need to reexplore the bypass because of residual valve leaflet requiring a venotomy for valve lysis, valvulotome injury, torsion of the vein conduit, anastomotic stricture, formation of platelet aggregates on the endothelial flow surface, or replacement of a sclerotic, varicose, or small-diameter vein, with a free vein segment harvested from elsewhere. Modification techniques include vein patch angioplasty, primary repair, resection and venovenostomy, and resection and interposition of a translocated vein graft into the in situ vein bypass. All of our patients were followed with a postoperative duplex surveillance protocol.

At the time of in situ bypass grafting, 23% of the 361 saphenous vein conduits required modification to successfully complete the procedure. The secondary procedure was performed to correct an inadequate vein in 10% of the bypasses and technical problems related to vein preparation or vascular construction in 13% (Table 1). The primary patency at 4 years for bypasses requiring modification was 50% which was significantly less than the rate of 70% for nonmodified bypass conduits. Also, the secondary patency for bypasses requiring modification was 72% which was significantly less than the patency for nonmodified bypass conduits, which was 84%. Forty percent of the in situ saphenous vein bypasses with modified conduits required revision in the postoperative period compared to 22% of the nonmodified conduits.

The decline in the secondary patency of the revised bypasses compared to the nonrevised bypasses was due to the poor patency of in situ conduits that were thrombosed at the time of revision. The secondary patency rate for bypasses patent at the time of revision was equivalent to the bypasses never undergoing revision. The secondary patency rate for revised thrombosed bypasses was 47% at 4 years, a level comparable to other reports.[4, 5] The poor outcome of procedures on thrombosed conduit veins coupled with the excellent patency of patent bypass revisions underscores the importance of monitoring the graft hemodynamics with a surveillance protocol in order to detect the failing bypass prior to thrombosis. As the number of technical errors decreased with additional surgical experience, the quality of the vein has emerged as the most important factor determining the need for modification of the bypass conduit. We define a good-quality vein as a thin-walled vein, greater than 2 mm internal diameter, with or without a bifurcated segment, that has a glistening endothelial flow surface. If a technical error occurs or if a poor-quality segment of vein is identified, the short segment of abnormal vein can be modified and the in situ technique maintained for the remainder of the bypass. Intraoperative modification of the in situ conduit should result in normal blood flow hemodynamics if early bypass patency is to be expected.[6] Long-term patency is dependent on careful postoperative hemodynamic surveillance to identify and correct new lesions which can develop.

The long-term patency of vein bypasses constructed by both in situ and reversed techniques is decreased when the ipsilateral saphenous vein is inadequate and requires modification. In a recent series of reversed vein

TABLE 1.

Modification of 86 in Situ Saphenous Vein Conduits Performed to Correct Inadequate Veins (37 of 361, 10%) or Technical Failure of Adequate Veins (49 of 361, 13%)

Lesion	Vein Patch	Primary Repair	Resection Venovenostomy	Interposition Vein Segment	Totals
Adequate vein					
Vein injury	9	19	1	—	29
Anastomotic stenosis	3	1	—	1	5
Retained valve	4	—	—	—	4
Bypass torsion	2	—	2	—	4
Platelet aggregates	4	—	—	—	4
Low-flow state	—	—	—	3	3
					49
Inadequate vein					
Sclerotic segment	8	—	2	12	22
Previously utilized	—	—	—	7	7
Small diameter	—	—	1	4	5
Varicosity	1	2	—	—	3
					37

grafts, Taylor et al.[3] reported that the primary patency of grafts with inadequate ipsilateral saphenous vein (68%) was significantly decreased compared to grafts with adequate ipsilateral saphenous vein (80%). The secondary patency of grafts with inadequate vein (77%) was also decreased compared to grafts with adequate vein (84%), but the two were not statistically compared. Similarly, a significant decline was documented in this series with the use of an inadequate vein that underwent modification. The in situ technique has the advantage of utilizing the ipsilateral saphenous vein (90%) more frequently in comparison to the reversed vein grafts (55%).[3] The reason for this difference in vein utilization is unclear, but is probably related to the use of smaller-diameter veins for the in situ bypass. The ability to utilize the ipsilateral saphenous vein for the length of the bypass can significantly decrease the number of conduits requiring modification and preserves the contralateral saphenous vein for bypass of the opposite extremity (performed in 9% of patients in our series).

INFLOW ARTERY REVISION

Occlusive or aneurysmal disease of the femoral artery may require vascular repairs to make this vessel suitable as an inflow source of a femoral distal graft. Femoral artery repairs also adversely affect the long-term patency of distal bypasses. In our series, severe atherosclerotic disease of the common femoral artery was present in 12% of cases and was treated by endarterectomy, patch angioplasty, or replacement with an interposition prosthesis to complete the proximal anastomosis. The primary patency at 3 years was significantly lower for bypasses originating from diseased inflow arteries requiring reconstruction (45%) compared to bypasses for inflow arteries not reconstructed (69%). The secondary patency at 3 years was not significantly decreased for the bypasses originating from a reconstructed inflow artery (76%) compared to bypasses from inflow arteries not reconstructed (89%). Revision of the in situ saphenous vein bypasses was not significantly different for those with (34%) and without (25%) a reconstructed inflow artery. However, 53% of the revisions on bypasses with reconstruction of the inflow artery were to correct a problem with the conduit reconstruction, compared to 82% of the revisions on bypasses with no reconstruction of the inflow artery. In the follow-up period, in situ bypass revision for anastomotic or outflow artery stenosis was significantly more frequent for bypasses of reconstructed inflow arteries (16%) compared to bypasses originating from nonreconstructed inflow arteries (4.5%). Decline in primary patency was not due to failure of the reconstruction of the inflow artery, but was associated with the severity of the preexisting atherosclerotic disease of the patient undergoing bypass. The secondary patency was maintained with bypass surveillance and elective revision.

EFFECT OF POSTOPERATIVE REVISION ON PATENCY

The secondary patency at 4 years was significantly lower for bypasses undergoing prior revision (68%) compared to nonrevised bypasses (88%). The decline in secondary patency for revised bypasses was due primarily to the poor patency of bypasses that were thrombosed at the time of revision (47%) compared to the patency of bypasses patent at the time of revision (93%). Secondary graft patency after revision of the patent bypasses was equivalent to the secondary patency rate of bypasses that never required revision.

GRAFT THROMBOSIS PRIOR TO REVISION

An interesting correlation was the effect of graft thrombosis on the development of aneurysm vein conduit degeneration. Aneurysm degeneration of saphenous vein grafts is an infrequent late finding with only 29 cases described in the literature.[7-13] We found 8 such grafts in a series that evaluated 72 lower extremity grafts functioning for at least 5 years.[14] Two thirds (62%) of the grafts had become occluded and undergone either a thrombectomy or thrombolysis many months before the diagnosis of vein graft aneurysm. Three grafts with aneurysms had no history of occlusion and two of these were reversed saphenous vein grafts. We postulate a transmural ischemic injury can occur at the time of graft thrombosis or vein retrieval. This alters the integrity of the vein graft wall, which predisposes to subsequent aneurysm formation. Vein graft aneurysms have been described as atherosclerotic in nature, but this may be a result of an ongoing repair of ischemic injury rather than the primary cause of the aneurysm.

EFFECT OF GRAFT REVISION ON LONG-TERM FUNCTION

Long-term graft structure is affected by postoperative revisions. Approximately one half (53%) of the grafts in our series, followed at least 5 years, had undergone at least one revision either to repair the conduit or to maintain inflow or outflow. These revised conduits contained a majority of the significant graft-threatening lesions detected on follow-up, whereas grafts that had never been modified tended to be normal in appearance. During the early postoperative period all revisions involved the conduit and were necessary to correct technical errors such as retained valves, arteriovenous (AV) fistulas, twisted graft, and the use of an unsuitable vein segment. Between 1 and 24 months after operations grafts were usually revised because of stenotic lesions at the anastomosis and valve sites. This tended to portend future problems and only 17% of these conduits were normal by color duplex ultrasonography at late follow-up. After 2 years the grafted extremities were more affected by the ongoing atherosclerotic process. Progression of inflow and outflow disease necessitated two thirds of the late revisions.

SURGEON EXPERIENCE

In order to determine the effect of surgeon experience on graft patency, the first 179 cases, which represents our experience from 1981 to 1985, were compared to the subsequent 182 cases, which was our experience from 1986 to 1989, to identify variables that have improved with increasing surgical experience. A comparison of the two time intervals revealed no significant difference in the number of diabetic patients, indications for surgery, total number of conduits undergoing modification, the vein diameter of the conduits, the inflow artery, the outflow artery, or the number of bypasses undergoing revision (Table 2). A significant decrease in the number of technical errors encountered in preparing the saphenous vein conduit for in situ bypasses is documented for the latter half of the experience (Table 3). The primary patency improvement for the second half compared to the first half of the experience was not statistically significantly different. The secondary patency rate was significantly improved from the latter half of the series compared to the first half. The secondary patency rate of the revised bypasses at 3 years was not significantly different for the latter half (86%) compared with the first half (80%) of experience. The number of bypasses thrombosed at the time of revision decreased for the second half compared to the first half but was also not significantly different. The secondary patency at 3 years of the bypasses not undergoing revision did significantly improve in the latter half (97%) compared to the first half (83%) of the experience.

The primary patency for the second half of the series was equivalent to the primary patency in a recent series of reverse vein bypass grafts reported by Taylor and his group from the University of Oregon.[3] Patency rates were associated with a significant improvement in surgical tech-

TABLE 2.

Comparison of Clinical and Anatomic Factors Between the First 179 Cases (1981–1985) and the Subsequent 182 Cases (1986–1989) of In Situ Saphenous Vein Bypasses*

	No. of Bypasses (%)	
Factor	1981–1985	1986–1990
Diabetes mellitus	75(42)	81(45)
Tobacco use	149(42)	155(44)
Indication		
Critical limb ischemia	169(94)	166(91)
Popliteal artery aneurysm	8(5)	7(4)
Claudication	2(1)	9(5)
Conduit		
Modified	50(29)	36(20)
No modification	124(71)	145(80)
Vein diameter		
<3.0 mm	6(5)	8(10)
3.0–3.9 mm	48(44)	27(35)
≥4.0 mm	56(51)	42(55)
Inflow artery		
Diseased/reconstructed	16(9)	22(13)
No reconstruction	157(91)	153(87)
Outflow artery		
Popliteal	56(31)	59(32)
Tibial	123(69)	123(68)
Bypass revision	55(31)	40(22)

*From Bergamini TM, Towne JB, Bandyk DF, et al: *J Vasc Surg* 1991; 13:137–147. Used by permission.

TABLE 3.

Technical Errors Encountered in Performing the In Situ Saphenous Vein Bypass Comparing the First 179 Cases (1981–1985) to the Subsequent 182 Cases (1986–1989)

Technical Error	1981–1985	1986–1989
Valvulotome injury	20	9
Anastomotic stenosis	5	0
Bypass torsion	5	0
Residual valve leaflet	4	0
Total (%)*	34 (18)	9 (5)

*Total number of technical errors for the first half compared to the second half is significantly different, $P = .0001$ (chi-square analysis).

nique, vein preparation during the bypass, and a decrease in the number of technical errors. Long-term patency of the in situ saphenous vein bypass was improved by meticulous technique and increasing surgical experience.

VEIN SIZE

In order to assess the effect of vein diameter on bypass patency, in 187 bypasses in which operative angiograms were available the vein diameters were measured and stratified according to diameter.[15] In ten patients, the vein diameter was 2.0 to 2.9 mm; in 73 grafts were 3.0 to 3.9 mm, and in 98 they were greater than 4 mm. No vein less than 2 mm in diameter was used. The 30-day patency of veins less than 3 mm was less, but long term there was no difference between the three groups, demonstrating that long-term patency was not affected by vein diameter. Leather et al.[16] also noted no difference in patency for vein grafts less than 3 mm. Wengerter et al.,[17] on the other hand, reported significantly decreased patency rates for reversed veins less than 3 mm compared with reversed vein grafts with greater diameters.

LOCATION OF INFLOW VESSEL AND OUTFLOW VESSEL

The site of the inflow artery did not affect secondary patency of the in situ bypasses. This observation is consistent with the results of vein bypasses reported by Leather and Wengerter and colleagues.[16, 17] The primary and secondary patency rates also were not significantly different for the tibial compared to the popliteal artery. In this series the site of the distal anastomosis was the above-knee popliteal artery in 2%, the below-knee popliteal artery in 29%, and the tibial artery in 68%. This is at variance with the work of Taylor and his group[3] who report a significant decrease in primary patency for reverse vein grafts to the infrapopliteal artery (69%) compared to the below-knee popliteal artery (80%). The secondary patency for reversed vein grafts to infrapopliteal arteries (77%) was also decreased compared to below-knee popliteal arteries (86%), but the two were not statistically compared. A significant decrease in cumulative patency for reversed vein grafts compared to the in situ bypass to the tibial outflow artery has also been noted by Rutherford et al.[18]

Factors not significantly affecting the primary and secondary in situ patency were diabetes, tobacco use, bifurcated saphenous vein, and the site of the inflow or outflow artery. The bypass patency rates at 4 years for diabetic tobacco users (86%), diabetic nontobacco users (92%), nondiabetic tobacco users (85%), and nondiabetic nontobacco users (83%) were not significantly different. This is similar to work reported by Shah et al.[19] By contrast, the long-term patency for reversed saphenous vein grafts was significantly affected by the presence or absence of diabetes in reports by Taylor et al.,[3] Cutler et al.,[20] and Reichle et al.[21] A bifurcated saphenous vein was used in 21 cases. The long-term patency of the bypasses with bifurcated veins was equivalent to bypasses performed with adequate, nonbifurcated ipsilateral saphenous vein.

STATUS OF RUNOFF BED

We have been unable to determine any discriminant effect of the status of the pedal arch on the success of distal bypass grafting. A series of 77 consecutive peroneal artery bypasses performed between 1981 and 1990 demonstrated that the presence of a patent dorsalis or posterior tibial artery on the intact pedal arch did not significantly influence primary or secondary patency.[22] The 5-year secondary patency rates for patients with a patent dorsalis pedis or posterior tibial arch ankle was 88%. The inability to develop outflow assessment scores which predict the success of lower extremity bypass has been confirmed by the results of Synn and Shortell and co-workers.[23, 24] To date there is no preoperative or intraoperative evaluation that reliably predicts which bypass grafts are going to be successful.

REFERENCES

1. Bergamini TM, Towne JB, Bandyk DF, et al: Experience with in situ saphenous vein bypasses during 1981 to 1989: Determinant factors of long-term patency. *J Vasc Surg* 1991; 13:137–147.
2. Leather RP, Shah DM, Chang BB, et al: Resurrection of the in situ saphenous vein bypass: 1000 cases later. *Ann Surg* 1988; 208:435–442.
3. Taylor LM, Edwards JM, Porter JM: Present status of reversed vein bypass grafting: Five-year results of a modern series. *J Vasc Surg* 1990; 11:193–206.
4. Whittemore AD, Clowes AW, Couch NP, et al: Secondary femoropopliteal reconstruction. *Ann Surg* 1981; 193:35–42.
5. Belkin M, Donaldson MC, Whittemore AD, et al: Observations on the use of thrombolytic agents for thrombotic occlusion of infrainguinal vein grafts. *J Vasc Surg* 1990; 11:289–296.
6. Schmitt DD, Seabrook GR, Bandyk DF, et al: Early patency of in situ saphenous vein bypasses as determined by intraoperative velocity waveform analysis. *Ann Vasc Surg* 1990; 4:270–275.
7. Davidson ED, DePalma RG: Atherosclerotic aneurysm occurring in an autogenous vein graft. *Am J Surg* 1972; 124:112–114.
8. DeWeese JA: Aneurysms of venous bypass grafts in the lower extremities. *J Cardiovasc Surg* 1973; 14(suppl):271–273.
9. De La Rocha AG, Peixoto RS, Baird RJ: Atherosclerosis and aneurysmm formation in a saphenous vein-graft. *Br J Surg* 1973; 60:72–73.
10. Sassoust G, Moreau J, Courchia G, et al: Deterioration of in-situ vein bypasses: Anatomic study of 11 cases. *Ann Vasc Surg* 1988; 2:345–348.
11. Kelly PH, Julsrud JM, Dyrud PE, et al: Aneurysmal rupture of a femoropopliteal saphenous vein graft. *Surgery* 1990; 107:468–470.
12. Peer RM, Upson JF: Aneurysmal dilatation in saphenous vein bypass grafts. *J Cardiovasc Surg* 1990; 31:668–671.
13. Straton CS, Beckmann CF, Jewell ER: Aneurysm formation in distal saphenous vein bypass grafts as a cause of graft failure. *Cardiovasc Intervent Radiol* 1991; 14:167–269.
14. Reifsnyder T, Towne JB, Seabrook GR, et al: Biologic characteristics of long-term autogenous vein grafts: A dynamic evolution. *J Vasc Surg* 1993; 17:207–217.
15. Towne JB, Schmitt DD, Seabrook GR, et al: The effect of vein diameter on patency of in situ grafts. *J Cardiovasc Surg* 1991; 32:192–196.
16. Leather SP, Shah DM, Karmody AM: Intrapopliteal arterial bypass for limb

salvage: Increased patency and utilization of the saphenous vein use "in situ." *Surgery* 1981; 90:1000–1008.

17. Wengerter KR, Veith FJ, Gupta SK, et al: Influence of vein size (diameter) on infrapopliteal reversed vein graft patency. *J Vasc Surg* 1990; 11:525–531.
18. Rutherford RB, Jones DN, Bergentz SE, et al: Factors affecting the patency of infrainguinal bypass. *J Vasc Surg* 1988; 8:236–246.
19. Shah DM, Chang BB, Fitzgerald KM, et al: Durability of the tibial artery bypass in diabetic patients. *Am J Surg* 1988; 156:133–135.
20. Cutler BS, Thompson JE, Kleinsasser LJ, et al: Autologous saphenous vein femoro-popliteal bypass: Analysis of 298 cases. *Surgery* 1976; 79:325–331.
21. Reichle FA, Rankin KP, Tyson RR, et al: Long-term results of femoro-popliteal bypass in diabetic patients with severe ischemia of the lower extremity. *Am J Surg* 1979; 137:653–656.
22. Plecha EJ, Seabrook GR, Bandyk DF, et al: Determinants of successful peroneal artery bypass. *J Vasc Surg* 1993; 17:97–106.
23. Synn AL, Hoballah JJ, Sharp WJ, et al: Vein bypass to the peroneal artery for lower extremity tissue loss: Are there angiographic predictors of failure? *Am J Surg* 1992; 164:276–280.
24. Shortell CK, Ouriel K, DeWeese JA, et al: Peroneal artery bypass: A multifactorial analysis. *Ann Vasc Surg* 1992; 6:15–19.

PART II

Alternative Autogenous Conduits

Current Practices of Arterial Bypass With Arm Veins

George Andros, M.D.
Medical Director, Vascular Laboratory, St. Joseph Medical Center, Burbank, California

Peter A. Schneider, M.D.
Private Practice, Burbank, California

Robert W. Harris, M.D.
Private Practice, Burbank, California

B ypass grafting of arterial occlusions has been the major catalyst in the development of infrainguinal arterial surgery. Reversed greater saphenous vein has many advantages and few limitations. Inevitably, however, some vein bypass grafts fail: when they do, short of using the contralateral greater saphenous vein, no equivalent substitute conduit is readily available for repeat vascularization. The quest for alternative grafts has ranged from the bovine carotid artery and Sparks Mandrit to Dacron fabric tube grafts, expanded polytetrafluoroethylene (EPTFE), and human umbilical veins. Recognition of the deficiencies of the various prostheses coincided with a renewed interest in an all-autogenous revascularization approach.[1] This policy of avoiding synthetic grafts has spawned an awareness that strategic considerations of revascularization are at least as important as the nature of the bypass graft itself. The use of arm veins now stands as one of the central components to an effective program of primary and repeat revascularization of the ischemic lower extremity. However, the role of these grafts and their natural history was uncertain 25 years ago when their use was first described.

BACKGROUND

Kakkar and Tsapogas[2] first described the use of arm veins in infrainguinal revascularization with a series of seven patients and experimental studies on the length and bursting strength of the cephalic vein. Able to withstand a bursting pressure of 200 to 400 mm of Hg, half that of the greater saphenous vein, arm veins were shown to be sufficiently long and strong for femoropopliteal revascularization. These findings did not go unnoticed and were quickly seized upon by many innovative vascular surgeons.[3-8] Their reports confirmed the published report of Kakkar,[9] that cephalic veins and other arm veins were certainly a highly desirable alternative to the greater saphenous vein. Gradually, arm veins emerged, after greater saphenous veins, as the autogenous conduit of choice.

Advances in Vascular Surgery, vol 2
© 1994, Mosby–Year Book, Inc.

Responding to the negative report of Shulman and Badrey,[10] in which the authors noted aneurysmal dilation and mediocre long-term patency for arm vein bypass grafts, we reported our long-term results in 1984 with experience dating back to 1969.[11] As our use of arm veins increased, we investigated the natural history of these translocated veins and found them to resemble the greater saphenous vein with regard to late secondary degenerative changes.[12] Aneurysmal dilation was a rare finding, but fibrostenotic lesions probably resulting from myointimal hyperplasia were found to be the most common secondary abnormality in arm vein grafts; these lesions usually occurred within the first 2 years of implantation. Since the early reports, we have now performed more than 400 arm vein bypass grafts and find them an indispensable part of our leg revascularization program. In this chapter we describe current practices regarding their use as developed since 1969.

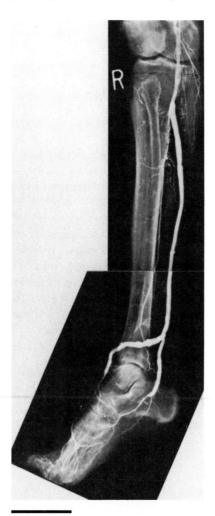

FIGURE 1.
Popliteal-to-dorsalis pedis and medial plantar artery bifurcated bypass composed of nonreversed basilic cephalic vein. The patient was a 62-year-old diabetic woman with gangrene of the first toe and the heel.

INDICATIONS

Arm veins are indicated for arterial reconstruction when a substitute for the greater saphenous vein is necessary.[11, 12] The most common reasons for using an arm vein are the unavailability of the greater saphenous vein because of a previous bypass graft in the leg or the coronary circulation, stripping for treatment of varicose veins, varicose dilation, or postthrombotic damage. Peripheral arterial applications to which arm vein bypasses can be applied encompass virtually all clinical conditions amenable to saphenous vein bypass grafting. These include primary and repeat bypass grafts originating at or near the common femoral artery and extending as far as the plantar and dorsal pedal arteries[13] (Fig 1). Additionally, we have used arm veins for upper extremity bypass grafting, subclavian brachial artery revascularization,[14] and renal artery bypass.[15] In the last circumstance, grafts have originated from branches of the celiac artery.

ANATOMY AND GRAFT CONFIGURATIONS

Since the report of Kakkar much has been learned about the applied anatomy of arm vein bypasses.[16] Beginning with the cephalic vein, we have extended the use of arm veins to all upper extremity veins including the entire forearm and arm cephalic vein, the median antecubital vein, and the forearm and arm basilic veins.[17]

Arm vein segments of differing length may be required for a variety of uses. Inflow and outflow jump grafts to existing grafts need only be 15 to 30 cm in length.[18, 19] These can normally be obtained by harvesting a segment of cephalic or basilic vein from either the arm or forearm. Of course, this requirement can also be met by the lesser saphenous vein.[20] Full-length bypass grafts are often necessary for reoperative surgery, usually repeat bypass to infrapopliteal vessels.[21, 22] Consequently, long grafts measuring 45 to 60 cm or more may be required. These are constructed either as single lengths or as composite grafts made up of multiple segments of arm vein or greater or lesser saphenous vein or a combination of these.[23] The clinical experience of some workers has suggested that forearm cephalic, and to a lesser extent basilic veins are more often diseased and unusable.[24] This leaves the upper arms as the more reliable source of available vein segments.

Over the last several years, the importance of the medial upper arm veins, the subfascial often-paired brachial and the more superficial basilic, has become well established.[13] Anatomic variations and inconsistencies occur frequently[25]; the median antecubital vein may continue cephalad into either vein. In our experience, when the basilic vein is large, the brachial veins are small and not always paired; if the basilic vein is small or absent, there is usually a single large unpaired brachial vein. De Frang et al.[22] have accurately observed that the basilic veins may be the last remaining usable autogenous veins, yet when they are harvested from both arms and spliced end to end the resulting graft will extend from the common femoral artery to the infrapopliteal arteries. The forearm basilic vein is quite posterior and surprisingly often is spared from intravenous infusion and puncture-induced damage. Attempts at harvesting this segment are usually rewarded with an additional 15 to 25 cm of usable vein 3 to 4 mm in diameter.[16] There are two caveats to the use of the full-length basilic veins. First, they should be implanted "non-reversed" valve-incised; second, special care is required to incise valve cusps because they can be unexpectedly tough and resistant to lysis with the retrograde valvulotome.[13] Fortunately, because arm veins are thin the valve and the valvulotome can be seen through the wall; this visibility facilitates precise valve lysis.

If the median antecubital vein segment is intact, it can be harvested in continuity with the cephalic and basilic (or brachial) veins to create a single long conduit that will extend from the common femoral artery to the mid-leg infrapopliteal arteries. LoGerfo et al.[26] have reported using this sequence of segments with the basilic vein proximally, whereas Grigg and Wolfe[27] have advised the reverse. In both instances, the proximal vein valves are competent and must be incised. Of the two configurations, we prefer placing the basilic vein proximally. However, in more than 25 attempts to construct this so-called U-shaped graft we have had to resect the median antecubital portion because of endoluminal scarring more than half of the time. Moreover, in five of the cases in which the median anticubital segment was retained because it appeared to be disease-free, that portion of the arterialized vein has gone on to develop myointimal fibrous changes. Harvest of both basilic and cephalic veins in their entirety with the median antecubital segment has been performed many times without resulting edema or wound complications. For more than 10 years it has been our policy to evaluate routinely arm vein with duplex ultrasonography in all patients suspected of requiring autogenous graft when the saphenous veins are known to be unavailable.[28]

OPERATIVE TECHNIQUES

Before the advent of preoperative duplex assessment of arm veins, our practice was to begin harvesting the cephalic vein in the anatomic snuff box; the dissection then continued proximally directly over the vein.[16] We now begin the dissection over that portion of the vein where it was demonstrated ultrasonographically to be patent, continuous, nondiseased, compliant, and greater than 2 mm in diameter.[28] Unroofing is begun with a no. 15 scalpel blade and continued with scissors. The technical aspects of the technique have been described elsewhere.[13, 29] After the vein is completely exposed there remains a thin covering layer of transparent tissue which helps to prevent desiccation. This gossamer tissue is not incised until the entire vein is exposed and the segments to be harvested have been selected. Inspection of the vein with a proximal tourniquet is useful; likewise, the ability of the vein to fill, distend, empty, and refill during in situ distention helps to identify the usable disease-free segment. Areas which appear to be narrow, white, and fibrotic, speckled or thickened, will invariably have a compromised lumen occluded by synechial webs; these segments should be excluded from the final conduit.[23] Marcaccio et al.,[24] using angioscopy, resected and revised nearly two thirds of veins. Analogously, angioscopy has been posited as a means of upgrading greater saphenous veins for use with bypasses.[30] Porter[31] upgraded up to 25% of arm vein bypasses by resecting abnormal segments; this percentage approximates our own. Most workers agree that intraluminal webs and synechiae are a potential nidus for delayed fibrous stricture in the arterialized vein.

After harvesting, veins can be further assessed by transillumination, palpation, or notation of resistance to the passage of an 8F pediatric feeding tube. There have been no reports of intraluminal ultrasound to scrutinize potentially damaged arm veins. On occasion, we have detected luminal irregularity with the retrograde Leather valvulotome while incising vein valves in nonreversed conduits. Great care is taken to moisten the surface of the vein with saline as it is being harvested and prepared. Compositing to create long grafts from veins of disparate sources has become an increasingly important part of arm vein revascularization technique.[22, 23] Creation of grafts with more than four segments, however, is seldom warranted. Composite grafts are prepared over a stent using 7-0 nonabsorbable suture (Prolene) with gentle traction on the two sutures to prevent pursestringing of the anastomosis.

Arm vein implantation is similar to that of saphenous veins. The proximal anastomosis is constructed first; all constricting adventitial bands are incised and unsecured branches ligated or sutured. The graft is then flushed to assess adequacy of pulsatile flow and passed through the prepared tunnel to the outflow artery, and the distal anastomosis completed. We have been impressed by the frequency of proximal anastomotic intimal hyperplasia when the anastomosis originates from a Dacron graft and believe therefore that extraordinary efforts should be made to originate grafts from autogenous tissue.[32] Because of our experience with the in situ bypass technique, our initial preference for using only orthotopic tunnels has been modified; medial and lateral subcutaneous tunnels have been found to be satisfactory and are used if deep tunneling is contraindicated. A further advantage of superficial tunnels is that they allow patients to palpate their own grafts on a daily basis. If there is any change in the quality of the pulse, they are instructed to inform their vascular surgeon immediately.

PREOPERATIVE ENHANCEMENT

In addition to preoperative duplex evaluation, some workers have attempted to enhance cephalic veins with the construction of a Cimino fistula as first described over 20 years ago.[33] In the only large series employing arterialization of arm veins,[34] 35 fistulas were created in 34 patients; 23 patients were deemed to have marginal arm veins based on physical examination. Preoperative phlebography was performed prior to an end-to-side anastomosis either to the radial or brachial artery. After 10 to 14 days of maturation, the cephalic veins were harvested for lower extremity grafting. The late failure rates among patients receiving preliminary fistulas was equivalent to the rates in patients who did not receive fistulas. This finding is consistent with the angioscopic observations of Marcaccio et al.[24] The authors concluded that creation of an arterial venous fistula added nothing to the usability of the cephalic veins.

Rather than attempting to enhance the diameter and wall characteristics of the cephalic vein, we recommend preoperative assessment and preservation. Although we rely heavily on preoperative duplex assessment, both arms are also visually scrutinized in a warm room with and without tourniquets, dependency, and exercise. In fat arms with obscured veins, we have regularly observed that the obesity that often masks the arm vein also reduces the risk of damage from repeated vein puncture or intravenous infusion. Likewise, tattooing appears not to damage arm veins. On the contrary, nursing personnel seem reluctant to puncture veins through tattoos and this serves to protect them. We have not performed preoperative or intraoperative phlebography.

Preoperative vein preservation may be even more important than accurate preoperative assessment. The person who stands to gain the most and thus is most responsible for the preservation and protection of arm veins against venipuncture-related damage is the patient. Those with known arteriosclerotic cardiac or peripheral vascular disease should be informed that, at some time in the future, they may require a bypass graft. They and their families should be advised that in the 5% to 20% of patients in whom the saphenous vein is inadequate, an alterative autogenous conduit will be required. Education is particularly important for patients who have had previous bypass grafting, superficial phlebitis, or varicose veins. Venipuncture must be done with small needles (no larger than 19Fr) using the median antecubital vein remote from the cephalic vein. Alternatively, veins on the dorsum of the hand can be used for venipuncture or short-term infusion. For prolonged intravenous infusions a central venous catheter is recommended. The education program for floor nurses, intravenous technicians, and anesthesiologists in helping to preserve veins must be ongoing. Once patients are in the hospital, arm veins are further protected by placing conspicuous admonishments in the chart, on the patient's door, and on the bed. The patient's arms are wrapped with gauze on which is written "NO VENIPUNCTURES." A sedated patient hoping that his or her arm veins will be usable is no match for a determined phlebotomist with a mission. Arm vein preservation will improve the surgeon's yield of serviceable conduits but it is also one of the most underappreciated aspects of their use.

NATURAL HISTORY

Natural history studies of arm vein grafts consist of life table analysis of patency, serial angiography, and duplex ultrasound surveillance.[12, 35-38] Most current reports have documented a patency approximating that of saphenous veins (Table 1). Meaningful comparison of primary and secondary patency rates from series to series is problematic because some series combine first-time operations with multiple repeat operations and single-length grafts with composites, both autogenous and autogenous-prosthetic. Most authors discriminate between grafts terminating in the popliteal artery and those extending to infrapopliteal vessels. The most common secondary lesions are myointimal fibrostenoses both within the body of the graft and at the proximal and distal anastomoses that develop within the first 18 months postimplantation. In our series of 56 patients who underwent 73 angiograms, symptomatic and asymptomatic lesions were found. As Shulman and Badrey[10] observed, some grafts become aneurysmal, but this finding occurs infrequently and largely in patients undergoing bypass for popliteal aneurysms. Mild enlargement of 18% of

TABLE 1.

Results of Arm Vein Graft Patency: Recent series

Series	Patients/Grafts	Patency			Comment
		1 yr	3 yr	5 yr	
Andros et al.[12]	142/160	P 84	75	68	First bypass of the
		S 87	78	70	leg; angiographic survey
Balshi et al. [38]	38/41	P 72			
		S 82			
Sesto et al.[34]	34/35	P 49	40		Cephalic vein
		S 68	44		enhancement with Cimino fistula; 12 of 35 composites; graft dilatation observed
Harward et al.[37]	43/43	P 67	49		Preoperative duplex
		S 74	64		ultrasonography of arm veins; infrapopliteal bypass in 79% of cases
Marcaccio et al.[24]	104/109	P 71			Intraoperative
		S 78			angioscopy of arm vein to revise or resect diseased vein in 66% of cases
Chalmers et al.[36]	40/42	P 51			Postoperative
		S 85			duplex surveillance to detect patency-threatening lesions

*P = primary patency; S = secondary patency.

grafts has been noted. The importance of this finding is uncertain since arm vein bypass grafts tend on average to be 6 to 7 mm in diameter prior to implantation. Hence, a small amount of dilation may confer the appearance of graft ectasia, especially when compared with the average arterialized saphenous vein.

Postoperative saphenous vein surveillance has successfully identified "failing grafts" which are losing hemodynamic effectiveness usually because of a single short focal lesion. Identification and correction of these lesions reconfers durable patency to otherwise satisfactory grafts. Chalmers et al.[36] using postoperative graft surveillance techniques developed to identify failing saphenous vein bypasses, have prospectively studied 42 arm vein bypass grafts up to 5 years (mean, 17 months) postoperatively.

Their data suggested that duplex surveillance detected the lesions occurring within the first year; surprisingly, two grafts proceeded to unheralded occlusion despite being subjected to the surveillance protocol. Although their excellent secondary patency results suggest that careful postoperative follow-up can improve long-term results, the effectiveness of postoperative arm vein duplex surveillance remains to be corroborated. Nevertheless, it appears to be a worthwhile procedure because many of these patients have little remaining conduit for a repeat revascularization.

MANAGEMENT OF GRAFT COMPLICATIONS

Diffuse aneurysmal dilation is perhaps the most frustrating mechanism of arm vein bypass failure to manage. Although focal aneurysms have

23 MAR 1993

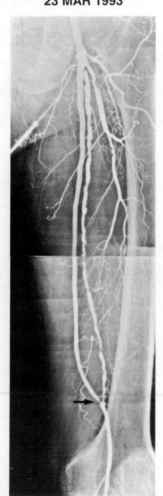

FIGURE 2.

Left common femoral-to-above-knee popliteal artery bypass with reversed cephalic vein: distal anastomotic myointimal hyperplasia 7 months after graft implantation.

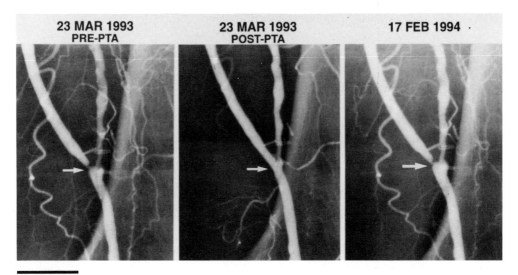

FIGURE 3.

23 MAR 1993: Stenotic lesion. *23 MAR 1993:* Appearance of anastomosis immediately after balloon angioplasty which restored popliteal and pedal pulses. *17
FEB 1994:* Symptomatic recurrent stenosis 11 months later. The lesion was successfully repaired with vein patch angioplasty.

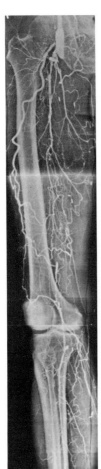

FIGURE 4.

Thrombosed common femoral-to-infrageniculate popliteal artery
nonreversed valve-incised arm and forearm basilic vein bypass 13
months after implantation.

been observed, diffuse enlargement seems to occur most commonly in younger patients operated on for popliteal aneurysm. Only if patients become symptomatic because of repeated atheroembolism or graft occlusion is graft replacement contemplated. In the absence of other available conduit, the surgeon may consider the lesser saphenous vein, superficial femoral vein or a synthetic conduit such as human umbilical vein (Dardik) or polytetrafluoroethylene (PTFE). The availability of replacement conduits is obviously constricted.[21, 22] As a result, we eschew popliteal aneurysm repair in asymptomatic patients under the age of 50 years.

Grafts failing because of proximal neointimal anastomotic fibrostenosis are treated with inflow jump grafting,[18] patch angioplasty,[35] and occasionally transposition angioplasty[39] in patients whose grafts originate from the common femoral artery; distal anastomotic lesions are treated most often with distal jump grafting.[19] Balloon angioplasty is rarely effective[40] (Figs 2 and 3). In contrast, fibrostenosis at venovenous anastomoses for composite graft construction appears to be more amenable to balloon dilation and we attempt this procedure once before resorting to open revascularization. We have treated several arm vein bypass grafts with thrombolysis and have found this to be an effective therapy. Our longest time interval between thrombosis and lytic therapy is approximately 50 days (Fig 4). This graft was successfully lysed over 6 hours using pulse-spray high-dose thrombolytic therapy (Fig 5). The unmasked long fibrointimal retrogeniculate lesion was rebypassed with the contralateral basilic vein and has achieved satisfactory durable patency. It is a daunting truism that the utilization of arm veins for bypass grafting taxes the patience and resourcefulness of the vascular surgeon; likewise, further graft failure imposes continuing demands to employ innovative therapy, particularly in the absence of any other available autogenous bypass conduits.

CURRENT CHALLENGES

The modern all-autogenous approach to infrainguinal revascularization is a mosaic of elements including endovascular surgical techniques, endarterectomy, "redo" operative procedures, very distal bypass, in situ bypass grafting, and the use of alternative autogenous conduits.[1] Current series have emphasized that both cephalic and basilic veins are important sources of alternative conduits. Although it is unlikely that this question will be subjected to prospective comparison, our clinical experience suggests that the veins are equivalent. Good results with either vein will be enhanced by preoperative duplex ultrasonography vein assessment, intraoperative assessment including angioscopy in selected cases, postoperative graft surveillance, and graft salvage with techniques developed for saphenous vein graft. Similarity of arm veins to leg veins has thus far been limited to clinical studies. Little is known about the biological properties of arm veins; new research initiatives to increase our knowledge of the vein in situ as well as after arterialization may help to improve our algorithms for their clinical application.

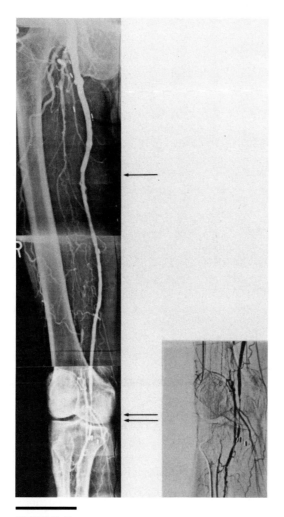

FIGURE 5.

Graft was thrombosed for 50 days and urokinase thrombolysis unmasked extensive distal anastomotic myointimal hyperplasia (*double arrows*). *Single arrow* indicates a small amount of residual thrombus which was successfully lysed.

REFERENCES

1. Donaldson MC, Whittemore AD, Mannick JA: Further experience with an all-autogenous tissue policy for infrainguinal reconstruction. *J Vasc Surg* 1993; 18:41–48.
2. Kakkar VV, Tsapogas MJ: The use of the cephalic vein as a peripheral vascular graft. *Br J Surg* 1968; 55:384.
3. Vellar IDA, Doyle JC: The use of cephalic and basilic veins as peripheral vascular grafts. *Aust N Z J Surg* 1970; 40:52–57.
4. Stipa S: The cephalic and basilic veins in peripheral arterial reconstructive surgery. *Ann Surg* 1972; 175:581–587.
5. Bernhard VM, Ashmore CSD, Evans WE, et al: Bypass grafting to distal arteries for limb salvage. *Surg Gynecol Obstet* 1972; 135:219–224.
6. Clayson KR, Edwards WH, Allen TR, et al: Arm veins for peripheral arterial reconstruction. *Arch Surg* 1976; 111:1276–1280.

7. Campbell DR, Hoar CS Jr, Gibbons GW: The use of arm veins in femoral-popliteal bypass grafts. *Ann Surg* 1979; 190:740–744.

8. Graham JW, Lusby RJ: Infrapopliteal bypass grafting: use of upper limb vein alone and in autogenous composite grafts. *Surgery* 1982; 91:646–649.

9. Kakkar VV: The cephalic vein as a peripheral vascular graft. *Surg Gynecol Obstet* 1969; 128:551–556.

10. Schulman ML, Badrey MR: Late results and angiographic evaluation of arm veins as long bypass grafts. *Surgery* 1982; 92:1032–1041.

11. Harris RW, Andros GA, Dulawa LB, et al: Successful long-term limb salvage using cephalic vein bypass grafts. *Ann Surg* 1984; 6:785–792.

12. Andros G, Harris RW, Salles-Cunha S, et al: Arm veins for arterial revascularization of the leg: Arteriographic and clinical observations. *J Vasc Surg* 1986; 4:416–427.

13. Andros G, Harris RW: The place of arm veins in arterial revascularization, in Bergan JJ, Yao JST (eds): *Arterial Surgery: New Diagnostic and Operative Techniques.* Orlando, Fla,. Grune & Stratton, 1988, pp 523–539.

14. Harris RW, Andros G, Dulawa L, et al: Large-vessel arterial occlusive disease in symptomatic upper extremity. *Arch Surg* 1984; 119:1277–1282.

15. Andros G, Harris RW, Salles-Cunha SX: Arm veins as arterial autografts, in Rutherford RB (ed): *Vascular Surgery,* col 1, ed 3. Philadelphia, WB Saunders, 1989, pp 434–449.

16. Andros G, Harris RW, Dulawa LB, et al: The use of cephalic vein as a conduit, in Greenhalgh RM (ed): *Vascular Surgical Techniques.* London, Butterworths, 1984, pp 169–176.

17. Andros G, Salles-Cunha SX, Harris RW: Arm veins for arterial reconstruction, in Ernst CB, Stanley JC (eds): *Current Therapy in Vascular Surgery,* ed 2. Philadelphia, BC Decker, 1991, pp 505–512.

18. Smith CR, Green RM, DeWeese JA: Pseudoocclusion of femoropopliteal bypass grafts. *Circulation* 1983;(suppl 2):11–88.

19. Andros G, Harris RW, Dulawa L, et al: Patency of femoropopliteal and femorotibial grafts after outflow revascularization (jump grafts) to bypass distal disease. *Surgery* 1984; 96:878–885.

20. Weaver FA, Barlow CB, Edwards WH, et al: The lesser saphenous vein: Autogenous tissue for lower extremity revacularization. *J Vasc Surg* 1987; 5:687–692.

21. Harris RW, Andros G, Salles-Cunha SX, et al: The totally autogenous venovenous composite bypass grafts. *Arch Surg* 1986; 121:1128–1132.

22. De Frang RD, Edwards JM, Moneta GL, et al: Repeat leg bypass after multiple prior bypass failures. *J Vasc Surg* 1994; 19:268–277.

23. Harris RW, Andros G, Dulausa LB, et al: Totally autogenous venovenous composite bypass grafts: Salvage of the almost irretrievable extremity. *Surgery* 1986; 100:822-827.

24. Marcaccio EJ, Miller A, Tannenbaum GA, et al: Angioscopically directed interventions improve arm vein bypass grafts. *J Vasc Surg* 1993; 17:994–1004.

25. Sladen JG, Reid JDS, Riggs MO: Harvest of brachio-basilic vein complex for arterial bypass. *J Cardiovasc Surg* 1992; 33:169–171.

26. LoGerfo FW, Paniszyn CW, Menzvian J: A new arm vein graft for distal bypass. *J Vasc Surg* 1987; 5:889–891.

27. Grigg MJ, Wolfe JHN: Combination reversed and non-reversed upper arm vein for femoro-distal grafting. *Eur J Vasc Surg* 1988; 2:49–55.

28. Salles-Cunha S, Andros G, Harris RW, et al: Preoperative noninvasive assessment of arm veins to be used as bypass grafts in the lower extremities. *J Vasc Surg* 1986; 3:813–816.

29. Andros G, Harris RW, Dulawa L, et al: The use of arm veins as lower-extremity

arterial conduits, in Kempczinski RF (ed): *The Ischemic Leg.* St Louis, Mosby—Year Book, 1985, pp 419–438.

30. Panetta T, Marin M, Veith F, et al: Unsuspected preexisting saphenous vein disease: An unrecognized cause of vein bypass failure. *J Vasc Surg* 1992; 15:102–112.
31. Porter JM: Alternatives to saphenous vein for lower extremity bypass. Postgraduate course. American College of Surgeons spring Meeting, April 1994.
32. Andros G, Salles-Cunha SX, Harris RW, et al: Arm veins for arterial reconstructive surgery: A twenty-three-year experience, in Yao JST, Pearce WH (eds): *Long-Term Results in Vascular Surgery.* Norwalk, Conn, Appleton & Lange, 1993, pp 247–258.
33. Beals RL: Surgically created arteriovenous fistula to augment the cephalic vein: Use as an arterial bypass graft. *N Engl J Med* 185:29, 1971.
34. Sesto ME, Sullivan TM, Hertzer NR, et al: Cephalic vein grafts for lower extremity revascularization. *J Vasc Surg* 1992; 15:543–549.
35. Whittemore AD, Clowes AW, Couch NP, et al: Secondary femoropopliteal reconstruction. *Ann Surg* 1981; 193:35–42.
36. Chalmers RTA, Hoballah JJ, Kresowik TF, et al: The impact of color duplex surveillance on the outcome of lower limb bypass with segments of arm veins. *J Vasc Surg* 1994; 19:279–288.
37. Harward TRS, Coe D, Flynn TC, et al: The use of arm vein conduits during infrageniculate arterial bypass. *J Vasc Surg* 1992; 5:420–427.
38. Balshi JD, Cantelmo NL, Menzoian JO, et al: The use of arm veins for infrainguinal bypass in end-stage peripheral vascular disease. *Arch Surg* 1989; 124:1078–1081.
39. Andros G, Harris RW, Dulawa LB, et al: Transposition angioplasty: A technique for the correction of proximal anastomotic neointimal hyperplasia in femorodistal bypasses. *Surgery* 1988; 103:698–700.
40. Whittemore AD, Donaldson MC, Polak JF, et al: Limitations of balloon angioplasty for vein graft stenosis. *J Vasc Surg* 1991; 14:340–345.

Lesser Saphenous Vein as an Alternative Conduit

Benjamin B. Chang, M.D.
Assistant Professor of Surgery, Department of Vascular Surgery, Albany Medical College, Albany, New York

Dhiraj M. Shah, M.D.
Professor of Surgery, Department of Vascular Surgery, Albany Medical College; Chief, General Surgery, Albany Medical Center, Albany, New York

R. Clement Darling III, M.D.
Assistant Professor of Surgery, Department of Vascular Surgery, Albany Medical College, Albany, New York

Robert P. Leather, M.D.
Professor of Surgery, Department of Vascular Surgery, Albany Medical College, Albany, New York

---

A rterial bypass operations of many kinds are often most successfully completed with the use of autogenous vein, usually from the greater saphenous vein. However, in cases in which the greater saphenous vein is not available, whether from congenital atresia, previous phlebitis, stripping, or use in arterial reconstruction, alternative conduits must be used. Artificial prosthetic grafts are useful for femoropopliteal bypasses to the above-knee segment, but perform poorly when used in infrageniculate reconstructions.[1, 2] The contralateral greater saphenous vein is the most convenient alternative conduit available for these reconstructions, but is also subject to limited availability. Arm veins are readily available and can be used with fairly good results in many cases.[3, 4] The lesser saphenous vein (LSV) is another often overlooked alternative autogenous conduit that provides good-quality vein for reconstructive procedures.[5–7] Herein we describe our experience with the use of the LSV as an arterial bypass conduit.

ANATOMIC STUDIES

Over the past 7 years, a total of 524 LSVs have been imaged with duplex ultrasound. The use of duplex ultrasound in defining preoperative venous anatomy has been validated with the greater saphenous vein.[8] As the LSV was imaged, a map of the vein was drawn on the overlying skin, with care taken to note important features such as varicosities, closed loops, recanalization, and significant branching. One hundred eighty-seven of these veins were later explored at the time of surgery and the operative findings were noted and correlated with the preoperative imaging data.

Of 187 LSVs explored at the time of surgery, preoperative imaging provided accurate information in 177 cases (94.7%). In two cases the LSV was not imaged preoperatively but was present operatively. In three cases the LSV was absent operatively in spite of imaging data to the contrary. In two cases, the LSV was believed to be thrombosed preoperatively but was patent at the time of operation. In both of these cases the wall of the vein was partially calcified. In three cases the LSV was found to be re-canalized and unusable at the time of surgery in contrast to the imaging report.

The LSV is pictured in Figure 1. This vein arises from the lateral plantar vein and may be found just posterior to the lateral malleolus. Crossing the Achilles tendon just above the level of the malleoli, the LSV rises along the posterior aspect of the leg, usually with the sural nerve. The LSV usually terminates as it joins the popliteal vein at the knee crease, although it was found to enter the deep venous system above the knee

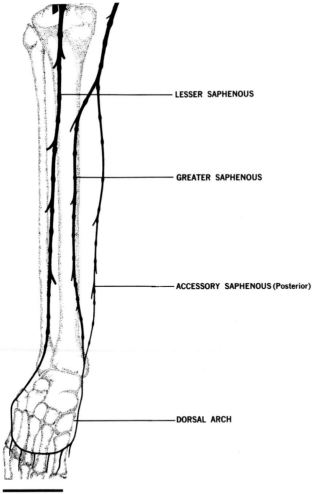

FIGURE 1.

Normal anatomy of the lesser saphenous vein.

joint in 33 of 524 (6.3%) LSVs imaged. In the lower two thirds of the leg, the LSV runs in the subcutaneous tissue superficial to the deep fascia. In the proximal leg the LSV runs deep to the fascia.

In 30 cases the LSV was not detectable (5.7%). Forty-one LSVs were found to ramify into surgically unusable branches distally at or just above the malleoli (7.8%). The LSV was thrombosed in 19 cases (3.6%).

At the time of operation, LSVs were distended with arterial pressure and their diameter measured. The mean external diameter of the LSVs explored was 4.13 ±0.66 mm. Duplex ultrasound did not reliably predict vein diameter as the vein diameter is obviously larger when distended under pressure at the time of surgery. The LSV was absent in 5 of 187 cases (2.3%) and too small to be used (less than 3.0 mm outer diameter) in 9 (4.8%). Two LSVs were not used because of extensive varices and three were not used owing to recanalization. Therefore, 10.2% of LSVs were not usable as arterial bypass conduits at the time of surgery (5% of the greater saphenous vein is unusable).

The length of usable LSV has been measured by others. In the study of Rutherford et al.,[6] the average usable length of LSV was 37.4 cm. In our series, the average length of the LSV from the popliteal vein to its crossing of the Achilles tendon was 28.6 ±4.2 cm. The differences in the LSV length in the two series can be attributed to differences in harvest methods.

Qualitatively, the LSV differs only slightly from the greater saphenous vein. The wall of the LSV is similar to that of the greater saphenous vein and is more substantial than the typical arm vein. The LSV does tend to have more small branches than an equivalent length of greater saphenous and has more valves.

METHODS OF HARVEST

The posterior position of the LSV makes harvesting this vein somewhat difficult. The ideal method of harvest varies depending on the vagaries of the particular case. The patient can be placed in a prone position and the incision made over the LSV directly.[5] This is most useful when using the LSV for a reconstruction such as a popliteal aneurysm in which the operation can be completed with the patient in the prone position. If the vein is first harvested in this position and the patient repositioned, there will be an inordinate delay in arterializing the LSV; the increased ischemic injury to the vein can be potentially harmful.

Alternatively, the limb may be flexed at the knee and externally rotated and the incision placed directly over the LSV. This conveniently exposes the midportion of the LSV. However, it is difficult to harvest the extreme ends of the LSV unless the assistant holds the leg up in the air and the operator works looking upward at the popliteal fossa. In addition, such a stocking-seam incision is not useful for completing the remainder of the reconstruction and a second incision must be made medially or laterally and parallel to access the greater saphenous vein and the tibial and peroneal arteries.

Finally, a third strategy for harvesting the LSV may be used.[7, 9] This involves making a medial calf incision usually over the greater saphe-

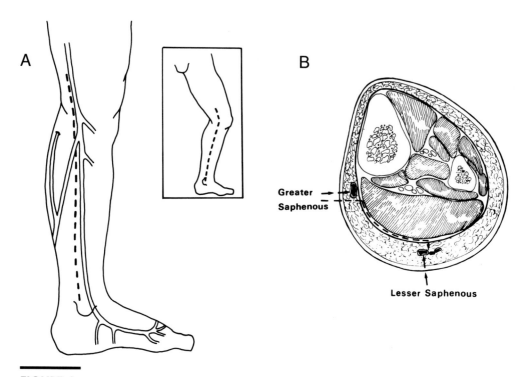

FIGURE 2.

A, incision for lesser saphenous vein harvest. **B,** plane of dissection for lesser saphenous vein harvest.

nous vein (Fig 2,A). The skin, subcutaneous tissue, and deep fascia are all divided along this line. Subsequently a full-thickness skin and fascial flap is elevated posteriorly until the LSV is exposed in the flap (Fig 2,B). The vein may then be dissected out with the operator looking downward at the vein. Harvesting of the proximal end of the LSV may be done up to the popliteal vein with this method. Harvest of the LSV for the distal few centimeters still requires the assistant to hold the leg up and for the operator to approach the LSV and lateral plantar vein laterally while looking upward.

The utility of this method of vein harvest is that a single incision may be used to expose the tibial arteries, greater saphenous, and LSV. Harvesting the LSV is made easier because the surgeon looks downward at the LSV. If the LSV is being harvested for use in coronary bypass procedures, circumferential preparation of the legs is unnecessary.

Care must be taken in performing this type of harvest in that vascular pedicles from the gastrocnemius to the flap should be preserved when possible. Those that are divided should be carefully secured to ensure meticulous hemostasis. A 10-mm Jackson-Pratt drain is inserted through a separate stab wound to drain the space between the flap and the muscle. This is done to prevent the formation of a hematoma or seroma leading to flap necrosis. Patients are also kept at bed rest for 24 to 48 hours to help stabilize the flap. Earlier in this series there were five cases of flap hematoma leading to varying degrees of flap necrosis. This has been avoided over the past 4 years by uniformly draining the flap.

USE OF THE LESSER SAPHENOUS VEIN AS AN ARTERIAL BYPASS

The LSV is an often-overlooked source of autogenous vein that should be held in greater esteem by vascular surgeons. Use of preoperative imaging, either venography or, preferably, duplex ultrasound, is very useful in allowing the surgeon to plan the procedure before the actual operation. Accurate information as to the presence or absence and the general configuration of the LSV can be expected well over 90% of the time with experienced ultrasound operators.

The principal limitation to the use of the LSV as an arterial bypass conduit is its length. When harvested from a medial flap approach, an average of 29 cm of LSV is available. If a second incision is used to harvest the distal LSV and lateral plantar vein, usually over 40 cm of usable vein is obtainable. On the other hand, 7.8% of LSVs ramify into small, unusable branches in the lower third of the leg. Usually only 20 to 24 cm of vein is available in these cases. Over a 7-year period, 190 LSVs in 183 patients (114 male, 76 female) were utilized in lower extremity arterial bypass procedures.

In general, the LSV can be used to perform an entire bypass or be spliced to other lengths of vein to complete the reconstruction. The LSV is usually of sufficient length to complete a femoral-to-above-knee popliteal artery bypass in most cases. In addition, bypasses to the below-knee popliteal artery and proximal tibial arteries may be completed with one LSV if the distal extension of the LSV is harvested. It should also be remembered that the LSV terminates at a point above the knee crease in 6.3% of cases; this extra length can be used for bypass procedures. Bypasses completed with a single LSV are listed in Table 1.

It is noted that the largest group of these bypasses in this series are below-knee popliteal artery-to-tibial artery bypasses. Twelve of these bypasses were completed with an in situ technique (Fig 3). Use of the LSV as an in situ bypass has been reported previously.[9] This is most easily performed when the distal anastomosis is above the level of the malleoli. All but one of these bypasses are still open (mean follow-up, 30.7 months). It should be remembered that only a relatively short length of the LSV is left "in situ" in this type of reconstruction. It is difficult to

TABLE 1.

Bypasses Completed With a Single Lesser
Saphenous Vein

Bypass	n
Popliteal-tibial in situ	12
Popliteal-tibial reversed	22
Popliteal-tibial nonreversed, excised	20
Femoral—above-knee popliteal	10
Femoral—below-knee popliteal	14
Femorotibial	7
Total	85

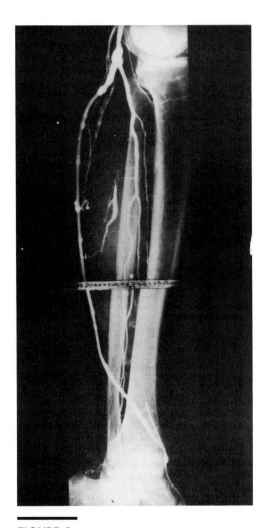

FIGURE 3.
Popliteal-to-anterior tibial in situ bypass with lesser saphenous vein.

recommend the use of the LSV preferentially as an in situ conduit with the limited data available.

The LSV may also be excised for use as an arterial conduit. The vein may be reversed or nonreversed. We tend to reverse veins that do not taper appreciably, whereas veins that do taper are anastomosed proximally and the valves incised with the modified Mills valvulotome.[10] Approximately half of excised LSVs were used in a reversed configuration in this series. Patency rates for bypass procedures completed with a single LSV are shown in Table 2.

The second major group of bypasses utilizing the LSV as an arterial conduit are those reconstructions in which the LSV is spliced to other conduits to complete the procedure. As can be seen in Table 3, six of these bypasses consisted of a proximal femoral-to-above-knee popliteal artery bypass of polytetrafluoroethylene (PTFE) and completion of the reconstruction with a popliteal-to-distal artery bypass with LSV. These sequential bypasses function better than composite or prosthetic bypasses

TABLE 2.

Lesser Saphenous Vein Bypasses

Interval (m.)	Grafts at Risk	Occlusions	Intervals Patency	Cumulative Patency
Primary patency				
0–1	85	6	0.925	0.925
2–12	69	5	0.909	0.841
13–24	36	4	0.862	0.725
25–36	18	1	0.923	0.669
37–48	7	0	1.000	0.669
49–60	5	1	0.778	0.520
Secondary patency				
0–1	85	6	0.925	0.925
2–12	69	4	0.927	0.857
13–24	36	0	1.000	0.857
25–36	18	0	1.000	0.857
37–48	7	0	1.000	0.857
49–60	5	0	1.000	0.857

TABLE 3.

Bypasses Completed With Other Conduits*

Bypass	n
Femoral–above-knee popliteal PTFE+ popliteal-tibial LSV	6
Greater saphenous vein in situ + LSV	24
Autogenous vein conduits	
Two pieces	12
Three pieces	5
Four pieces	4
Five pieces	1
Total	52

*PTFE = polytetrafluoroethylene; LSV = lesser saphenous vein.

to the below-knee vessels.[11, 12] In two of these cases, the expanded PTFE bypass became occluded while the LSV remained patent. These were both recovered with a proximal rebypass with expanded PTFE. The remaining four are still patent (mean follow-up, 28.8 months).

The remainder of bypasses in the second group consisted of autogenous conduits completed with one or both LSVs. This group may be subdivided into those in which the use of the LSV as part of an excised spliced vein bypass was preplanned (Fig 4). Of the 22 bypasses in this group, both LSVs were used in six cases, three in conjunction with two or three pieces of greater saphenous or arm veins to complete the bypass. In the other three, two LSVs were sufficient to complete the entire bypass. Of the spliced, excised vein bypasses, five have become occluded (mean follow-up, 26.2 months).

In 24 cases, the LSV was used to complete a bypass, primarily using the greater saphenous vein in situ. Use of the LSV in these cases was planned in 9 cases and unplanned in 15. In the former group, previous

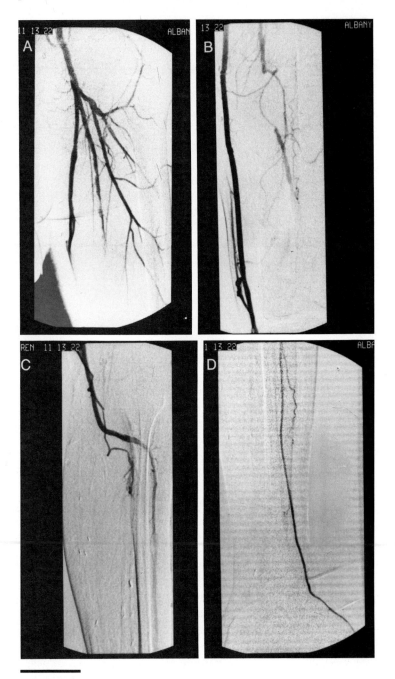

FIGURE 4.
Femoral-to-anterior tibial bypass **(A)** with reversed lesser saphenous vein **(B)**, orthograde greater saphenous vein **(C)**, and reversed greater saphenous vein **(D)**.

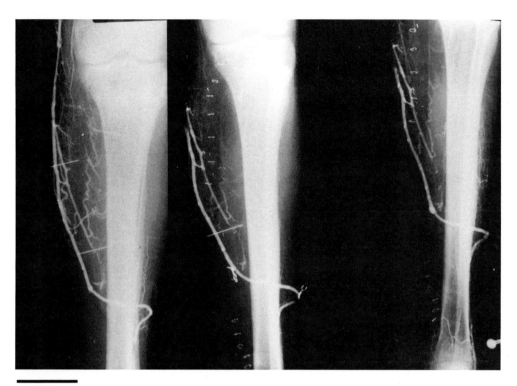

FIGURE 5.
Femoral-to-anterior tibial in situ bypass completed with translocated, excised lesser saphenous vein.

harvest of the distal greater saphenous for coronary artery bypass allowed for in situ preparation of the greater saphenous vein to the knee, with the distal portion of the bypass completed with reversed or orthograde LSV.

In 15 cases, the LSV was used to complete an in situ bypass when the greater saphenous vein unexpectedly proved to be inadequate or (more often) there was a segmental injury to the greater saphenous vein either proximally or distally in the preparation of the vein (Fig 5). In these cases, the LSV was explored through a medial subfascial flap incision and harvested for use as a conduit. The use of the LSV as a means of completing a difficult distal bypass is an especially important use of the LSV that all surgeons should recognize and utilize.

A third major group of cases in which the LSV was used consisted of cases in which a preexisting vein graft developed a stenosis or in which progression of proximal or (more often) distal disease decreased limb perfusion (Table 4). The LSV was used to patch or segmentally replace a vein graft stenosis in 18 cases. A jump graft from a more proximal artery to a preexisting vein graft was performed in 3 cases. In 26 cases, the LSV was anastomosed to a preexisting vein graft and then to a more distal tibial artery.

Use of the LSV in reoperation or revision is especially helpful to the surgeon as most of the time only one leg need be prepared and completion of the bypass is usually straightforward.

Finally, at least 58 LSVs have been used by the cardiac surgery ser-

TABLE 4.
The Lesser Saphenous Vein in Revision of a Preexisting Vein Graft

Revision	n
Midgraft stenosis	
Patch	5
Segmental replacement	13
Inflow artery stenosis	
Segmental replacement	3
Outflow artery/graft stenosis	
Segmental replacement	26
Total	47

vice for coronary artery bypass procedures. They have been taught the medial flap method of LSV harvest and now routinely use it in cases in which the greater saphenous vein is inadequate.[13]

DISCUSSION

The greater saphenous vein remains the conduit of choice for most infrainguinal bypass procedures. This is supported by extensive clinical studies documenting the superiority of the greater saphenous vein over prosthetic conduits, especially for longer tibial bypasses.[1, 2] In particular we favor the use of the greater saphenous vein in situ whenever possible. However, the ipsilateral greater saphenous vein can be unavailable in up to 45% of cases in selected series.[14] In such cases, the contralateral greater saphenous vein is preferred, especially if there is no appreciable occlusive disease in the donor leg. Use of this vein in a reversed or nonreversed position can be expected to obtain acceptable results.[14, 15]

The LSV is therefore of secondary utility to the vascular surgeon. In primary procedures, it is especially well suited for popliteal-based short bypasses. In general, the results of these bypasses are quite good.[16–18] The LSV is also usually long enough to perform femoral-to-popliteal bypasses, especially to the above-knee segment. Thus, if the surgeon so wants, the LSV may be used instead of prosthetic conduits in this situation.

The LSV may also be useful in a primary or redo procedure as part of a longer, autogenous conduit. While the performance of such spliced vein bypasses in our series has been acceptable, there has been little attention paid to this type of reconstruction, although mention of it has been made by others.[14] We believe that in this situation a spliced vein bypass functions better than a prosthetic or composite bypass.

The LSV is of particular use in reoperative procedures. Many of the LSVs used in our series served to perform short bypasses to, from, or within a preexisting vein bypass. The LSV in these cases is invaluable as it provides an autogenous, ipsilateral conduit that is almost always long enough to complete the reconstruction. In cases where the original bypass has failed completely, the LSV and residual greater saphenous vein may be spliced to complete most bypasses to the lower leg.

Finally, in cases where the greater saphenous vein is being prepared for use as a bypass conduit, the LSV is invaluable in providing autogenous vein to replace sections of the conduit that are injured or are in other ways inadequate for use. The knowledge that the LSV is available as a "bailout" in times of trouble we find very reassuring.

Use of the LSV in these cases may be preferable to the use of arm veins. Although arm veins can be used with acceptable results, harvest usually requires a second operative field and general anesthesia and patients often do not like the idea of long scars on their arms. In addition, arm veins are typically quite flimsy and are more difficult to work with than the more substantial LSV which resembles very closely the greater saphenous vein in its handling qualities.

REFERENCES

1. Bergan JJ, Veith FJ, Bernhard VM, et al: Randomization of autogenous vein and polytetrafluoroethylene grafts in femoral-distal reconstruction. *Surgery* 1982; 92:921–930.
2. Veith FJ, Gupta SK, Ascer E, et al: Six year prospective multicenter randomized comparison of autologous saphenous vein and expanded polytetrafluoroethylene grafts in infrainguinal arterial reconstructions. *J Vasc Surg* 1986; 32:104–114.
3. Andros G, Harris RW, Salles-Cunha SX, et al: Arm veins for arterial revascularization of the leg: Arteriographic and clinical observations. *J Vasc Surg* 1986; 4:416–427.
4. Sesto ME, Sullivan TM, Hertzer MR, et al: Cephalic vein grafts for lower extremity revascularization. *J Vasc Surg* 1992; 15:543–549.
5. Weaver FA, Barlow CR, Edwards WH, et al: The *lesser saphenous vein*: Autogenous tissue for lower extremity revascularization. *J Vasc Surg* 1987; 5:687–692.
6. Rutherford RB, Sawyer JD, Jones DN: The fate of residual saphenous vein after partial removal or ligation. *J Vasc Surg* 1990; 12:422–426.
7. Chang BB, Paty PSK, Shah DM, et al: The lesser saphenous vein: An underappreciated source of autogenous vein. *J Vasc Surg* 1992; 15:152–157.
8. Leopold PW, Shandall AA, Kupinski AM, et al: Role of B-mode venous mapping in infrainguinal in situ vein-arterial bypasses. *Br J Surg* 1989; 76:305–307.
9. Shandall AA, Leather RP, Corson JD, et al: The use of the short saphenous vein in situ for popliteal to distal artery bypass. *Am J Surg* 1987; 154:240–244.
10. Sottiurai VS: Nonreversed translocated vein bypass. *Semin Vasc Surg* 1993; 6:180–184.
11. Flinn WR, Ricco J-B, Yao JST, et al: Composite sequential grafts in severe ischemia: A comparative study. *J Vasc Surg* 1984; 1:449–454.
12. McCarthy WJ, Pearce WH, Flinn WR, et al: Long-term evaluation of composite sequential bypass for limb-threatening ischemia. *J Vasc Surg* 1992; 15:761–770.
13. Chang BB, Ferraris VA, Sadoff J, et al: Alternate conduits for coronary revacularization: A novel approach for harvest of the lesser saphenous vein. *J Cdiovasc Surg* 1993; 1,3:280–284.
14. Taylor LM, Edwards JM, Porter JM: Present sttus of reversed vein bypass graing: Five-year results of a modern series. *J Vasc Surg* 1990; 11:193–205.

15. Bandyk DF, Schmitt DD, Seabrook GR, et al: A comparison of in situ and reversed saphenous vein bypasses: The impact of a surveillance protocol and elective revision. *J Vasc Surg* 1989; 9:286–296.
16. Wengerter KR, Yang PM, Veith FJ, et al: A twelve-year experience with the popliteal-to-distal artery bypass: The significance and management of proximal disease. *J Vasc Surg* 1992; 15:143–151.
17. Cantelmo NL, Snow JR, Menzoian JO, et al: Successful vein bypass in patients with an ischemic limb and a palpable popliteal pulse. *Arch Surg* 1986; 121:217–220.
18. Schuler JJ, Flanigan DP, Williams LR, et al: Early experience with popliteal to infrapopliteal bypass for limb salvage. *Arch Surg* 1983; 118:472–476.

Composite Prosthetic-Vein Grafts

Walter J. McCarthy, M.D.

Assistant Professor of Surgery, Division of Vascular Surgery, Northwestern University Medical School, Northwestern Memorial Hospital, Chicago, Illinois

Paula K. Shireman, M.D.

General Surgery Resident, Department of Surgery, Northwestern University Medical School, Northwestern Memorial Hospital, Chicago, Illinois

L ittle evidence supports the use of prosthetic material for bypass below the knee joint when sufficient autogenous venous conduit is available. Thus an underlying premise of the following material is that adequate vein for bypass is somehow limited. This circumstance is not common, and a diligent search for upper extremity vein and a familiarity with the lesser saphenous vein expand the surgeon's reconstructive horizon considerably. Nevertheless, patients will occasionally be encountered for whom long segments of graft material are needed and in whom the greater saphenous vein has been previously used for coronary or leg bypass. For example, reconstruction to the dorsalis pedis might be necessary in the setting of a recently failed distal in situ vein graft. The use of composite techniques might, in this case, provide relief of ischemia to prevent amputation and sufficient long-term patency for a reasonable outcome from such a complicated and expensive hospitalization.

Composite bypass grafting is defined here as the use of two separate materials to complete a femoral-to-distal reconstruction. The word *composite* is sometimes used to refer to an all-autogenous venovenous reconstruction, but not in this chapter. Background rationale and techniques are presented for the use of composite grafts, composite sequential grafts, and the use of distal vein patches with prosthetic material, which are perhaps the most abbreviated form of composite grafting.

COMPOSITE GRAFTS

The concept of using prosthetic material and a portion of distal autogenous conduit for femoral bypass was first proposed by Deterling in 1958.[1] In this operation the proximal prosthetic anastomosis at the femoral artery is followed by an intermediate anastomosis to autogenous vein, allowing the vein to cross the knee. The venous conduit is then anastomosed to a popliteal or tibial vessel. Dale et al.[2] reported a favorable laboratory experience with this configuration in 1962, but were disappointed with the subsequent clinical performance of the composite graft. Using a combination of Teflon and vein in patients, Dale and colleagues reported that only 1 of these 16 bypass grafts remained patent beyond 1 year. Their article, entitled "Failure of Composite (Teflon and Vein) Grafting in Small Human Arteries," was published as a reappraisal and retraction of the earlier laboratory work.[2] This early discontent effectively subdued publication related to composite grafting techniques for nearly a decade, until DeLaurentis and Friedmann[3] and Linton and Wirthlin[4] reported more impressive patency rates. Linton and Wirthlin's report in 1973 compared the patency of 40 composite Dacron-vein grafts with 5-year patency of 53% to 345 all-venous grafts with 5-year patency approximating 70%.[4] The composite technique represented a significant improvement over all-Dacron grafting for small vessel bypass. By 1975 Lord et al.[5] had developed a refined technique for the intermediate anastomosis. They proposed an end-to-side intermediate anastomosis between the Dacron and saphenous vein. At the completion of the end-to-side venous anastomosis the blind cuff was ligated adjacent to the Dacron heal. They also favored anchoring the intermediate anastomosis to the deep fascia to avoid "angulation, rotation, kinking, etc.," and placing the venous half of the composite graft across the knee joint where it might better handle repeated flexion. Lord and colleagues reported a 60% 2-year patency rate.[5]

A significant contribution to the development of composite grafting was made by Snyder et al.[6] of Norfolk, Virginia, in the early 1980s. They initially reported on 69 composite grafts using polytetrafluoroethylene (PTFE) material with vein as compared to 89 bypasses of PTFE material alone. Though follow-up was limited, the composite graft patency at twelve months was superior with 71%, as compared to 50% in the all-PTFE group. This group's enthusiasm for composite grafting led to a combined paper with surgeons from the University of Erlangen in Nuremberg, Germany.[7] PTFE-vein composite grafts (208 cases) were compared with all-PTFE bypasses (235 cases), and mean follow-up of 15.8 months was achieved. Life table analysis led to some interesting conclusions. The composite PTFE-vein series was similar in patency to all-PTFE, about 50% at 3 years, when used in the femoropopliteal position. However, if the analysis focused on grafts anastomosed distally to tibial runoff vessels the composite was clearly superior. Composite grafts had a 53% patency at 3 years, compared to 33% in the all-PTFE group. The Norfolk surgical experience preferred a widely spatulated intermediate prosthetic-vein anastomosis dubbed "the hand clasp anastomosis."[6]

Recent work of interest includes that presented by Holdsworth et al.[8] from the York District Hospital, England. Completed in 1989, this experience outlines 42 patients who required femoral–below-knee popliteal bypass for claudication (45%) or rest pain (55%). These authors used PTFE anastomosed to nonreversed saphenous vein which required lysis of the venous valves. The advantage of the nonreversed veins, they speculate, is to allow a better size match between the 6-mm PTFE material and the vein at the intermediate anastomosis. In addition, the vein was arranged so that it would cross the knee. The 12- and 18-month patency rates were 84% and 79%, respectively.

Why is this operation not used more frequently? Few surgeons would claim any experience with this technique despite the previously mentioned generally optimistic short-term patency results. The reasons for this are multiple and somewhat irrational. Many among us remember the atrocious patency rates of Dale et al.[2] (15 of 16 failed in 1 year) reported over 30 years ago and may not be familiar with more current reports from lesser-known surgical personalities. However, Linton and Wirthlin's 53% 5-year patency is quite respectable. Second, extended patency is really not known. All of the previously mentioned studies have mean follow-ups between 11 and 15 months. Even in the face of patient loss to follow-up and mortality, this short length of time is inadequate to establish long-term patency. Careful reporting will achieve at least a 36- to 48-month mean follow-up in most distal bypass series. Perhaps if careful long-term follow-up would clearly define patency, this procedure would seem more appealing to surgeons. Despite its theoretic and conceptual attractiveness, wholehearted endorsement of composite bypass grafting must not be given until long-term patency rates are established.

TECHNIQUES FOR COMPOSITE BYPASS

Combining all the advantages of the previously reported techniques the modern approach to composite bypass would utilize a 6 mm-diameter PTFE graft for the proximal conduit, anastomosed end-to-side to the common femoral artery. Autogenous vein consisting of part of the greater or lesser saphenous vein would then be anastomosed to the PTFE graft using a very generous spatulated end-to-end anastomosis. The vein should not be reversed to allow a better size match between conduits. The placement of this intermediate anastomosis would preferentially allow the vein to cross the knee joint. The prosthetic graft should be anchored with suture to convenient fascia in the above-knee location to limit motion of the graft and perhaps reduce kinking in the early postoperative period prior to complete incorporation of the bypass graft. Anticoagulation with heparin in the postoperative period and then with warfarin sodium (Coumadin) indefinitely seems advisable in patients without high risk for bleeding complications.

COMPOSITE SEQUENTIAL BYPASS

Composite sequential bypass for completing femoropopliteal or femorotibial bypass is also defined as combining prosthetic material and autogenous vein. The difference between composite sequential and composite grafting is that the composite sequential configuration provides an intermediate arterial anastomosis, usually at the above- or below-knee popliteal level. Many variations of this concept are useful including external iliac-to-popliteal-tibial bypass, femorotibial-to-tibial bypass, or femoro to femoral with popliteal bypass. This grafting technique is recommended only when autogenous vein is insufficient to complete the desired arterial reconstruction. Theoretical advantages include a venous-to-distal arterial anastomosis which may limit intimal hyperplasia despite the use of short segments of vein (Fig 1). In addition, the intermediate anastomosis at the popliteal level creates a point of fixation for the vein-to-artery anastomosis which limits rotation and kinking. Finally, the in-

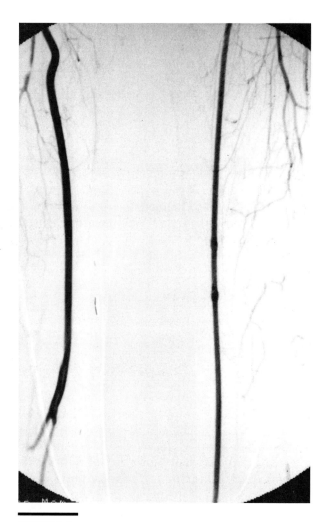

FIGURE 1.

This patient required distal bypass after having had previous greater saphenous vein removal for coronary bypass and contralateral femoral-distal in situ reconstruction. Composite sequential grafting was employed for successful limb salvage.

termediate arterial anastomosis will usually increase the flow through the prosthetic graft limb and possibly enhance its patency.

In 1971, DeLaurentis and Friedmann[3] reviewed their experience with femoropopliteal and tibial bypass for the New England Surgical Society. Seventy-four reconstructions were appraised in many innovative configurations, including the orientation we would now term *composite sequential*. They called this operation the "double bypass" and used it as a method of solving the problem of inadequate greater saphenous vein length. Dacron graft material was used for the proximal portion of the reconstruction. The vein segment was anastomosed to the popliteal artery just distal to the Dacron–popliteal artery anastomosis. All three of these double bypasses were functioning well at 3 months of follow-up.

In 1976 the *British Journal of Surgery* published Bliss and Fonseka's[9] interpretation of the "hitchhike graft," which emulated the experience of DeLaurentis and Friedmann.[9] Sixteen cases were described using 6-mm Dacron velour prosthesis along with autogenous vein. The authors performed an endarterectomy of the popliteal artery and then anastomosed Dacron proximally and vein distally to a single longitudinal popliteal arteriotomy (Fig 2). They reported 11 out of 16 functional grafts after 2 to 4 months of follow-up.

Rosenfeld et al.[10] in 1981, reported a large collection of composite sequential, femoropopliteal, and femorotibial bypasses. They combined work performed at the Pennsylvania Hospital with the ongoing efforts of Friedmann in Springfield, Massachusetts and reviewed 55 reconstructions. Thirty-three were femoropopliteal-to-popliteal grafts and 22 were anastomosed distally to a tibial vessel (Fig 3). In this series the proximal

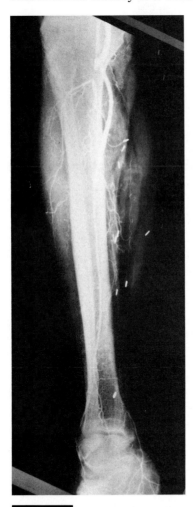

FIGURE 2.

Intermediate anastomosis to the popliteal artery does not require the usual standards of runoff. There is only a limited retrograde perfusion from the below-knee popliteal anastomosis in this patient. The cephalic vein was used to complete the bypass to the perineal artery. Clips document the previous harvest of greater saphenous vein for past coronary artery bypass.

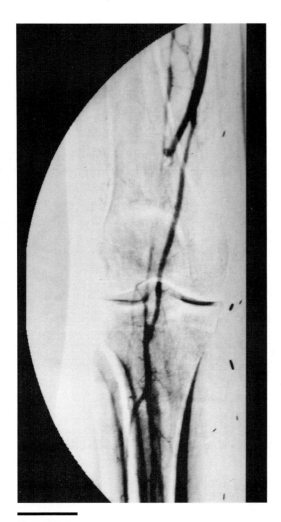

FIGURE 3.

Composite sequential technique has been used successfully in the below-knee popliteal position. Here the 6-mm PTFE material is anastomosed to the above-knee popliteal, and lesser saphenous vein is used for the distal limb to the below-knee popliteal artery.

graft material was either Dacron or PTFE. The authors reported that the patency rates were similar regardless of whether the distal anastomosis was at the tibial or popliteal level. With the femoropopliteal bypass the 12-, 24-, and 48-month patencies were 66%, 58%, and 48%, respectively. For the femorotibial bypass the 12-, 24-, and 48-month patencies were 65%, 59%, and 42%, respectively. This report convincingly supported the extended patency potential of the composite sequential configuration.

In the late 1970s there was considerable interest in composite sequential grafting at Northwestern University in Chicago. Flinn et al.[11] presented outcomes for 40 bypasses with intermediate anastomosis to the Central Surgical Association in 1980. At that time there was interest in using a intermediate side-to-side anastomosis termed a "kiss-and-run" bypass, and 30 of 40 grafts reported on were of this configuration. Most of the kiss-and-run operations were entirely of PTFE material, but several were all-autogenous vein. In their report, nine cases were in the configuration of composite sequential and were found to perform well with a limb salvage rate at 18 months of 76%. This paper helped to define the role of a side-to-side popliteal anastomosis. It seemed to offer little advantage for an all-prosthetic reconstruction as flow through the distal segment was probably reduced. This information was helpful in that side-to-side anastomosis at the popliteal for femorotibial prosthetic grafting has been largely abandoned in recent years.

The next publication from Chicago on this topic was by Verta,[12] who had been a co-author of Flinn's 1980 paper. Verta analyzed 54 patients from his practice placing vein grafts to very distal tibial vessels preferentially. A respectable mean follow-up of 26.4 months was reported and the patency rates at 2 and 4 years were 81% and 72%, respectively. Flinn et al.[13] then presented material to the Midwest Vascular Surgical Society in 1983; 30 composite sequential bypasses were highlighted. The 1- and 2-year patency rates of 93% and 80% endorsed the reliability of this configuration.

The composite sequential bypass has remained a useful tool at Northwestern, even with the current greater emphasis on all-venous reconstruction. Careful preoperative duplex scanning, to identify various arm vein sources and lesser saphenous vein, has allowed most patients to have all-venous conduit for tibial bypass. However, if only short segments of vein can be procured, rather than performing an all-PTFE femorotibial bypass, composite sequential grafting is often utilized. The most recent Northwestern experience was presented to the Midwestern Vascular Surgical Society in 1991.[14] Only operations with the proximal anastomosis from the common femoral artery and an intermediate above- or below-knee anastomosis with venous tibial grafting were reviewed. Other configurations such as femorotibial-tibial grafting were not reported. Sixty-seven

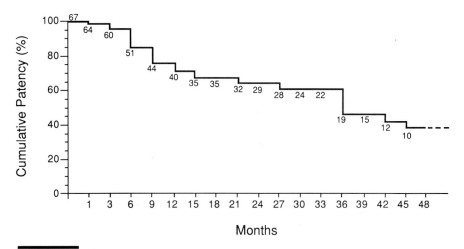

FIGURE 4.

Cumulative life table primary patency. The standard error remains less than 10% until after 48 months. (From McCarthy WJ, Pearce WH, Flinn WR, et al: *J Vasc Surg* 1992; 15:761–770. Used by permission.)

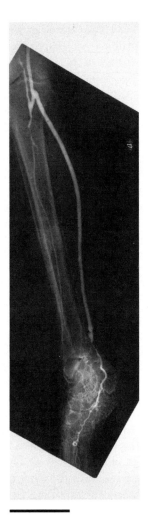

FIGURE 5.

The lesser saphenous vein can be used to advantage with composite sequential reconstruction. Here, anastomosis from the below-knee popliteal prosthetic PTFE graft to the far distal posterior tibial artery allows limb salvage. (From McCarthy WJ, Pearce WH, Flinn WR, et al: *J Vasc Surg* 1992; 15:761–770. Used by permission.)

reconstructions were identified and followed. The mean follow-up was 33 months with a range of 6 to 91 months. With this large number a significant life table analysis to 48 months was possible. A cumulative life table primary patency of 72% at 1 year, 64% at 2 years, and 48% at 3 years was identified (Fig 4). In this series the intermediate anastomosis was placed above the knee in 44 patients, allowing the venous extension to cross the knee. The intermediate anastomosis was below the knee in 23 patients. Patencies were reviewed in an attempt to compare these two groups. A trend without statistical significance favored placing the intermediate popliteal anastomosis above the knee. This arrangement has at least two conceptual advantages. First, the vein graft probably tolerates knee flexion better than prosthetic material. Second, if the intermediate anastomosis is below the knee it is closer to the runoff bed of the tibial extension graft. This produces more competitive flow between the two anastomoses for the distal runoff. In this series an extension graft of greater saphenous vein was used for 57 patients and lesser saphenous was utilized for 10 (Fig 5). Distal anastomosis was to the anterior tibial artery in 19, the posterior tibial artery in 26, and the perineal artery in 21 patients. There was no difference in patency rate between these three tibial runoff vessels. The oldest patent graft in this series was found to be functioning well 91 months after initial placement. Limb salvage was 84% at 2 years and 70% at 4 years. During the 7-year follow-up period for 67 operations there were 28 graft occlusions. Fifteen were managed by reoperation. One patient after graft occlusion was without significant rest pain and was managed without reoperation. However, 12 patients were found to have no viable distal runoff vessels requiring 11 below-knee amputations and one above-knee amputation.

SURGICAL TECHNIQUE FOR SEQUENTIAL BYPASS

Exposure of the popliteal and tibial bypass is the same as for other femoral procedures and anatomic rather than subcutaneous tunnels are preferred. An effort to place the intermediate PTFE femoropopliteal anastomosis above the knee seems advantageous. Popliteal vessels with very poor runoff are still acceptable recipient vessels and endarterectomy has been used successfully to enhance the local anastomosis. However, it is generally not advisable to explore popliteal segments not visualized by angiography. The venous segment can be taken from lesser saphenous, residual greater saphenous, or arm venous conduit, and may be used reversed or, more frequently in the orthograde configuration with valve lysis by a valvulotome. The venous anastomosis is placed end to side on the proximal PTFE graft material and can be located directly over the distal PTFE hood. An ellipse of PTFE material is removed from the proximal graft with a No. 11 scalpel blade.

Angiography is routinely performed with a catheter placed in the PTFE graft material. Usually a single injection will visualize the intermediate and distal anastomosis. Occasionally, if the popliteal runoff is of high quality and low resistance, the contrast will preferentially flow through this route necessitating a clamp placed across the intermediate anastomosis to allow better visualization of the distal vein anastomosis. Although its efficacy is unsubstantiated by any clinical trial, use of postoperative anticoagulation with heparin and long-term anticoagulation with warfarin seems to be advantageous in this patient group.

DISTAL PROSTHETIC GRAFT VEIN PATCH AND COLLARS

In an attempt to prevent intimal hyperplasia from occluding the distal end of prosthetic grafts, several simple innovations have been recently introduced. Two separate techniques, both requiring only several centimeters of useful vein, will be described.

The Miller Collar has been used for the prosthetic-to-popliteal and tibial bypass.[15] The procedure entails harvesting a length of arm vein, or residual greater or lesser saphenous vein sufficient to circumferentially surround the distal anastomosis. The vein is opened along its length and a suture line is constructed around the distal arteriotomy. The suture line is brought to its conclusion with an anastomosis of the two venous ends to form a cylindrical collar. Next, the prosthetic graft hood is sewn to the venous collar in the usual way. Although conclusive long-term patency results are not yet available, anecdotally, its utility seems promising. We have noted a marked redundancy of the anastomosis if the full width of saphenous vein is used for the collar. It may, therefore, be better to trim larger-caliber veins longitudinally in some cases. There is also a concern that laminated thrombus will form in this large anastomosis, as it does, for example, in popliteal aneurysms. Anticoagulation with warfarin over the long term therefore seems reasonable.

Another variation of distal patching is the Taylor Patch.[16] This configuration requires even less viable vein material than the Miller Collar. A standard prosthetic distal anastomosis is planned. The distal half of the prosthetic-to-arterial suture line is not used and the graft toe is removed. In addition, a wedge-shaped portion of the prosthetic material is removed from the graft hood. To fill this defect, a diamond-shaped vein patch is then placed so that the entire distal half of the anastomosis is completed with vein material. While our anecdotal experience with this configuration has been favorable, the flexibility of the distal anastomosis in some cases seems to cause some local side-to-side kinking. Again, anticoagulation with long-term warfarin seems advisable.

These two patching techniques are of interest in the consideration of composite bypass grafting because they represent perhaps the simplest form of a composite graft. They do not address the issue of prosthetic material crossing the knee joint, but may help with the onset of intimal hyperplasia.

CONCLUSIONS

Faced with the situation where limb salvage requires a femoral-distal bypass graft without sufficient autogenous vein, the surgeon may reasonably resort to composite grafting techniques. Strictly composite grafts combining prosthetic material with an end-to-end prosthetic venous anastomosis have been used for over 35 years. However, no large series with sufficient long-term follow-up has been reported to allow precise evaluation and endorsement of this technique. On the other hand, the composite sequential graft which incorporates an intermediate popliteal anastomosis, while somewhat complicated technically, has a more established track record. Patency rates approaching 100 months have been reported with this technique. In addition, innovations involving vein patch of the distal-prosthetic anastomosis have recently been proposed. These are essentially the simplest form of composite grafting and may be useful to enhance graft patency in these difficult situations.

REFERENCES

1. Deterling RA: Experience with permanent by-pass grafts in treatment of occlusive arterial disease. *Arch Surg* 1958; 76:247–260.

2. Dale WA, Pridgen WR, Shoulders HH: Failure of composite (Teflon and vein) grafting in small human arteries. *Surgery* 1962; 51:258–262.

3. DeLaurentis DA, Friedmann P: Arterial reconstruction about and below the knee: Another look. *Am J Surg* 1971; 392–397.

4. Linton RR, Wirthlin LS: Femoropopliteal composite Dacron and autogenous vein bypass grafts. *Arch Surg* 1973; 107:748–753.

5. Lord JW Jr, Sadranagani B, Bajwa G, et al: New technique for construction of composite Dacron vein grafts for femoro-distal popliteal bypass in the severely ischemic leg. *Ann Surg* 1975; 181:670–675.

6. Snyder SO Jr, Gregory RT, Wheeler JR, et al: Composite grafts utilizing polytetrafluoroethylene-autogenous tissue for lower extremity arterial reconstructions. *Surgery* 1981; 90:881–888.

7. Gregory RT, Raithel D, Snyder SO Jr, et al: Composite grafts: An alternative to saphenous vein for lower extremity arterial reconstruction. *J Cardiovasc Surg* 1983; 24:53–57.

8. Holdsworth PJ, Riddell PS, Leveson SH: Distal femoropopliteal bypass using a composite graft of PTFe and non-reversed saphenous vein. *Ann R Coll Surg Engl* 1989; 71:4–6.

9. Bliss BP, Fonseka N: "Hitch-hike" grafts for limb salvage in peripheral arterial disease. *Br J Surg* 1976; 63:562–564.

10. Rosenfeld JC, Savarese RP, Friedmann P, et al: Sequential femoropopliteal and femorotibial bypasses: A ten-year follow-up study. *Arch Surg* 1981; 116:1538–1543.

11. Flinn WR, Flanigan DP, Verta MJ Jr, et al: Sequential femoral-tibial bypass for severe limb ischemia. *Surgery* 1980; 88:357–365.

12. Verta MJ Jr: Composite sequential bypasses to the ankle and beyond for limb salvage. *J Vasc Surg* 1984; 1:381–386.

13. Flinn WJ, Ricco JB, Yao JST, et al: Composite sequential grafts in severe ischemia: A comparative study. *J Vasc Surg* 1984; 1:449–454.

14. McCarthy WJ, Pearce WH, Flinn WR, et al: Patency potential of composite sequential femoral bypass, in Yao JST, Pearce WH (eds): *Long-Term Results in Vascular Surgery.* Norwalk, Conn, Appleton & Lange, 1993, pp 267–271.

15. Miller JH, Foreman RK, Ferguson L, et al: Interposition vein cuff for anastomosis of prosthesis to small artery. *Aust N Z J Surg* 1984; 54:283–285.

16. McFarland RJ, Taylor RS: Une amélioration technique d'anatomose des prosthèses artérielles fémoro-distales. *Phlebologie* 1988; 41:229–233.

PART III

Endovascular Techniques

Infrainguinal Percutaneous Transluminal Balloon Angioplasty

Maria G.M. Hunink, M.D., Ph.D.*

Associate Professor of Sciences, Department of Health Sciences, Faculty of Medicine, University of Groningen; Decision Office for Medical Technology Assessment, Academic Hospital Groningen, Groningen, The Netherlands; Department of Health Policy and Management, Harvard School of Public Health, Boston, Massachusetts

Michael F. Meyerovitz, M.D.

Associate Professor of Radiology, Department of Radiology, Harvard Medical School; Co-Director, Cardiovascular and Interventional Radiology, Brigham and Women's Hospital, Boston, Massachusetts

P ercutaneous transluminal angioplasty (PTA) of the superficial femoral and popliteal arteries has become an accepted and widely practiced form of therapy for claudication and critical ischemia resulting from focal stenoses and short-segment occlusions of the superficial femoral and popliteal arteries. With advancement in balloon and wire technology, PTA is also becoming more frequently used for short focal stenosis of the tibial and peroneal arteries. There has been a proliferation of devices to cut, pulverize, burn, evaporate, or in some other way destroy atherosclerotic stenoses or occlusions. As yet, none of these devices has been proven to have any long-term benefits over balloon PTA for the majority of atherosclerotic lesions. The Simpson Atherocath (an atherectomy device with a side-cutting chamber to remove relatively small amounts of plaque or intimal flaps) is valuable for certain indications such as very eccentric stenoses, for cutting out intimal flaps,[1] and possibly for vein graft stenoses.[2] However we cannot currently recommend this device for most angioplasties in view of its expense, the requirement for a larger sheath size, and because of conflicting reports on long-term patency.[2, 3] In view of this and because of space limitations, this chapter focuses only on balloon PTA.

*Supported by a PIONIER grant from The Netherlands Organization for Scientific Research.

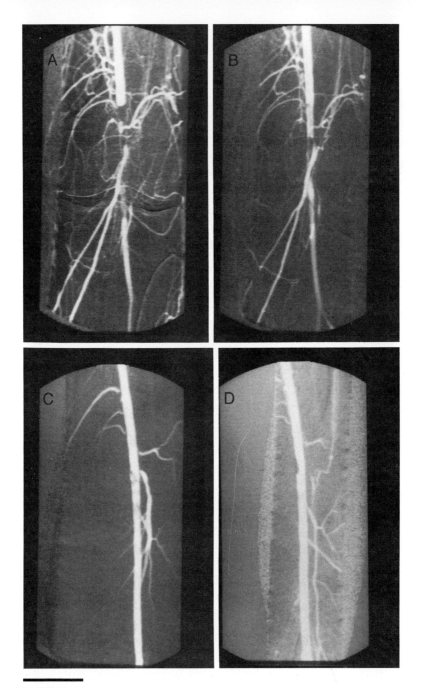

FIGURE 1.

A, digital subtraction arteriogram (DSA) of the left popliteal artery in a 60-year-old man with a 5-month history of gradually increasing left leg claudication. There is a 6-cm occlusion of the popliteal artery with reconstitution of the popliteal artery at the level of the knee joint via collaterals. **B,** repeat DSA after 10 mg of recombinant tissue plasminogen activator (Activase, Genentech Inc., South San Francisco, Calif.) was pulse-sprayed into the occluded segment over 20 minutes. There is now decreased thrombus present as well as some antegrade flow. **C,** after continuous infusion of Activase into the popliteal artery at 4 mg/hr for 3.5 hours, the thrombus has been lysed revealing an underlying 1-cm long eccentric stenosis. **D,** following angioplasty of the popliteal artery stenosis with a 5-mm balloon, there is minimal residual stenosis.

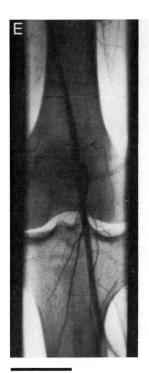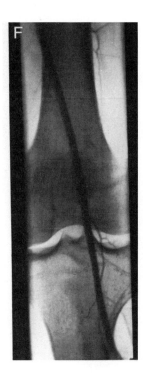

FIGURE 1 (cont.).

E, 2 years later a repeat arteriogram for recurrent claudication reveals a focal 1-cm popliteal artery stenosis at the same site as the previous stenosis. **F,** following repeat balloon angioplasty, this time with a 6-mm balloon, there is no significant residual stenosis.

INDICATIONS

The Standards of Practice Committee of the Society of Cardiovascular and Interventional Radiology has published guidelines for PTA based on lesion morphology.[4] Their suggested indications for femoropopliteal PTA are as follows: (a) PTA is the procedure of choice for single stenoses or occlusions up to 3 cm in length that do not involve the origin of the superficial femoral artery or the distalmost region of the popliteal artery (Fig 1,E); (b) single stenoses or occlusions 3 to 10 cm in length, and lesions up to 3 cm in length that are heavily calcified or multiple are well suited for PTA, although this is not necessarily the procedure of choice (Figs 2 and 3); (c) lesions greater than 10 cm long, 3- to 10-cm lesions involving the distal popliteal artery, and multiple 3- to 5-cm lesions are generally not good candidates for PTA if there is a good surgical alternative; (d) complete common or superficial femoral artery occlusions and complete popliteal and proximal trifurcation occlusions are unsuitable for PTA unless there is no surgical alternative.

For infrapopliteal angioplasty, the suggested indications are as follows: (a) PTA is the procedure of choice for single focal tibial or peroneal stenoses that are 1 cm or less in length; (b) Multiple focal tibial or peroneal stenoses that are 1 cm or less in length or one or two focal stenoses involving the tibial trifurcation are well suited for angioplasty al-

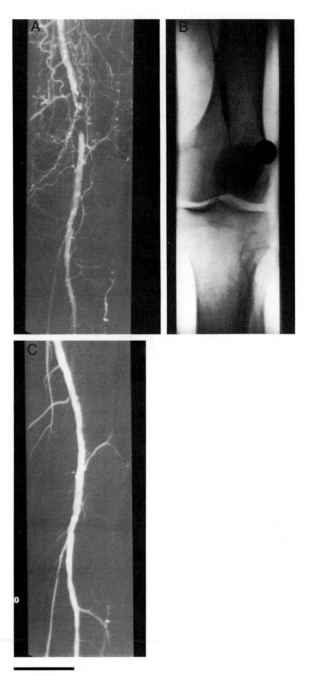

FIGURE 2.

A, arteriogram on this 75-year-old, insulin-dependent diabetic man with foot pain and a left toe ulcer reveals a 3-cm complete occlusion of the popliteal artery. There are numerous small collaterals around the occlusion. **B,** a 5-mm-diameter balloon was inflated across the occluded segment. **C,** following the balloon angioplasty, a repeat arteriogram reveals an irregular but patent popliteal artery with no significant residual stenosis and good antegrade flow. Note the absence of collaterals compared to 2**A.**

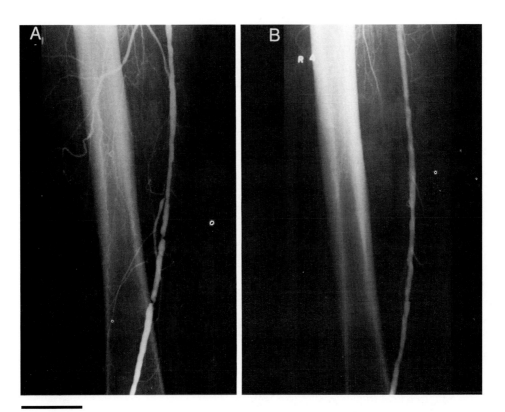

FIGURE 3.

A, arteriography in this 39-year-old woman with right leg rest pain reveals two focal stenoses in the distal superficial femoral artery. **B,** following angioplasty with a 5-mm-diameter balloon, there are only minor residual stenoses present in the superficial femoral artery.

though this is not necessarily the procedure of choice (Fig 4); (c) 1- to 4-cm stenoses and 1- to 2-cm tibial or peroneal occlusions or extensive involvement of the trifurcation are not generally good candidates for angioplasty if there is a good surgical alternative; (d) Tibial or peroneal occlusions greater than 2 cm in length and diffusely diseased infrapopliteal arteries are unsuitable for PTA unless there is no surgical alternative.

While the aforementioned indications suggested are fairly widely accepted as reasonable, they are in some instances arbitrary in that limited data exist on long-term outcomes. This is particularly true in infrapopliteal angioplasty. In addition, some (including us) would argue that superficial or femoral artery occlusions of 7 to 10 cm are not well suited to angioplasty alone because of poor long-term results. In order to improve these long-term results, superficial femoral and popliteal artery occlusions greater than 3 cm in length (even if they are chronic in nature) may be treated by initial thrombolysis in order to reveal a shorter underlying focal stenosis that may be treated by angioplasty[5, 6] (see Fig 1).

TECHNICAL CONSIDERATIONS

Infrainguinal PTA is usually most easily performed from an ipsilateral approach. On occasion a contralateral approach is advantageous, as when

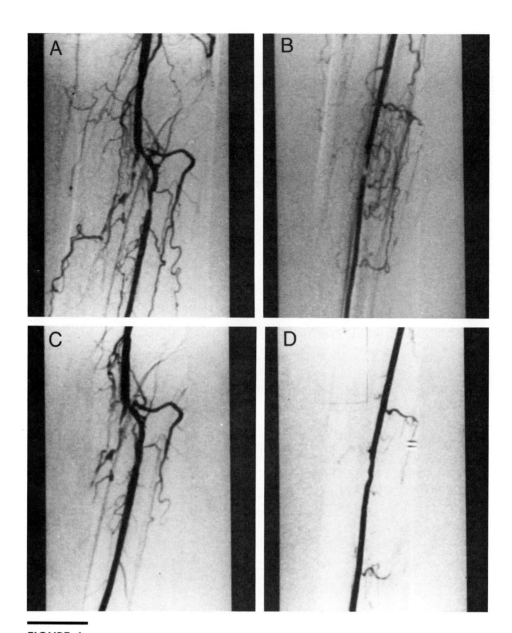

FIGURE 4.

A and **B,** arteriography in this 75-year-old man with an ischemic left foot ulcer reveals two focal stenoses in the left anterior tibial artery. The ankle-brachial index (ABI) was 0.57. **C** and **D,** following angioplasty of the anterior tibial artery stenoses with a 3-mm-diameter balloon, there has been marked arteriographic improvement in luminal caliber. The ABI after angioplasty was 1.0.

the infrainguinal lesion is in the common femoral artery or in the proximal superficial femoral artery close to the common femoral bifurcation. A contralateral approach may also be preferentially utilized when the superficial femoral artery has an unusually high origin or when iliac and femoral or popliteal lesions are to be treated by angioplasty at the same sitting. In these instances, a long curved polyethylene sheath placed from the contralateral side with its distal end over the aortic bifurcation may facilitate the PTA. In general, however, a contralateral approach increases the technical difficulties encountered in common and external iliac as well as infrainguinal PTA. This is particularly true the more distal the PTA site in the lower extremity.

After localizing the skin puncture site under fluoroscopy, an antegrade puncture of the common femoral artery is made using the Seldinger technique. It is particularly important to identify under fluoroscopy the correct skin level for the puncture as the inguinal crease is variable in location and cannot be relied on for this purpose. Once the common femoral artery has been entered with the needle, a curved guidewire that has torque control is manipulated under fluoroscopy into the superficial femoral artery, and an arterial sheath (usually 6F in diameter) is inserted over the guidewire. The sheath will not only facilitate multiple balloon exchanges while minimizing arterial entry site trauma but also allow for contrast medium and vasodilator injections.

An arteriogram (usually digital subtraction) is performed by injecting contrast medium through the arterial sheath. This will give excellent definition of the arterial stenosis or occlusion and allow for identification of runoff vessels if these have not previously been demonstrated. The next step is to cross the stenosis or occlusion with a guidewire, choices of which are becoming almost endless with multiple manufacturers each having a range of guidewires on the market. Most stenoses can be crossed with some type of torquable guidewire while occlusions can often be crossed with a hydrophilically coated wire even when other wires fail. For superficial femoral or popliteal artery lesions, a wire 0.035-in. in diameter is usually used, while for tibial or peroneal lesions a 0.016- or 0.018-in. wire is usually used.

Once the lesion has been crossed, a bolus of 5,000 units of heparin is given intravenously (or intraarterially). For stenoses in smaller arteries, particularly tibial and peroneal arteries, the intraarterial administration of vasodilators is important to counteract spasm. We usually use 100-μg boluses of intraarterial nitroglycerin for this purpose because of its efficacy and safety, and because multiple boluses can be given. A balloon catheter is then positioned over the guidewire, across the stenosis, and inflated until the waist in the balloon disappears. The balloon is sized to match the normal luminal diameter of the artery being dilated. The most common balloon diameter for a superficial femoral artery is 6 mm and for tibial vessels 3 mm, although there is obviously individual variation. For a femoropopliteal lesion the balloon is usually mounted on a 5F shaft, whereas for tibioperoneal lesions the shaft size is under 5F. For extremely high-grade lesions through which a standard balloon will not pass, a balloon mounted directly onto a guidewire will usually pass across the stenosis owing to the very low deflated profile of this type of device. Balloon inflation is for approximately 1 minute and one or several inflations may be necessary.

Following balloon inflation, the balloon is withdrawn leaving the guidewire in place and a repeat digital subtraction arteriogram is performed through the arterial sheath. If the appearances are satisfactory, the guidewire is withdrawn and a completion arteriogram is performed. We

TABLE 1.
Morbidity and Mortality of Angioplasty (Given as Percentages of the Number of Procedures Performed*), Ordered by Increasing Percentage of Procedures Performed for Ischemia

Reference	Procedures	Femoropopliteal† (%)	Mean Age (yr)†	Critical Ischemia† (%)	Morbidity†‡ (%)	Major Morbidity†‡ (%)	Mortality (%)
Morse et al.[7]	500	NA	66	NA	8.8	NA	0.8
Henriksen et al.[8]	86	36	58	0	10.5	NA	0.0
Hunink et al.[9]	72	100	63	0	1.4	1.4	0.0
Johnston[10]	984	26	60	13	9.5	0.8	0.4
Capek et al.[11]	217	100	64	26	8.8	1.4	1.4
Belli et al.[12]	1642	54	NA	26	2.6	0.2	0.1
Wilson et al.[13,14]	129	38	61	27	20.9	NA	0.0
Jeans et al.[15]	500	51	64	38	NA	NA	2.0
Hasson et al.[16]	202	44	63	41	21.8	4.0	5.9
Weibull et al.[17]	134	15	66	43	20.9	8.2	2.2

Walden et al.[18]	69	33	62	55	15.9	2.9	1.4
Milford et al.[19]	27	100	65	93	11.1	3.7	7.4
Hunink et al.[9]	54	100	67	100	20.4	10.9	1.8
Jørgenson et al.[20]	92	61	67	100	10.9	NA	0.0
Jones et al.[21]	92	61	67	100	7.6	NA	2.2
Range	27–1,642	15–100	58–67	0–100	1.4–21.8	0.2–10.9	0–7.4
Pooled (±SE)§	4,800	49(±20)	63(±1)	30(±21)	8.1(±0.4)	1.3(±0.2)	0.9(±0.1)

*Percentages may differ from those published in the original papers; adjustments were made when figures were reported as percentages of patients instead of procedures and where the employed morbidity definitions did not conform to ours.

†NA = not available.

‡Major morbidity included nonfatal cardiac, pulmonary, and cerebrovascular complications; bowel ischemia; sepsis; and renal failure. Morbidity included major morbidity and hematomas, wound infections, thromboses, dissections, and emboli. Mortality was procedure-related, in hospital, or overall 30-day mortality.

§The pooled results, and standard errors, give the probability of the event and associated variability in the *average* study population. The standard error does *not* indicate the variability across studies, because the case mix differs across studies.

remove the arterial sheath when the activated coagulation time is under 180 seconds. Once hemostasis has been achieved, an overnight intravenous heparin infusion is started if there is a significant angioplasty site dissection on the completion arteriogram, if the initial lesion was an occlusion, or if angioplasty was performed for an infrapopliteal lesion.

Intravascular ultrasound is being utilized in some centers to try to obtain more information about lesion morphology and to visualize the postangioplasty appearance, in particular the presence of dissection and intimal flaps. While these devices probably allow this to be done more accurately than with arteriography, they suffer the disadvantage of adding considerable time and expense to the procedure, without proven benefit. At this point in time we believe intravascular ultrasound is more useful as a research tool than as a clinical device.

COMPLICATIONS

INCIDENCE

The overall incidence of complications following femoropopliteal PTA is approximately 8% (range, 1.4%–21.8%) of procedures performed (Table 1). Major morbidity, including nonfatal cardiac, pulmonary, and cerebrovascular complications; bowel ischemia; sepsis; and renal failure, occurs on average in 1.3% (range, 0.2%–10.9%) of procedures (see Table 1). Mortality, reported as procedure-related, in hospital or overall 30-day mortality, occurs on average in 0.9% (range, 0%–7.4%) of procedures. The incidence of complications following infrapopliteal PTA is, given the limited number of series, impossible to quantify but probably not very different from that following femoropopliteal PTA.

Complications requiring treatment occur in 2.0% to 2.5% of procedures performed.[22] Major local complications include acute occlusion (2%–5%), distal embolization (2%), false aneurysm (0.3%–2.0%), arteriovenous (AV), fistula (0.1%–0.3%), arterial rupture (0.3%–13.0%), and amputation (0.2%).[17, 22–24] Arterial rupture is usually due to an oversized balloon. Predisposing to arterial rupture are steroid medication and underlying vascular abnormalities.[24] Minor local complications include hematoma (2%–4%), guidewire perforation without bleeding (0.3%), dissection extending beyond the PTA site (1%–4%), and balloon rupture.[17, 22–24]

MANAGEMENT

Occlusion (abrupt closure) of the artery during or after angioplasty may result from spasm, thrombosis, or dissection.[23, 24] Spasm is, of course, usually easily dealt with by giving intraarterial vasodilators such as nitroglycerin, and this should be the first line of treatment for any abrupt closure. The next line of treatment is usually repeat balloon dilation, and if the standard inflation time does not lead to lasting patency, the balloon may be inflated for a more prolonged period (5–20 minutes) in the hope of "tacking up" any intimal flaps against the arterial wall. If this does not work and the occlusion appears on the arteriogram to be due to dissection, the intimal flap may be excised using the Simpson Athero-

Moving?

I'd like to receive my *Advances in Vascular Surgery* without interruption.
Please note the following change of address, effective:

Name: _____

New Address: _____

_____

City: _____ State: _____ Zip: _____

Old Address: _____

_____

City: _____ State: _____ Zip: _____

Reservation Card

Yes, I would like my own copy of *Advances in Vascular Surgery*. Please begin my subscription with the current edition according to the terms described below.* I understand that I will have 30 days to examine each annual edition. If satisfied, I will pay just $69.95 plus sales tax, postage and handling (price subject to change without notice).

Name: _____

Address: _____

City: _____ State: _____ Zip: _____

Method of Payment
○ Visa   ○ Mastercard   ○ AmEx   ○ Bill me   ○ Check (in US dollars, payable to Mosby, Inc.)

Card number: _____ Exp date: _____

Signature: _____

LS-0909

---

*Your *Advances* Service Guarantee:*

When you subscribe to *Advances*, we'll send you an advance notice of future volumes about two months before they publish. This automatic notice system is designed to take up as little of your time as possible. If you do not want *Advances*, the advance notice makes it quick and easy for you to let us know your decision, and you will always have at least 20 days to decide. If we don't hear from you, we'll send you the new volume as soon as it's available. And, of course, *Advances* is yours to examine free of charge for 30 days (postage, handling and applicable sales tax are added to each shipment.).

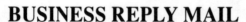

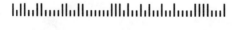
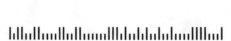
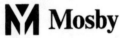

Mosby

Dedicated to publishing excellence

cath.[1] If, on the other hand, the appearance on the arteriogram resembles thrombosis, intraarterial thrombolytic therapy with recombinant tissue-type plasminogen activator or urokinase may be undertaken provided there are no contraindications to thrombolysis.[25] Sometimes, however, it may be difficult to distinguish between thrombosis and dissection as the cause of the occlusion and in some cases both of these mechanisms may play a role. The last line of therapy for abrupt closure is placement of an arterial metallic stent, if such be available. To date, no arterial stent has been approved by the U.S. Food and Drug Administration for use in infrainguinal arteries although clinical trials with the Schneider Wallstent are underway. Experience in Europe, however, indicates that the long-term patency of femoropopliteal lesions treated with stents is suboptimal and that the use of these devices should be limited to failed angioplasty.[26-29]

If a small and insignificant distal embolization occurs, systemic heparinization is acceptable. Significant emboli may be aspirated with a large-bore nontapered catheter, or percutaneous or surgical embolectomy, or thrombolysis may be performed. If acute ischemia develops, urgent removal is necessary to avoid a compartment syndrome or limb loss.

A false aneurysm or AV fistula at the entry site may be treated with ultrasound-guided compression, under adequate sedation and pain control.[30] If unsuccessful, surgical intervention is required. Arterial rupture with extravasation may be treated by occluding the rupture site with a PTA balloon (or Stack balloon to maintain distal flow) for 20 minutes.[24] If after two attempts control of bleeding is not obtained, urgent surgical intervention is necessary.

Balloon rupture is generally insignificant. The balloon catheter should be removed through a sheath.

PATENCY RESULTS

REPORTING PATENCY RESULTS

Standards have been published for reports on patency after vascular interventions. Briefly these standards are[31, 32]:

1. An improvement of ankle-brachial index (ABI) of greater than 0.10 with relief of symptoms is considered a success.[32] During follow-up a decrease in ABI of greater than 0.15 compared with the maximum early post-PTA ABI, or recurrence of symptoms, is considered a failure.
2. The initial success rate should be reported and initial failures are included in the patency analysis.[31, 32] (Note that if initial failures are not included in the results, the patency among all patients undergoing intervention may be derived by multiplying by the initial success rate.)
3. Primary patency refers to those vessels that remain patent without further intervention. Secondary patency refers to all vessels that remain patent, with or without additional angioplasty procedures.
4. Patency results should be analyzed and reported using actuarial life table or Kaplan-Meier analysis, reporting the number of limbs at risk in each interval during follow-up.[31, 32]

RANDOMIZED CONTROLLED TRIALS

Only two randomized controlled trials (RCTs) comparing PTA to another treatment have been published. In an RCT comparing PTA and supervised exercise,[33] 36 patients with unilateral claudication (due to infrainguinal or aortoiliac disease) were randomized. Significantly more patients undergoing supervised exercise stopped smoking, confounding the results. The ABI increase after 3 to 9 months was 0.21 with PTA and 0 with exercise. However, with exercise the claudicating and maximum-walking distance increased progressively, while in all PTA patients this was limited at 12 months by contralateral disease. Note that exercise also prevents and treats contralateral disease while PTA was performed unilaterally in this trial. In the second RCT, comparing PTA and bypass,[13, 14] 97 patients with femoropopliteal lesions were randomized. No difference was demonstrated between femoropopliteal PTA and bypass, with 5-year primary patencies of 59% and 55% respectively. The majority of the femoropopliteal interventions in the randomized trial (71/97, or 73%) were performed for claudication, as opposed to limb-threatening conditions such as rest pain, ischemic ulcers, or gangrene. Results were stratified for the site of the lesion but not for other known risk factors predictive of long-term failure such as the indication (critical ischemia vs. claudication), lesion type (occlusion vs. stenosis), and the bypass material used (polytetrafluoroethylene [PTFE] vs. saphenous vein).

FEMOROPOPLITEAL ANGIOPLASTY

A published literature review and meta-analysis on the results of femoropopliteal angioplasty combined results of procedures performed in the 1970s and early 1980s.[34] Unfortunately, this meta-analysis included papers that were not strictly selected and employed different definitions of patency,[32] and other than stratifying patency by indication, did not examine risk factors predictive of long-term failure. More recently another literature review and meta-analysis were performed of studies pertaining to conventional balloon angioplasty of femoropopliteal arterial disease published between January 1985 and January 1993.[35] The methods and results of the meta-analysis are summarized here.[35, 36] Studies included in the baseline analysis did the following:

- Conformed or could be adapted to the published standards for such reports[31, 32]
- Defined patency as maintenance of hemodynamic improvement
- Were sufficiently detailed to allow for stratification over subgroups at varying risk for long-term patency
- Specified the number of subjects at risk during follow-up or reported the standard errors of patency rates

Of 66 papers that were reviewed, 11 studies (Table 2) were included. Studies varied in their definition of patency success; the baseline analysis includes only the 7 studies that required hemodynamic improvement (see Table 2). In a sensitivity analysis (i.e., a "what-if" analysis) 4 studies with the more lenient criteria were also included. For reports which did not conform to the set standards (see Table 2) the data were adjusted by (1) estimating the cumulative patency from a published figure that presented the results of a life table or Kaplan-meier analysis specifically for femoropopliteal procedures, (2) estimating the number of patients at risk during follow-up from the reported standard error using the inverse of the Peto formula,[41] and (3) adjusting the reported patency to include initial failures.

The effect of different covariates, i.e., patient characteristics that have significant prognostic value in predicting failure, was modeled using a method previously described.[36] The method combines failure time data (from life tables or patency curves) from different studies with adjustment for covariates. It is based on the proportional hazards model and actuarial life table approach. The underlying assumption is that the variation across studies may in part be explained by heterogeneity of the case mix. The method entailed the following steps:

1. The available data were summarized in the form of life tables.
2. The effective sample size was calculated for each interval (i.e., the sample size was adjusted for subjects withdrawn or lost to follow-up).
3. All patients subjected to intervention were included in the meta-analysis, which therefore also included the immediate technical failures.
4. Based on a published proportional hazards model of follow-up data after angioplasty, two covariates that predicted failure were identified: lesion type (occlusion vs. stenosis; hazard rate ratio = 2.7 [95% confidence interval (CI) 1.3−5.6]) and indication for the procedure (critical ischemia vs. claudication; hazard rate ratio = 2.0 [95% CI 1.2−3.3]).[9]
5. The subgroup with claudication and a stenosis had the lowest risk for failure and was chosen as the reference stratum.
6. Hazard rate ratios for the other strata were calculated from the published hazard rate ratios.[9]
7. The results from one paper, reported as secondary patency instead of primary patency,[40] were adjusted downward. Primary patency was the endpoint used throughout the meta-analysis.
8. Six of the 11 studies were not fully stratified with respect to the covariates: for these studies the initial distribution of subjects across risk subgroups and effective sample size in each subgroup in each interval were estimated.
9. The adjusted data were combined to estimate the hazard rate of the reference stratum during each interval.
10. The hazard rate and patency curve for every stratum at varying risk for failure was calculated using the hazard rate ratios.
11. Finally, sensitivity analysis ("what if?" analysis) was performed by repeating the analysis

    a. Including all angioplasty studies irrespective of the criteria used for patency.
    b. Varying the estimated number of patients withdrawn and lost to follow-up.

TABLE 2.
Review of the Results of Femoropopliteal Angioplasty of Studies Reporting Cumulative Patency Determined With a Life Table or Kaplan-Meier Analysis*†

Reference	n	Isch (%)	Occl (%)	Poor (%)	Success†	Type of Patency	Patency (%)						
							Initial	1 yr	2 yr	3 yr	4 yr	5 yr	±SE#
Gallino et al.[37]	289	39	41	41	Hem	Primary‡	87	62	61	60	58	58	±3
Johnston[10]	254	20	39	36	Hem	Primary§	96	63	53	51	44	38	±4
Capek et al.[11]	217	26	32	40	Hem	Primary‡§**	89	56	51	49	48	42	±4
Hunink et al.[9]	131	42	10	45	Hem	Primary	95	57	50	45	45	45	±5
Jørgenson et al.[20]	58	100	62	59	Hem	Primary‡	64	40	33	25	25	NA	±8
Henriksen et al.[8]	31	0	42	NA	Hem	Primary‡	77	47	41	41	41	NA	±10
Walden et al.[18]	23	65	71	71	Hem	Primary‖	91	68	68	NA	NA	NA	±10

Jeans et al.[15]	190	49	66	37	S/H	Primary‡	82	48	43	42	41	41	±4
Krepel et al.[38]	164	10	23	NA	S/H	Primary‖	88	71	68	62	62	62	±4
Samson et al.[39]	89	90	0	NA	S/H	Primary	92	50	46	46	46	NA	±7
Murray et al.[49]	93	34	40	NA	S/H	Second‖††	81	64	62	49	49	49	±7
Wilson[13,14]¶	49	28	NA	NA	Hem	Primary	71	62	59	59	59	NA	±7

*From Hunink MGM, Wong JB, Donaldson MC, et al: *Med Decis Making* 1994; 14:71–81. Used by permission.

†NA = no available; Isch = critical ischemia; occl = occlusion; poor = poor runoff; Hem = Maintenance of hemodynamic improvement was required for success; S/H = Maintenance of either symptomatic or of hemodynamic improvement was considered a success. The baseline analysis is based on the 1,003 subjects from the seven studies that required hemodynamic improvement for success and reported the percentage of subjects with critical ischemia and occlusions. The studies using symptomatic or hemodynamic criteria for success were included in the sensitivity analysis.

‡Patency was estimated from a published figure specifically of femoropopliteal angioplasty, based on life table or Kaplan-Meier analysis.

§Number at risk during follow-up were estimated from the reported standard error using the inverse of the Peto formula.[31]

‖Reported patency was adjusted to include initial failures.

¶The results of the study by Wilson et al.[13] have been added for comparison because this is the only randomized controlled trial available, but have not been included in the analysis because the distribution of lesion type is not available.

**Eight percent were redilations. Both primary and secondary patency were reported. The hazard ratio for secondary patency was calculated from this study.

††Thirteen percent were redilations. Only secondary patency was reported.

‡‡To avoid cluttering the table we tabulated only the standard error of the last patency available (calculated with the Greenwood formula from the reported data).

c. Analyzing the data with a jackknife-type of procedure (i.e., the analysis was repeated multiple times, each time removing a single study from the baseline group of studies).

d. Using lesion type and runoff as significant covariates predictive of failure.[36]

Table 2 summarizes the angioplasty reports that were sufficiently detailed for inclusion in the meta-analysis. Five-year patency in these reports ranges from 38% to 62%. However, one study reports a 4-year patency of 25%,[20] implying that the 5-year patency in this study could never have been higher, and thus the inferred 5-year patency range is broader, i.e., 25% to 62%. First, the life table data were pooled without adjustment for covariates which yielded a 5-year cumulative primary patency of 45% (±2%). These pooled unadjusted patency results do not reflect the variation of results across subgroups at varying risk for failure. Using the described method the life table data were adjusted and pooled. The pooled adjusted life table data for the reference group (i.e., the subgroup with claudication and a stenosis) are presented in Table 3. The primary patency curves for various risk groups defined by indication and lesion type were derived from the adjusted life table (Fig 5). After adjustment for covariates the 5-year cumulative primary patency ranged from 68%, performed for claudication with a stenosis, to 12%, performed for critical ischemia with an occlusion (Table 4).

Including the four angioplasty papers with the more lenient criteria for patency did not change the results substantially. The results were also insensitive to varying estimates of the number of subjects lost to follow-up and withdrawn. The jackknife sensitivity analysis gave a range of values within 2 SE of the baseline value (see Table 4). An alternative model used

TABLE 3.
Life Table of the Primary Patency of Angioplasty Adjusted to the Reference Group (Claudication and Stenosis; Hazard Rate Ratio=1.0), Including the Range of Values Found in the Sensitivity Analysis for this Group*†

Interval (yr)	n	Censored	Failures	Patency(%)	SE	Range
0−0‡	1,003	71	50	100		
0−0.5	882	72	89	95	1	94−95
0.5−1.0	721	49	52	85	1	83−86
1.0−2.0	620	45	24	79	1	76−80
2.0−3.0	551	150	11	75	2	72−78
3.0−4.00	390	60	11	74	2	70−76
4.00−5.00	319	138	11	71	2	66−75
5.00+	170			68	2	62−73

*Data from Hunink MGM, Wong JB, Donaldson MC, et al: *Med Decis Making* 1994; 14:71−81.
†n = the number of limbs at risk at the beginning of the interval; Censored = the number withdrawn and lost to follow-up; Patency = cumulative patency at the beginning and during the interval, i.e., determined by the failures during the previous interval; SE = standard error.
‡The first interval (0−0) is used to denote the immediate technical and clinical failures.

TABLE 4.

Five-Year Cumulative Primary Patency Results, Standard Error (SE), and Range in Sensitivity Analysis, for Angioplasty Performed for Femoropopliteal Lesions Depending on Lesion Type and Indication, or Depending on Lesion Type and Runoff*

Risk Factors	Five-Year Primary Patency (%)	
	Baseline (SE)	Sensitivity Analysis
Pooled, unadjusted	45 (±2)	39–47
Baseline model		
Stenosis and claudication	68 (±2)	62–73
Stenosis and critical ischemia	47 (±10)	38–53
Occlusion and claudication	35 (±14)	27–43
Occlusion and critical ischemia	12 (±12)	7–18
Alternative model		
Stenosis and good runoff	60(±2)	56–64
Stenosis and poor runoff	40 (±7)	35–45
Occlusion and good runoff	45 (±7)	40–50
Occlusion and poor runoff	24 (±9)	19–29

*Data from Hunink MGM, Wong JB, Donaldson MC, et al: *Med Dec Making* 1994; 14:71–81. Hunink MGM, Wong JB: *Med Dec Making* 1994; 14:59–70.

lesion type (occlusion vs. stenosis) and runoff (good [two or three vessels] vs. poor [none or one vessel]) as covariates,[36] including only those studies that specified these covariates. The alternative model yielded a similar set of patency curves (Fig 6) (see Table 4) as the baseline analysis.

INFRAPOPLITEAL AND BYPASS GRAFT ANGIOPLASTY

Reported initial clinical success (angiographically a residual stenosis of less than 20%–50% and symptomatic improvement) of infrapopliteal and bypass graft PTA ranges from 67% to 95%.[42–50] Only a limited number of series reporting long-term follow-up after infrapopliteal PTA have been published (Table 5). The case mix of the study populations and the definitions used in these reports vary enormously, thus precluding a meaningful meta-analysis of the results. In general, the long-term results of bypass graft PTA are poor (18% 4-year patency), unless the lesion is single (59%, 4-year patency).[42] This is also reflected in the series by Brown et al.[43] who reported a 3-year patency of 43%, while 42% of their angioplasty procedures were interventions on bypass grafts. The highest reported long-term patency after infrapopliteal PTA is 65% 3-year patency.[44, 45] Reported 2-year limb salvage rates among patients with infrapopliteal lesions treated for critical ischemia are 72% to 77%.[46, 47]

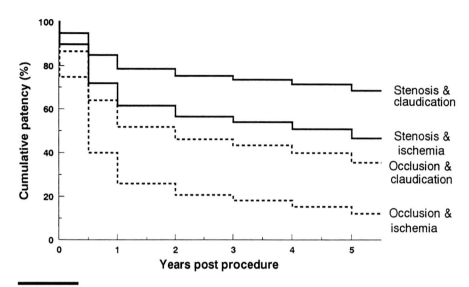

FIGURE 5.

Cumulative primary patency curves for femoropopliteal angioplasty depending on lesion type and indication. Note that the curves start at a point less than 1 because of immediate technical and clinical failures (From Hunink MGM, Wong JB, Donaldson MC, et al: *Med Decis Making* 1994; 14:71–81. Used by permission.)

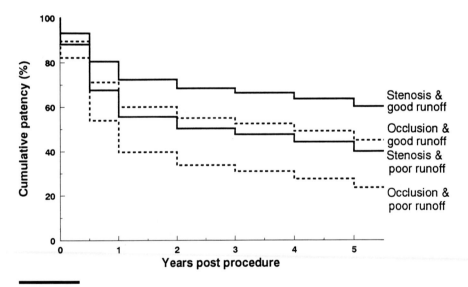

FIGURE 6.

Cumulative primary patency curves for femoropopliteal angioplasty depending on lesion type and runoff. Note that the curves start at a point less than 1 because of immediate technical and clinical failures. (From Hunink MGM, Wong JB: *Med Decis Making* 1994; 14:59–70. Used by permission.)

TABLE 5.
Review of the Results of Infrapopliteal and Bypass Angioplasty of Studies Reporting Cumulative Patency or Limb Salvage Determined With a Life Table or Kaplan-Meier Analysis*‡

Reference	No. of PTAs	No. of Patients	Isch (%)	Bypass (%)	Success	Type of Patency	Patency (%)				
							Initial†	1 yr	2 yr	3 yr	4 yr
Whittemore et al.[42]	54	30	43	100	Hem‡	Primary	70	36	25	18	18
Brown et al[43]	55	40	84	42	Sym§	Primary‖	84	50	43	43	NA
Horvath et al.[44]	103	71	42	0	Ag¶	NA	93	80	75	65	NA
Flueckiger et al[45]	125	91	44	0	Ag¶	NA	90	77	71	64	NA
Schwarten[46]	146	90	100	8	LS	LS	87	77	72	NA	NA
Saab et al.[47]	17	13	100	0	LS	LS	86	77	77	NA	NA

*NA = not available; Isch = critical ischemia; Bypass = % of procedures that were PTAs of bypass grafts; LS = limb salvage.
†Earliest clinical success rate available.
‡Hem = Maintenance of hemodynamic improvement was required for success.
§Sym = Limb salvage and no rest pain was required for success.
‖Reported cumulative patency or limb salvage was adjusted to include initial failures. Patency was estimated from a published figure based on life table or Kaplan-Meier analysis.
¶Ag = Patency was determined angiographically. Angiography was performed if a recurrence was suspected on the basis of clinical symptoms of noninvasive studies. Exact selection criteria for performing angiography were not stated.

FINANCIAL CONSIDERATIONS

The costs of PTA have generally been considered to be much lower compared to those of bypass surgery. However, this is based on analyses performed 8 to 10 years ago (Table 6). More recent cost analyses have focused on bypass surgery and amputation, not on PTA.[56-58]

An analysis of hospital costs performed at the Brigham and Women's Hospital included all patients admitted to the Vascular Surgery Service for femoropopliteal PTA or bypass surgery or both, between October 1, 1985 and October 31, 1991.[55] Information was available on 255 admissions of 228 patients for bypass surgery and 82 admissions of 71 patients for PTA. Hospital costs included routine room and board, intermediate and intensive care room and board, operating room and nonprofessional anesthesia services, diagnostic angiography, interventional radiology, other diagnostic radiology services, clinical laboratory services, patient laboratory services (such as noninvasive testing), pharmacy and blood bank, and all other inpatient services immediately related to the admission. Professional fees, long-term costs (due to, e.g., failure of the procedure), and indirect costs (such as production loss during convalescence) were excluded from this analysis. Length of stay was determined as the number of days from date of admission to the date of discharge.

TABLE 6.
Review of Published Costs and Charges for PTA and Bypass Surgery*

Reference-Year, Cost/Charge Studied, Procedure	1990 U.S. Dollars†		PTA-Bypass Cost Ratio
	PTA	Bypass	
Doubilet & Abrams[51]: 1982, hospital charges, including diagnostic angiogram	3,318	17,829	19%
Wolf & McLean[52]: 1982, hospital charges, excluding diagnostic angiogram	17,354	55,449	34%
Kinnison et al[53]: 1983, hospital charges, excluding diagnostic angiogram	4,483	13,281	31%
Jeans et al.[54]: 1984, hospital costs, from U.K.,‡ including diagnostic angiogram	322	1,475	21%
Hunink et al.[55]: 1985–1991, hospital costs, including diagnostic angiogram	8,019	13,439	60%
Claudication	6,152	11,582	53%
Critical ischemia	11,353	15,059	75%

*Data from Hunink MGM, Donaldson MC, Cullen KA: *J Vasc Surg* 1994; 19:632-641.
†Converted to 1990 U.S. dollars using the medical component of the consumer price index (CPI) (source: Bureau of Labor Statistics, U.S. Department of Labor).[59]
‡1984 pounds were converted to 1984 dollars at an exchange rate of 1.336 (source: International Monetary Fund).

Overall, PTA cost $8,019 (SD $5,753) and bypass surgery $13,439 (SD $6,791), a significant difference (P=.0001) (see Table 6). Although 8 to 10 years ago the costs of PTA were 19% to 34% of the costs of bypass surgery, this study found that PTA currently costs on average 60% of the cost of surgery—a far less favorable ratio. For claudicators the mean hospital costs for PTA were significantly lower than those for bypass surgery, and PTA cost 53% of that of a graft (P=.0001). For critical ischemia the difference in costs was of borderline significance, PTA costing 75% of that of surgery (P=.08). Mean hospital costs and length of stay were highly correlated ($P^2=0.89$, P=.0001). The mean length of stay was significantly different for PTA compared to bypass surgery (4.2 vs. 11.3 days, P=.0001). For claudicators the mean length of stay was 1.8 vs. 9.3 days for PTA and bypass surgery respectively (P=.0001). For admissions for critical ischemia the difference in length of stay was of borderline significance (8.6 vs. 13.0 days, P=.05).

We attempted to explain why the ratio of PTA to bypass surgery increased over the past 10 years. Analysis of the costs of PTA vs. bypass surgery suggested that the cost of PTA increased $1,269 (SE $731) per year (P=.08) (Fig 7) while the cost of bypass surgery decreased approximately $370/yr. (not significant). Analysis of the cost components (see Fig

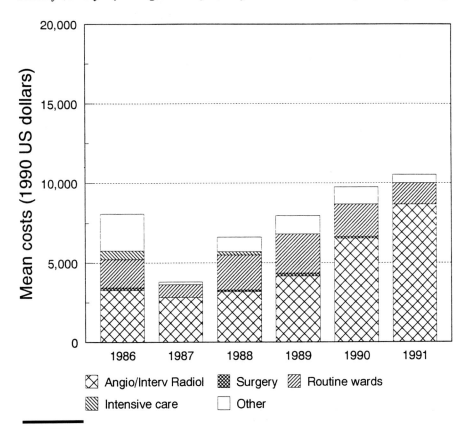

FIGURE 7.

Mean costs of PTA, expressed in 1990 U.S. dollars, for the years 1986–1991. (From Hunink MGM, Donaldson MC, Cullen KA: *J Vasc Surg* 1994; 19:632–641. Used by permission.)

7) suggested that the increase in cost for PTA was due to an increase in cost of the actual procedure, possibly explained by more expensive catheters and guidewires employed during PTA and the use of more expensive (low-osmolar) contrast agents. For bypass surgery, operating room expenses appeared more or less constant during the study period, the cost for diagnostic angiography increased, and costs for room and board decreased.

CONCLUSION

While the role of iliac PTA has been established, some questions still remain about the exact role of infrainguinal PTA. Current reports on the risks, efficacy, and costs of femoropopliteal and infrapopliteal PTA, based on strict outcome criteria and reporting standards, suggest selective use of infrainguinal PTA. A cost-effectiveness analysis comparing PTA with medical treatment and with bypass surgery may help elucidate the role of infrainguinal PTA.[51, 60–62] Such an analysis would need to be stratified for varying severity of disease. At the very least patients need to be stratified by indication, because revascularization performed for critical ischemia has a higher risk, yields lower long-term patency, and costs more than revascularization performed for claudication. However, many facts remain to be evaluated before a comprehensive reassessment and cost-effectiveness analysis of the treatment of infrainguinal peripheral arterial disease are feasible, including the long-term results of medical or conservative treatment and the improvement in quality of life following various forms of treatment.

REFERENCES

1. Maynar M, Reyes R, Cabrera V, et al: Percutaneous atherectomy as an alternative treatment for post-angioplasty obstructive intimal flaps. *Radiology* 1989; 170:1029–1031.
2. Kim D, Gianturco LE, Porter D, et al: Peripheral directional atherectomy: 4-year experience. *Radiology* 1992; 183:773–778.
3. Dorros G, Iyer S, Lewis R, et al: Angiographic follow-up and clinical outcome of 126 patients after percutaneous directional atherectomy (Simpson Athero-Cath) for occlusive peripheral vascular disease. *Cathet Cardiovasc Diagn* 1991; 22:79–84.
4. Standards of Practice Committee of the Society of Cardiovascular and Interventional Radiology: Guidelines for percutaneous transluminal angioplasty. *Radiology* 1990; 177:619–626.
5. Hess H, Mietaschk A, Bruckl R: Peripheral arterial occlusions: A 6-year experience with local low-dose thrombolytic therapy. *Radiology* 1987; 163:753–758.
6. Lammer J, Pilger E, Neumayer K, et al: Intraarterial fibrinolysis: Long-term results. *Radiology* 1986; 161:159–163.
7. Morse MH, Jeans WD, Cole SEA, et al: Complications in percutaneous transluminal angioplasty: Relationships with patient age. *Br J Radiol* 1991; 64:5–9.
8. Henriksen LO, Jørgensen B, Holstein PE, et al: Percutaneous transluminal angioplasty of infrarenal arteries in intermittent claudication. *Acta Chir Scand* 1988; 154:573–576.

9. Hunink MGM, Donaldson MC, Meyerovitz MF, et al: Risks and benefits of femoropopliteal percutaneous balloon angioplasty. *J Vasc Surg* 1993; 17:183–194.

10. Johnston KW: Femoral and popliteal arteries: Reanalysis of results of balloon angioplasty. *Radiology* 1992; 183:767–771.

11. Capek P, McLean CK, Berkowitz IID: Femoropopliteal angioplasty: Factors influencing long-term success. *Circulation* 1991; 83(suppl I):I-70–I-80.

12. Belli AM, Cumberland DC, Knox AM, et al: The complication rate of percutaneous peripheral balloon angioplasty. *Clin Radiol* 1990; 41:380–383.

13. Wilson SE, Wolf GL, Cross AP, et al: Percutaneous transluminal angioplasty versus operation for peripheral arteriosclerosis. Report of a prospective randomized trial in a selected group of patients. *J Vasc Surg* 1989; 9:1–9.

14. Wolf GL, Wilson SE, Cross AP, et al: Surgery or balloon angioplasty for peripheral vascular disease: A randomized clinical trial. *J Vasc Interv Radiol* 1993; 4:639–648.

15. Jeans WD, Armstrong S, Cole SEA, et al: Fate of patients undergoing transluminal angioplasty for lower-limb ischemia. *Radiology* 1990; 177:559–564.

16. Hasson JE, Acher CW, Wojtowycz M, et al: Lower extremity percutaneous transluminal angioplasty: Multifactorial analysis of morbidity and mortality. *Surgery* 1990; 108:748–754.

17. Weibull H, Bergqvist D, Jonsson K, et al: Complications after percutaneous transluminal angioplasty in the iliac, femoral, and popliteal arteries. *J Vasc Surg* 1987; 5:681–686.

18. Walden R, Siegel Y, Rubinstein ZJ, et al: Percutaneous transluminal angioplasty. A suggested method for analysis of clinical, arteriographic, and hemodynamic factors affecting the results of treatment. *J Vasc Surg* 1986; 3:583–590.

19. Milford MA, Weaver FA, Lundell CJ, et al: Femoropopliteal percutaneous transluminal angioplasty for limb salvage. *J Vasc Surg* 1988; 8:292–299.

20. Jørgensen B, Henriksen LO, Karle A, et al: Percutaneous transluminal angioplasty of iliac and femoral arteries in severe lower-limb ischemia. *Acta Chir Scand* 1988; 154:647–652.

21. Jones BA, Maggisano R, Robb C, et al: Transluminal angioplasty: Results in high-risk patients with advanced peripheral vascular disease. *Can J Surg* 1985; 28:150–152.

22. Becker GJ, Katzen BT, Dake MD: Noncoronary angioplasty. *Radiology* 1989; 170:921–940.

23. Gardiner GA, Meyerovitz MF, Stokes KR, et al: Complications of transluminal angioplasty. *Radiology* 1986; 159:208–210.

24. McDermott JC, Crummy AB: Complications of angioplasty, in Kadir S (ed): *Current Practice of Interventional Radiology*. Philadelphia, BC Decker, 1991, pp 57–61.

25. Kadir S: Angioplasty of superficial femoral artery stenoses and occlusions, in Kadir S (ed): *Current Practice of Interventional Radiology*. Philadelphia, BC Decker, 1991, pp 311–319.

26. Sapoval MR, Long AL, Raynaud AC, et al: Femoropopliteal stent placement: Long-term results. *Radiology* 1992; 184:833–839.

27. Zollikofer CL, Antonucci F, Pfyffer M, et al: Arterial stent placement with use of the Wallstent: Midterm results of clinical experience. *Radiology* 1991; 179:449–456.

28. Strecker EP, Hagen B, Liermann D, et al: Iliac and femoropopliteal vascular occlusive disease treated with flexible tantalum stents. *Cardiovasc Intervent Radiol* 1993; 16:158–164.

29. Do-dai-Do, Triller J, Walpoth BH, et al: A comparison study of self-

expandable stents vs balloon angioplasty alone in femoropopliteal artery occlusions. *Cardiovasc Intervent Radiol* 1992; 15:306–312.

30. Fellmeth BD, Roberts AC, Bookstein JJ, et al: Postangiographic femoral artery injuries: Nonsurgical repair with US guided compression. *Radiology* 1991; 178:671.

31. Rutherford RB, Flanigan DP, Gupta SK, et al: Suggested standards for reports dealing with lower extremity ischaemia. Prepared by the Ad Hoc Committee on Reporting Standards, Society for Vascular Surgery/North American Chapter, International Society for Cardiovascular Surgery. *J Vasc Surg* 1986; 4:80–94.

32. Rutherford RB, Becker GJ: Standards for evaluating and reporting the results of surgical and percutaneous therapy for peripheral arterial disease. *Radiology* 1991; 181:277–281.

33. Creasy TS, McMillan PJ, Fletcher EWL, et al: Is percutaneous transluminal angioplasty better than exercise for claudication?—Preliminary results from a prospective randomised trial. *Eur J Vasc Surg* 1990; 4:135–140.

34. Adar R, Critchfield GC, Eddy DM: A confidence profile analysis of the results of femoropopliteal percutaneous transluminal angioplasty in the treatment of lower-extremity ischaemia. *J Vasc Surg* 1989; 10:57–67.

35. Hunink MGM, Wong JB, Donaldson MC, et al: Patency results of percutaneous and surgical femoropopliteal revascularization procedures. *Med Decis Making* 1994; 14:71-81.

36. Hunink MGM, Wong JB: Meta-analysis of failure time data with adjustment for covariates. *Med Dec Making* 1994; 14:59-70.

37. Gallino A, Mahler F, Probst P, et al: Percutaneous transluminal angioplasty of the arteries of the lower limbs: A 5-year follow-up. *Circulation* 1984; 70:619–623.

38. Krepel VM, Van Andel GJ, Van Erp WFM, et al: Percutaneous transluminal dilatation of the femoropopliteal artery: initial and long-term results. *Radiology* 1985; 156:325–328.

39. Samson RH, Sprayregen S, Veith FJ, et al: Management of angioplasty complications, unsuccessful procedures and early and late failures. *Ann Surg* 1984; 199:234–240.

40. Murray RR, Hewes RC, White RI, et al: Long-segment femoropopliteal stenoses: Is angioplasty a boon or a bust? *Radiology* 1987; 162:473–476.

41. Harris EK, Albert A: *Survivorship Analysis for Clinical Studies*, New York, Marcel Dekker, 1991.

42. Whittemore AD, Donaldson MC, Polak JF, et al: Limitations of balloon angioplasty for vein graft stenosis. *J Vasc Surg* 1991; 14:340–345.

43. Brown KT, Moore ED, Getrajdman GI, et al: Infrapopliteal angioplasty: long-term follow-up. *J Vasc Interv Radiol* 1993; 4:139–144.

44. Horvath W, Oertl M, Haidinger D: Percutaneous transluminal angioplasty of crural arteries. *Radiology* 1990; 177:565–569.

45. Flueckiger F, Lammer J, Klein GE, et al: Percutaneous transluminal angioplasty of crural arteries. *Acta Radiol (Stockh)* 1992; 33:152–155.

46. Schwarten DE: Clinical and anatomical considerations for nonoperative therapy in tibial disease and the results of angioplasty. *Circulation* 1991; 83(suppl I):I-86–I-90.

47. Saab MH, Smith DC, Aka PK, et al: Percutaneous transluminal angioplasty of tibial arteries for limb salvage. *Cardiovasc Intervent Radiol* 1992; 15:211–216.

48. Casarella WJ: Percutaneous transluminal angioplasty below the knee: New techniques, excellent results. *Radiology* 1988; 169:271–272.

49. Dorros G, Lewin RF, Jamnadas P, et al: Below-the-knee angioplasty: Tibio-

peroneal vessels, the acute outcome. *Cathet Cardiovasc Diagno* 1990; 19:170–178.

50. Bakal CW, Sprayregen S, Scheinbaum K, et al: Percutaneous transluminal angioplasty of the infrapopliteal arteries: Results in 53 patients. *AJR* 1990; 154:171–174.

51. Doubilet P, Abrams HL: The cost of underutilization: Percutaneous transluminal angioplasty for peripheral vascular disease. *N Engl J Med* 1984; 310:95–102.

52. Wolf GL, McLean G: Comparison of the costs of bypass surgery and transluminal angioplasty for peripheral vascular disease. *Semin Intervent Radiol* 1984; 1:237–239.

53. Kinnison ML, White RI, Bowers WP, et al: Cost incentives for peripheral angioplasty. *AJR* 1985; 145:1241–1244.

54. Jeans WD, Danton RM, Baird RN, et al: A comparison of the costs of vascular surgery and balloon dilatation in lower limb ischaemic disease. *Br J Radiol* 1986; 59:453–456.

55. Hunink MGM, Donaldson MC, Cullen KA: Hospital costs of revascularization procedures for femoropopliteal arterial disease. *J Vasc Surg* 1994; 19:632-641.

56. Gupta SK, Veith FJ, Ascer E, et al: Cost factors in limb-threatening ischaemia due to infrainguinal arteriosclerosis. *Eur J Vasc Surg* 1988; 2:151–154.

57. Gupta SK, Veith FJ: Inadequacy of the diagnosis related group (DRG) reimbursements for limb salvage lower extremity arterial reconstructions. *J Vasc Surg* 1990; 11:348–357.

58. Cheshire NJW, Wolfe JHN, Noone MA, et al: The economics of femorocrural reconstruction for critical leg ischemia with and without autologous vein. *J Vasc Surg* 1992; 15:167–175.

59. Consumer Price Indexes, Bureau of Labor Statistics, US Department of Labor, in *The World Almanac and Book of Facts* 1992. Hoffman MS (ed). New York, World Almanac, Pharos Books, 1991, p 150.

60. Coffman JD: Intermittent claudication—be conservative. *N Engl J Med* 1991; 325:577–578.

61. Hunink MGM, Meyerovitz MF: Letter to the editor in response to Tunis SR, Bass EB, Steinberg EP: The use of angioplasty, bypass surgery, and amputation in the management of peripheral vascular disease. *N Engl J Med* 1992; 326:414.

62. Becker GJ, Ferguson JG, Bakal CW, et al: Angioplasty, bypass surgery, and amputation for lower extremity peripheral arterial disease in Maryland: A closer look. *Radiology* 1993; 186:635–638.

Intravascular Stents and Stented Grafts in the Treatment of Infrainguinal Occlusive Disease*

Michael L. Marin, M.D.
Division of Vascular Surgery, Department of Surgery, Albert Einstein College of
Medicine of Yeshiva University, Montefiore Medical Center, Bronx, New York

Frank J. Veith, M.D.
Division of Vascular Surgery, Department of Surgery, Albert Einstein College of
Medicine of Yeshiva University, Montefiore Medical Center, Bronx, New York

A dvances in vascular surgery have had a significant impact on limb preservation in patients with severe lower extremity arterial occlusive disease. Major amputation rates have continued to decline with the broader application of arterial bypass techniques, particularly to distal infrapopliteal arteries.[1] Vascular reconstructions have also been combined with other interventional strategies to further expand the limits of therapy for infrainguinal limb ischemia. Catheter-based techniques, including balloon angioplasty and rotational and directional artherectomy, have all been evaluated as methods to improve the therapeutic outcome of patients with lower extremity arterial occlusive disease.[2–7]

Despite the effectiveness of arterial bypass in the treatment of limb threatening ischemia, surgical complications in these often debilitated patients remain a difficult problem. Virtually all patients who undergo therapy for limb salvage have one or more comorbid medical illnesses. Coexisting diabetes, hypertension, and hypercholesterolemia predispose to perioperative complications including myocardial and cerebrovascular events. General anesthetic risks coupled with less severe problems, including wound complications from vein harvest sites, all add to the complexity of care of peripheral vascular disease patients.[1]

Improving care, decreasing complications, and intelligent reduction in healthcare spending have fueled progress in vascular interventional techniques. This chapter discusses the potential of intravascular stents and stent-grafts for the treatment of atherosclerotic infrainguinal occlusive disease.

*Supported by grants from the U.S. Public Health Service (HL 02990-01), the James Hilton Manning and Emma Austin Manning Foundation, the Anna S. Brown Trust, and the New York Institute for Vascular Studies.

INTRAVASCULAR STENTS IN THE TREATMENT OF INFRAINGUINAL OCCLUSIVE DISEASE

The use of intravascular stents for the treatment of arterial disease developed as a product of Dotter's early work on arterial angioplasty.[8] This work launched several investigations into the development of a variety of vascular stent designs. Intravascular stents may be divided into three types: (1) balloon-expandable, (2) self-expanding, and (3) thermal-expanding. Each of these designs has advantages and limitations which center on deliverability, biocompatibility, and versatility.

BALLOON-EXPANDABLE STENTS

Two principal designs of balloon-expandable stents are commercially available for the treatment of occlusive vascular disease. The Strecker stent (Boston Scientific, Boston, Mass.) is a balloon-expandable stent composed of a single metallic tantalum wire 0.1–0.15 mm in diameter knitted in a series of loosely connected loops which have an elastic property. It is flexible in the longitudinal and radial directions, and because of its tantalum construction it is extremely radiopaque. For insertion into the vascular system, the device is attached to an angioplasty balloon by silicon sleeves at either end of the balloon. During balloon inflation there is a shortening of these sleeves in the longitudinal direction, which results in their retraction from the stent (Fig 1). After experimental testing, the broadest clinical evaluations of the Strecker stent have been in the treatment of iliac artery stenoses. Limited applications of this stent in the femoropopliteal arteries have been accomplished in Europe but have not demonstrated clear benefit. Early occlusions after stent placement in the

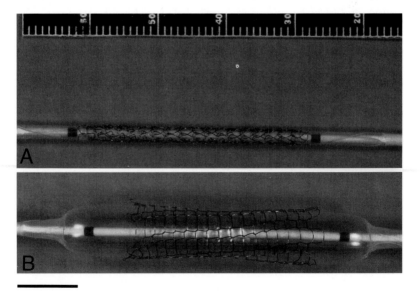

FIGURE 1.

The balloon-expandable Strecker stent. **A,** this tantalum wire stent is compressed onto a modified angioplasty balloon. **B,** following balloon inflation, the stent expands and conforms to the luminal surface of the artery.

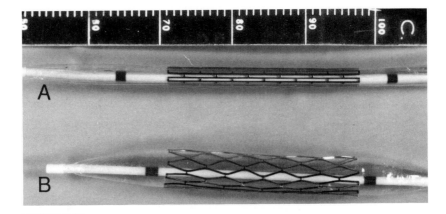

FIGURE 2.

The balloon-expandable Palmaz stent. This device is composed of a stainless steel tube which contains multiple rows of offset slots. For intravascular insertion it is mounted onto an angioplasty balloon (A). After balloon inflation (B), the steel framework of the stent deforms, permitting radial expansion.

superficial femoral system are frequent, and more work is needed prior to widespread clinical application.

Another balloon-expandable device is the Palmaz stent which has gained widest acceptance for the treatment of iliac angioplasty failure and recurrent iliac stenoses.[9] The Palmaz stent is constructed of stainless steel tubing which contains a variable number of slots arranged in offset rows. Inflation of the balloon causes a deformation of the malleable steel stent construction permitting the slot configuration to change to a diamond-shaped orientation (Fig 2). The newly formed wire mesh structure embeds into the wall of the artery, fixing the stent in position. Clinical trials have been conducted to evaluate these devices in the superficial femoral system.[10] Severely diseased inflow and outflow arteries frequently contribute to compromised blood flow through these stents when they are placed in the femoropopliteal arteries, resulting in a high rate of early occlusion. Thus the efficacy of balloon-expandable stenting in the femoral circulation has not as yet been confirmed.

SELF-EXPANDING STENTS

Self-expanding stents include those devices which are delivered to the site of disease in a compact form within a small-diameter introducer catheter. Once in appropriate position, the stent is released from the end of the catheter, allowing the stent to "spring" to a predetermined size. The Wallstent (Schneider, USA Inc., Minneapolis, Minn.) is a self-expanding device that has been used clinically since 1986. [11, 12] The Wallstent is composed of stainless steel wires which are woven into a criss-cross tubular pattern. The crossing points of the wires are not soldered to one another which allows the stent to self-expand and flex in the radial and longitudinal axes (Fig 3). The collapsed stent is introduced into the artery through a 5F to 9F catheter. Unconstrained stents vary from 3 to 10 cm in length. Clinical trials in the femoropopliteal system have had the same problems as balloon-expandable stents,[13] and have failed to dem-

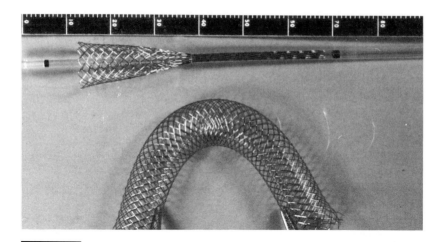

FIGURE 3.

The self-expanding Wallstent. Inside the introducer catheter, the Wallstent has a reduced profile *(solid arrow)*. When discharged from the introducer, the stent radially expands *(open arrow)*. The flexible construction of this stent permits acute bending without kinking *(curved arrow)*.

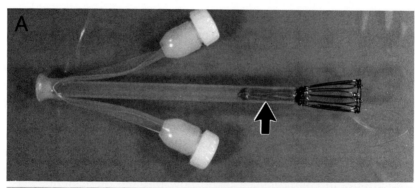

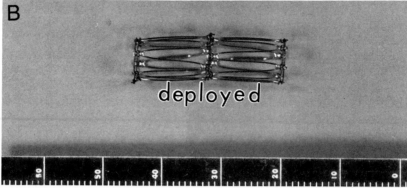

FIGURE 4.

The Gianturco wire stent. **A,** the Z-shaped bent-wire configuration permits this device to collapse into a small introducer catheter *(arrow)*, and also allows the stent to expand, exerting considerable radial force **(B).**

onstrate improved results with these devices when compared with standard balloon angioplasty techniques.[14]

Another important self-expanding stent device is the Gianturco wire stent (GWS) (Cook, Inc., Bloomington, Ind.), first used for malignant obstruction of the vena cava.[15] This stent is composed of stainless steel wire (0.45 mm in diameter) bent in a zigzag pattern (Fig 4). Several other stents have been developed recently, which appear to have been designed with a construction similar to the GWS, a device which produces sufficient radial force to secure the stent to the artery wall.[16, 17] When compressed, it can be introduced through a Teflon catheter measuring 8F to 12F. A coaxial pusher device expels the stent out of the catheter at the desired location. Although attempts to use this device in the infrainguinal location have been made, its use has been limited predominantly to larger vessels such as the vena cava. Currently, diameters between 15 and 40 mm are commercially available.

SHAPE MEMORY ALLOY STENTS (NITINOL)

The use of shape memory nitinol for stent design was first applied by Dotter et al.[18] and Cragg et al.[19] in animal investigations. Nitinol is a nickel-titanium alloy with unique thermal recovery properties. By annealing the metal at 500° C when it is constrained in a desired shape, it will "memorize" that shape. Cooling the wire in ice water transforms the alloy into a soft, easily deformed wire which can recall its "memorized" shape when warmed to its transition temperature (30–60° C). Once

NITINOL VASCULAR STENT

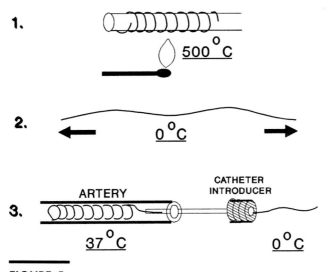

FIGURE 5.

Schematic drawing of the Nitinol Metal Memory Wire Vascular Stent. *(1.)* The wire is annealed at 500° C while snapped into a desired final coil configuration. *(2.)* The wire can then be cooled to 0° C at which time it may be deformed into any desired shape (straight for introduction into a Teflon catheter). *(3.)* After passing the cooled wire (0° C) through the introducer, it re-forms its original annealed shape (coil) within the warm (37° C) artery.

warmed, it will remain in its original annealed shape until it is recooled (Fig 5).

Marked intimal proliferation provoked by nitinol coils in iliac and femoral arteries of dogs has prevented broad clinical application of this device.[20] Recent work with a modified form of the nitinol alloy has improved the handling properties of the wire and appears to have decreased the extent of intimal proliferation seen in nitinol-stented vessels.[21] Clinical trials in the superficial femoral and popliteal arteries show some promise,[22] but additional improvements are needed.

COMBINATION STENT-GRAFTS IN THE TREATMENT OF INFRAINGUINAL OCCLUSIVE DISEASE

Intravascular stent and prosthetic graft technologies can be combined to form a minimally invasive, stented graft for endovascular arterial reconstruction. The conceptualization of the internal vascular bypass can be linked again to the work of Dotter[8] in the late 1960s when he proposed the possibility of creating an internal bypass graft fabricated from a vascular stent to treat aneurysms and traumatic arteriovenous fistulas. Further investigations in the 1980s defined the feasibility of using different graft and stent materials for endovascular bypasses.[18, 19, 23, 24] The first clinical trial using stent-graft technology was performed by Parodi and colleagues[25] in 1990 to repair an abdominal aortic aneurysm. Using a thin-walled Dacron graft and one or two modified Palmaz balloon-expandable stents, Parodi and his colleagues have been successful in excluding a variety of structurally different infrarenal aortic aneurysms with resulting thrombosis of the aneurysmal sac and a decrease in the overall size of the aneurysm.

At the Montefiore Medical Center Albert Einstein College of Medicine in New York, we have applied the concept of endoluminal bypass for the treatment of long-segment aortoiliac and femoropopliteal occlusive disease in limb-threatening ischemia.[26] Standard 6-mm and 5-mm polytetrafluoroethylene grafts are sutured to balloon-expandable Palmaz stents and mounted onto appropriately sized percutaneous transluminal angioplasty balloons. The stent-graft device is then inserted into a Teflon catheter which is used to deliver the stent-graft to the site of the arterial abnormality. With occluded femoropopliteal arteries, before placement of the stent-graft, the stenosed or occluded artery is predilated to 7 mm. These devices can be inserted percutaneously or by means of an arterial cutdown.[26, 27] Stents can be used to secure the proximal and distal portion of the graft, or, alternatively, one of the two ends of the graft can be directly anastomosed to the appropriate inflow or outflow artery at the site of insertion using standard suture anastomotic techniques.[26]

Preliminary results with endovascular femoropopliteal grafting by Cragg and Dake[27] By using a similar technique have been encouraging, demonstrating the feasibility of this technique. At our institution, we have successfully placed stented grafts to bridge long-segment femoropopliteal and aortoiliac occlusions to resolve severe limb-threatening ischemia and gangrene (Fig 6). Extension of these grafts to the below-

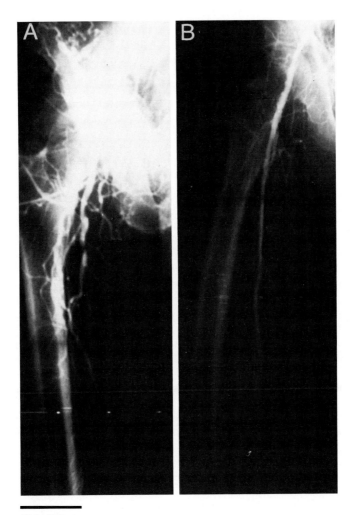

FIGURE 6.

A, preoperative arteriogram of a patient with a long segment occlusion of the superficial femoral artery (SFA) from its origin. **B,** following balloon angioplasty of the entire diseased segment, a polytetrafluoroethylene graft was endoluminally inserted creating a new flow surface within the SFA. A completion arteriogram demonstrates restored vascular continuity between the common femoral and the above-knee popliteal artery.

knee popliteal artery is also feasible. Successful treatment of a popliteal artery aneurysm using a stent-graft has also been accomplished by our group.[28] Additional developments in graft, stent, and introducer materials will undoubtedly expand the potential value of this minimally invasive technique. However, the durability of these procedures in comparison to standard bypass surgery must be established prior to wider use of these techniques.

REFERENCES

1. Veith FJ, Gupta SK, Wengerter KR, et al: Changing arteriosclerotic disease patterns and management strategies in lower-limb-threatening ischemia. *Ann Surg* 1990; 212:402–414.

2. Capek P, McLean GK, Berkowitz HD: Femoropopliteal angioplasty: Factors influencing long-term success. *Circulation* 1991; 83:170–180.

3. Johnston KW: Femoral and popliteal arteries: Reanalysis of results of balloon angioplasty. *Radiology* 1992; 183:767–771.

4. Vroegindeweij D, Kemper FJM, Tielbeek AV, et al: Recurrence of stenoses following balloon angioplasty and Simpson atherectomy of the femoro-popliteal segment. A randomised comparative 1-year follow-up study using colour flow duplex. *Eur J Vasc Surg* 1992; 6:164–171.

5. Perler BA, Osterman FA, White RI, Jr, et al: Percutaneous laser probe femoro-popliteal angioplasty: A preliminary experience. *J Vasc Surg* 1989; 10:351–357.

6. Lammer J, Pilger E, Karnel F, et al: Laser angioplasty: Results of a prospective, multicenter study at 3-year follow-up. *Radiology* 1991; 178:335–337.

7. Ahn S, Eton D, Yeatman LR, et al: Intraoperative peripheral rotary atherectomy: Early and late clinical results. *Ann Vasc Surg* 1992; 6:272–280.

8. Dotter CT: Transluminally-placed coilspring endarterial tube grafts: Long-term patency in canine popliteal artery. *Invest Radiol* 1969; 4:329–332.

9. Palmaz JC, Garcia O, Schatz RA, et al: Placement of balloon expandable intraluminal stents in iliac arteries: First 171 procedures. *Radiology* 1990; 174:969–975.

10. Henry M, Beron R, Chastel A: Endoprosthèsis vasculaires de Palmaz: Résultats préliminaires. *Presse Med* 1990; 19:1401–1402.

11. Joffre F, Puel J, Imbert C, et al: Use of a new type of self-expanding vascular stent prosthesis: Early clinical results. Presented at the 72nd Scientific Assembly of the Radiological Society of North America. Chicago, Nov 30, 1986.

12. Sigwart U, Puel J, Mirkovitch V, et al: Intravascular stents to prevent occlusion and restenosis after transluminal angioplasty. *N Engl J Med* 1987; 316:701–706.

13. Sapoval MR, Long AL, Ranaud AC, et al: Femoropopliteal stent placement: Long term results. *Radiology* 1992; 184:833–839.

14. Do D-D, Triller J, Walpoth BH, et al: A comparison study of self-expandable stents vs. balloon angioplasty alone in femoropopliteal artery occlusions. *Cardiovasc Intervent Radiol* 1992; 15:306–312.

15. Rösch J, Bedell JE, Putman J, et al: Gianturco expandable wire stents in the treatment of superior vena cava syndrome recurring after maximum-tolerance radiation. *Cancer* 1987; 60:1243–1246.

16. Chuter TAM, Green RM, Ouriel K, et al: Transfemoral endovascular aortic graft placement. *J Vasc Surg* 1993; 18:185–197.

17. Lazarus HM: Intraluminal graft device: System and method. US Patent (4,787,899 May 5, 1988).

18. Dotter CT, Buschmann RW, McKinney MK: Transluminal expandable nitinol coil stent grafting: Preliminary report. *Radiology* 1983; 147:259–260.

19. Cragg A, Lund G, Rysavy J, et al: Nonsurgical placement of arterial endoprostheses: A new technique using nitinol wire. *Radiology* 1983; 147:261–263.

20. Mass D, Demierre D, Deaton D, et al: Transluminal implantation of self-adjusting expandable prosthesis: Principles, techniques and results. *Prog Artif Org* 1983; 979–987.

21. Rabkin I, Novikova EG, Pronin AG, et al: Seven years experience with Rabkin technology Nitinol prostheses for vessels after balloon, laser, and rotor recanalization. *Med Radiol (MOSK)* 1991; 36:35-38.

22. Henry M, Rafael B: Initial clinical experience with the in stent Nitinol permanent and temporary stents. *Circulation* 1993; 88:I-586.

23. Balko A, Piasecki GJ, Shah DM, et al: Transfemoral placement of intralumi-

nal polyurethane prosthesis for abdominal aneurysm. *J Surg Res* 1986; 40:305–309.

24. Mirich D, Wright KC, Wallace S, et al: Percutaneously placed endovascular grafts for aortic aneurysms: Feasibility study. *Radiology* 1989; 170:1033.

25. Parodi JC, Palmaz JC, Baroné HD: Transfemoral intraluminal graft implantation for abdominal aortic aneurysms. *Ann Vasc Surg* 1991; 5:491–499.

26. Marin ML, Veith FJ, Panetta TF, et al: Transfemoral stented graft treatment of occlusive arterial disease for limb salvage: A preliminary report (abstract). American Heart Association 66th Annual Scientific Session, Nov 8–11, 1993.

27. Cragg AH, Dake MD: Percutaneous femoropopliteal graft placement. *Radiology* 1993; 187:643–648.

28. Marin ML, Veith FJ, Panetta TF: Transfemoral endoluminal stented graft repair of a popliteal artery aneurysm. *J Vasc Surg* 1994;19:754–757.

PART IV

Miscellaneous

Carotid Restenosis

Hugh A. Gelabert, M.D.
Assistant Professor of Surgery, Section of Vascular Surgery, University of California, Los Angeles, UCLA School of Medicine, Los Angeles, California

Wesley S. Moore, M.D.
Professor of Surgery, Chief, Section of Vascular Surgery, University of California, Los Angeles, UCLA School of Medicine, Los Angeles, California

---

T he recurrence of arterial stenosis following carotid endarterectomy is an infrequent but not uncommon event. While the implication of such a recurrence is still the substance of debate in the surgical literature, most surgeons clearly appreciate this event as a compromise of the original operation. The development of recurrent lesions suggests the return of some risk which the original endarterectomy was designed to avoid.

Recurrent carotid stenosis may be the result of a variety of lesions, principally including intimal hyperplasia or atherosclerosis. These recurrences may present either with or without symptoms, and their behavior usually is strikingly distinct according to the type of lesion involved. This difference in behavior accounts for the variety of management strategies proposed for these lesions. The most important areas of concern revolve about classification of the lesions and the criteria for intervention. Despite our recognition and study of these lesions during the past two decades, a clear appreciation of the natural history of the recurrent stenosis has only recently become available. From this, a rational approach toward evaluating the risk-benefit equation with regard to intervention or observation is beginning to take form.

The goals for vascular surgeons in confronting recurrent carotid stenosis are to understand how to prevent, how to identify, and how to effectively manage these problems. This understanding should be based on a clear definition of the natural history of the recurrent stenosis as well as the risk that the lesions present. Finally, insight into the pathophysiology and pathologic potential of these lesions allows an informed decision to be formulated regarding optimal management.

DEFINITIONS

Recurrent carotid stenosis may be defined by any one of a number of methods: anatomic, pathologic, and histologic. Anatomically, these lesions are identified as the reappearance of an intraluminal obstruction where an endarterectomy has been performed. While the recurrence of any intraluminal obstruction following a carotid surgical procedure is

Advances in Vascular Surgery, vol. 2
© 1994, Mosby–Year Book, Inc.

suggested by the name recurrent carotid stenosis, the term is reserved for a more specific use. As commonly used, recurrent carotid stenosis refers to those lesions which occur at the site of the endarterectomy and are consistent with the development of intimal hyperplasia or a recurrent atherosclerotic lesion. Implicit in this definition is the concept that a true recurrence develops over a period of time, that the growth of these lesions represents the consequence of a biologic process, and that the lesions develop following endarterectomy. The development of the recurrent lesion suggests rates of cell division and matrix deposition above the growth rates of the normal arterial wall. This is different from an early postoperative occlusion or residual stenosis which results from a technically inadequate operation.

Residual atherosclerotic plaque following inadequate endarterectomy is not considered a recurrent lesion. Such obstructions have come to be considered a persistence of the original lesion, usually reflecting the result of an inadequate surgical procedure. In a similar instance, most authors would not consider a residual common carotid plaque as a true recurrence. Finally, carotid artery thrombosis in the early postoperative period is not considered a recurrent stenosis. Such occlusions are likely related to technical difficulties with the endarterectomy and are not the result of fibrous plaque growth.

Implicit in the differentiation of a recurrent stenosis from a residual plaque is the concept of validation of the original endarterectomy and documentation of progression of the recurrent lesion. Validation of the immediate postoperative surgical result is accomplished either by arteriography or duplex scanning. It is important that studies obtained in the postoperative period be completed within the first 6 to 12 weeks following surgery; later studies may not be able to distinguish recurrent stenosis from persistent lesions because recurrent lesions may demonstrate rapid growth in this period. Progression of the lesion is most often demonstrated by the use of sequential postoperative duplex scanning.

Pathologically, the recurrent stenosis may be any one of several distinct lesions which accumulate within the carotid lumen following endarterectomy. Ultimately, these reduce to either intimal hyperplasia or recurrent atherosclerotic plaque. The gross pathologic examination of a recurrent carotid stenosis caused by intimal hyperplasia will identify the lesion as a firm, fibrous mass of tissue which partially or completely obstructs the carotid lumen. Histologically, the ultrastructure of hyperplastic lesions appears as collections of fibroblasts and matrix material beneath the intimal surface.[1-3] Atherosclerotic recurrences appear grossly and histologically as a typical atherosclerotic plaque: irregular surface, ulceration and pitting, hard calcific plaque, cholesterol deposits, and foam cells.[4]

DETECTION

The most common means for detection of recurrent carotid stenosis is the duplex scan. Alternatively, arteriography is considered the most reliable method of documenting an intraluminal obstruction of the carotid artery. Both of these techniques play complementary roles in defining the nature and pathologic potential of recurrent carotid stenosis.

DUPLEX SCAN

The duplex scan is a combination of two-dimensional B-mode ultrasonic imaging and Doppler analysis of blood flow velocity and turbulence. Lesions are identified on the basis of both the altered image of the artery as well as the corresponding alteration of the blood flow velocity. Blood flow alterations that serve to recognize recurrent stenosis include changes in flow velocity and the development of turbulent flow. The accuracy and sensitivity of duplex technology has been reported to be in the 90% to 95% range.[5] Additional information which may be obtained from a duplex scan includes B-mode imaging of plaque morphology, location, and composition.[1, 3, 6]

Because of availability and safety, duplex scanning has become the most common means of identifying and categorizing recurrent carotid lesions. Of particular importance are the criteria employed in identifying the recurrent lesions. The most reliably established classification of arterial stenosis based on Doppler criteria is that which identifies four principal categories of arterial stenosis: reductions in diameter of 0% to 19%, 20% to 59%, 60% to 79%, 80% to 99%, and occlusion.[7] The most reliable data from such duplex studies would be those that indicate a change from one category to another. Accordingly, a recurrent stenosis would be identified when a patient's scan indicates the presence of at least a 20% to 59% stenosis. Such low-grade stenoses present several problems. Identification may be inaccurate, their clinical significance is uncertain, and they are not hemodynamically significant. By consensus, only hemodynamically significant lesions are considered recurrent stenosis. While some authors may report lower-grade stenosis, the principal clinical concern is with more significant lesions. Accordingly, most authors have adopted the standard of defining a recurrence stenosis as one which causes more than a 50% reduction of arterial diameter.

A frequent use of duplex scanning is to detect progression of a given lesion. This is usually accomplished by periodically scanning a patient's arteries for signs of hemodynamic changes in carotid blood flow. The most common criterion employed in identifying progression of a plaque is increase in severity of the stenosis from one duplex category to another. Failure to advance in such a manner cannot reliably be considered progression. Important observations which should be made along with the recognition of increase in severity of the stenosis include the rate of progression of a stenosis and the period of time from the original operation. These observations may serve to provide insight into the nature of the plaque and hence into its pathologic potential.

In addition to detection of plaques and documentation of plaque growth, duplex scanning affords an opportunity to characterize the structure and constitution of the recurrent stenosis. Since different plaque constituents have differing ultrasonic signatures, these components may be generally distinguished on the basis of the B-mode images. The principal plaque characteristics which are recorded include heterogeneity, irregularity, and degree of calcification of the plaque. Some vascular laboratories have been able to identify important plaque features such as ulcerations, O'Donnell and associates[1] were able to identify four plaque ulcers and four intraplaque hemorrhages in a series of 26 recurrences. While promising, the reliability of this endeavor has not been widely reproduced. These characteristics suggest the nature of the recurrence: myointimal hyperplasia, recurrent atherosclerosis, or degenerating plaque with intraplaque hemorrhage.

RESIDUAL VS. RECURRENT DISEASE

The identification of any intraluminal lesion following carotid endarterectomy was once considered an indication of recurrence. While this is true generally, an important distinction should be made between recurrent stenosis and persistence of an intraluminal plaque. Persistent lesions are frequently the result of inadequate primary endarterectomy. These lesions represent a separate clinical and pathologic entity and should not be confused with recurrent stenosis. The recognition of persistent lesions has led to the realization that, in order to truly account for recurrent stenosis, some form of evaluation of the completed endarterectomy is necessary. This may include either an intraoperative completion arteriogram or an intraoperative completion duplex scan. Alternatively, these studies may be obtained in the early postoperative period.

The importance of a completion study is underscored by a report of the occurrence of late carotid restenosis presented by Bandyk and colleagues.[8] They noted that the incidence of restenosis following a normal completion study was 0%. When the completion study demonstrated an intraluminal defect, the incidence of significant restenosis rose to 21% at 2 years.[8] A similar phenomenon may explain the remarkably high incidence of severe recurrent stenosis reported by Ricotta and associates.[9] They identified 39 patients with late restenosis causing lumen reduction greater than 80%. The authors note that criteria for definition of recurrent and residual disease play a significant role in determining the subsequent fate of a late restenosis. Finally Hansen and colleagues[10] reported four postoperative carotid occlusions in a group of 232 patients. These occurred within 6 months of surgery. Three of the four occurred in the presence of a residual lesion. In a recent report from UCLA, it was noted that the incidence of postoperative neurologic symptoms was higher in patients who did not have completion arteriograms.[11] In a review of 268 carotid operations, the authors noted that neurologic events occurred in 5% of patients who did not have completion studies, whereas similar events occurred in only 2% of patients who did have completion arteriography.

A question which these studies present regards the significance of their results. How much disease detected on completion arteriography is sufficient to require reoperation? The same question arises with respect to defects identified on duplex scan. Interestingly, the answer to these questions is not well established. The criteria for intervention appear to be slightly different according to which study is used. Most lesions identified by completion arteriography require correction. Between one fourth and one half of defects identified by intraoperative duplex scan are corrected.[12]

In summary, duplex scanning offers a sensitive, convenient, and specific method of identifying recurrent carotid lesions. The duplex definition of recurrent lesions is based on ultrasonic detection of hemodynamic aberrations in the flow of blood through the carotid bifurcation. The initial postoperative duplex scan should be performed in order to document the adequacy of the endarterectomy. Later duplex scans may document the occurrence and progression of recurrent lesions. The B-mode characteristics provide insight into the composition of the recurrent plaque. Finally, the time between the original operation and the identification of the recurrence may provide insight into the pathologic nature of the lesion.

ARTERIOGRAPHY

Arteriography remains the gold standard against which all vascular imaging techniques are compared.[13] Because of its invasive nature and the potential for complications, postoperative arteriography is usually reserved for instances in which confirmation of a suspected lesion is required in planning reintervention. The value of arteriography is the detailed anatomic information which these studies provide. Arteriograms are the most accurate means of assessing the extent and severity of carotid lesions.

The role of arteriography in the management of recurrent carotid stenosis centers around the documentation of an adequate endarterectomy and the definition of a recurrent stenosis. Documentation of the success of the original operation may be achieved by either a completion intraoperative arteriogram or an early postoperative study. While some surgeons use intraoperative completion arteriography as a routine component of their surgical procedure, it has not been universally adopted. Alternatively, intraoperative duplex scanning has become a popular tool, frequently used in place of an intraoperative arteriogram. The advantage of intraoperative studies is the ability to correct any identified lesions before completion of the operation. Regardless of which study is used (arteriogram or duplex), a normal completion study is the most accurate assessment of technical success.

Early postoperative angiographic studies are used by some surgeons in place of completion arteriography.[14] The goal of such studies is to document the success of the operation. Additionally, a significant residual lesion may be identified and corrective action undertaken. The principal advantage of an early postoperative arteriogram is the ability to assess the patency of the arteries following surgery. The principal drawback is the invasive nature of this test. It requires the administration of radiopaque material by means of either an intravenous or an intraarterial canula. Postoperative arteriography is less convenient than noninvasive assessment and thus is not as frequently employed. Finally, as with any postoperative study, the possibility of returning a patient to the operating room because of a technically inadequate operation presents a significant problem.

A second role of arteriography in the management of recurrence stenosis is in the late evaluation of a suspected lesion. Arteriography is indicated in patients who develop postoperative neurologic symptoms, both to evaluate potential sources of the symptoms and to plan reoperation. In instances where a duplex scan suggests a recurrent stenosis, arteriography serves to confirm the suspected lesion. Because it is able to provide more exact anatomic detail than duplex scanning and is not so operator-dependent, arteriography is considered necessary in planning reoperative carotid procedures. It provides information regarding not only the extent and location of the recurrent plaque but will also inform the surgeon of anatomic variants which must be considered.

If a recurrent lesion is identified, arteriography may provide insight into the nature of such a lesion by suggesting possible origins of the new stenosis. The key radiologic feature is the location of the lesion with regard to the position of the original plaque. If the new lesion is located in the common carotid at the site of the proximal endpoint, then it may represent progression of the proximal carotid plaque rather than a true recurrence. Similarly, if the new lesion is located at the site of arterial clamping, then it may be related to a clamp injury to the normal artery. If the lesion is located at the bifurcation or the proximal internal carotid precisely where the endarterectomy occurred, then it may be a recurrence.

It should be noted that arteriographic identification of a lesion's genesis is based on deduction. Since the arteriographic silhouette of a hyperplastic recurrence may be identical to that of an atheromatous plaque, these cannot be reliably differentiated by contrast arteriography alone. Such distinctions must then be based on clinical data such as the suspected age of the lesion as well as its location.

In summary, completion arteriography is recommended as a routine measure to ensure an adequate operation as well as to allow correction of any residual lesions prior to completion of the original surgery. It serves both to clearly establish the technical success of the operation and to prevent reoperation for technical inadequacies. Late arteriographic studies are most often reserved for preoperative assessment of a suspected lesion and planning corrective intervention.

PATHOLOGY

The two principal pathologic entities involved in the development of recurrent carotid stenosis are myointimal hyperplasia and recurrent atherosclerosis.[4] Other causes of recurrent stenosis and recurrent neurologic symptoms include aneurysmal degeneration of the artery operated on, intraluminal thrombus, and extrinsic compression of the artery by surrounding scar. Of these, intimal hyperplasia and recurrent atherosclerosis are by far the most common.

INTIMAL HYPERPLASIA

Intimal hyperplasia is a proliferative lesion which consists primarily of myofibroblasts and matrix material. The lesions are thought to develop as a consequence of activation, migration, and replication of myocytes of the arterial wall. Presumably, the myocytes of the medial layers of the arterial wall exist in a quiescent state in the intact artery. This state is maintained by the interaction of the medial cells and the endothelial surface of the vessel. In the event of a disruption in the arterial wall, the endothelial surface is removed and the medical cells are stimulated by exposure and interaction with components of the blood as well as disinhibited by loss of endothelial contact. These myocytes then begin to replicate and migrate. As they do so, they dedifferentiate into polymorphous myofibroblasts. These cells are able to synthesize the collagenous matrix material which forms the background substance of the hyperplastic lesion. As the endothelial cells resurface the injured arterial wall, the dedifferentiated myofibroblasts will continue to proliferate and generate matrix. Cessation of these activities appears to vary between individuals, and the mechanisms which govern this process are not well understood. Some lesions progress to obliteration of the arterial lumen, while others progress to a given point and then become quiescent. Finally, some lesions may even regress with time. What determines which course the hyperplastic lesion will take is unknown.

The clinical effects of recurrent stenosis secondary to hyperplastic lesions are as varied as the courses of the lesions themselves. Hyperplastic lesions contrast sharply with primary or recurrent atherosclerotic lesions in their reduced potential for thromboembolization and plaque degeneration. The hyperplastic lesions are densely fibrous and homogeneous. Their surface is smooth and covered by endothelium. Thus these lesions do not afford the medium upon which surface thrombosis and thromboembolic phenomena may develop. The homogeneity and fibrous nature of hyperplastic lesions result in a dense, firm lesion which is not subject to the degenerative forces which operate upon atherosclerotic plaques. Accordingly, hyperplastic lesions do not develop intraplaque hemorrhages or ulceration as occurs with atherosclerotic plaques. This again reduces the pathologic potential of hyperplastic lesions.

ATHEROSCLEROSIS

Recurrent atherosclerotic lesions are thought to possess all of the thrombotic, embolic, and degenerative properties of primary atherosclerotic plaques. While genesis of these lesions is not well appreciated, one school of thought holds that recurrent carotid atherosclerotic plaques develop from precedent hyperplastic lesions. An alternative viewpoint is that recurrent atherosclerotic lesions develop in a manner similar to primary lesions: from an intact endothelium and a "normal" arterial wall. In either scenario, the remarkable fact of these recurrent atherosclerotic plaques is the time frame of their development. Most of these lesions develop within 3 to 7 years following the primary carotid endarterectomy. Typically, any recurrent carotid stenosis which is identified at a point beyond the initial 2 years after endarterectomy probably represents an atherosclerotic lesion.[4] Recurrent atherosclerotic plaques appear to demonstrate all of the characteristics of primary atherosclerotic lesions. Plaque degeneration, loss of endothelial cell function, genesis of atheroemboli, plaque ulceration, and intraplaque hemorrhage all appear to be properties of recurrent atherosclerotic lesions.

Atherosclerotic plaques demonstrate several distinct stages of growth and degeneration. These have been characterized as the early plaque, the mature plaque, and the senescent or degenerative plaque. As a plaque develops and matures, the accumulation of cholesterol and foam cells is followed by calcification of the plaque matrix and degeneration of the plaque itself. Plaque degeneration is thought to be the source of most cerebrovascular symptoms. The degenerative process involves two principal mechanisms: plaque erosion and intraplaque hemorrhage.

Plaque erosion occurs as a result of denudation of the overlying endothelial surface with exposure of the plaque substance to the flowing blood. This event triggers the accumulation of platelets and fibrin on the arterial wall. Once these aggregates achieve a critical size, they are dislodged by the flowing blood and become emboli. In instances where the plaque is composed of soft, heterogeneous material, the flowing blood may erode particles of the plaque itself leaving a residual plaque ulcer. Should this occur, then plaque emboli may generate cerebrovascular symptoms. As erosion of the plaque progresses, the excavated area provides a cul-de-sac in which larger platelet and fibrin aggregations may form. Thus, larger ulcers are more likely to cause symptoms than smaller ulcers both because more plaque material has been excavated and because the larger ulcer provides space for larger thrombi to form.

Intraplaque hemorrhage is thought to be an important mechanism by which plaques may rapidly enlarge and produce symptoms. The essential elements of intraplaque hemorrhage are thought to include necrosis of a portion of the plaque, loss of integrity of the vasa vasorum of the plaque, and bleeding into the plaque. The bleeding leads to rapid expansion of the plaque with concomitant loss of arterial lumen. Additionally, because of the rapid expansion of the underlying hematoma, the plaque may fracture. Plaque fracture leads to a break in the endothelial surface overlying the plaque and exposure of the plaque hematoma to the bloodstream. The factors which govern the occurrence of intraplaque hemorrhage are not well established. While antiplatelet agents such as aspirin have been thought to present a slightly increased risk of such events, this has not been conclusively established.

ETIOLOGY

A single cause of recurrent carotid stenosis has not been established. Despite the intense study of recurrent arterial stenosis over the course of the past two decades, most of the information that is available suggests several possible causes, but no single factor seems to be sufficient to explain these lesions. Like primary atherosclerosis, these lesions are probably the result of interaction of multiple factors which eventually channel through several pathways toward a common response to arterial injury.

Several risk factors have been associated with recurrent carotid stenosis. These include consumption of tobacco products, sex, age, size of arteries, hyperlipidemia, diabetes, and severe systemic atherosclerosis.[8, 9, 12, 15-18] These risk factors have been identified on the basis of clinical surgical series which detail the recurrence of carotid lesions and correlate the recurrent lesions with the clinical characteristics of the patients. The same risk factors associated with the development of atherosclerosis are also implicated in recurrent stenosis: hypertension, diabetes, lipid abnormalities, and use of tobacco. Arterial size and sex have also been identified as significant elements in recurrent stenosis. These latter two appear to be related factors: women tend to have small arteries. A final factor which must be taken into account is the adequacy of the endarterectomy: residual plaque predisposes to occlusion and progressive stenosis.

THEORIES OF ORIGIN

Several theories have been proposed to explain recurrent carotid stenosis, and they may be classified into several broad categories: the hemodynamic theories, the inflammatory cell theories, the peptide growth-stimulant theories, and the disinhibition theories.

The initiating event in the development of intimal hyperplasia in all instances appears to be some form of arterial injury. Following carotid endarterectomy, several injury mechanisms operate simultaneously: denudation, shear force, compression, and stretching of the arterial wall. The normal response to injury is the development of an inflammatory response with infiltration of inflammatory cells and cellular elements. The ultimate response to injury is the proliferation of fibroblasts and deposition of fibrous material. This culminates in the repair of injured structures by deposition of scar tissue. Thus viewed, both atherosclerosis and intimal hyperplasia may be variants of the normal repair mechanism as expressed in the arterial wall. Of note is the fact that while most wound healing and scar remodeling occur over a period of 6 months, hyperplastic lesions may progress over the course of years. This has led some to consider an ongoing stimulus for the progressive and sustained development of the hyperplastic lesions.

The inflammatory cell theory suggests that the development of the hyperplastic recurrent lesions is principally caused by the attraction and infiltration of inflammatory cells to the endarterectomy site. This attraction is mediated through a number of proposed mechanisms, including the release of cytokines from the denuded arterial wall, or from adherent platelets and leukocytes. The cytokines in turn attract inflammatory cells, such as the monocytes and polymorphonuclear leukocytes which are the mediators of inflammation. Once in the vicinity of the denuded artery, these inflammatory cells migrate into the subintima and media. There, they begin to undergo a series of alterations which result in both liberation of cytotoxic materials as well as the release of more cytokines. In combination, these events lead to the genesis of a new class of cells: the pluripotential mesenchymal cells of the arterial wall. While much debate has focused on the origin of these cells, they are considered likely to be derivatives of the smooth muscle cells of the arterial media. These cells become the myofibroblasts which migrate into the subintima and generate the matrix material which is characteristic of hyperplastic lesions.

A variant of the inflammatory cell theory, the peptide growth-stimulant theory, suggests that many of the cellular events which give rise to hyperplastic lesions are mediated by locally generated peptide growth factors.[17] Several peptide growth factors have been demonstrated to have a mitogenic effect on the smooth muscle cells of the arterial wall. Specific growth factors which have been implicated include platelet-derived growth factor (PDGF), monocyte-derived growth factor (MDGF), endothelial-derived growth factor (EDGF), and fibroblast-derived growth factor (FGF). Which of these growth factors are primarily implicated and which are innocent bystanders is not clearly established. The mechanisms regulating the production of the growth factors themselves also are unclear. Some are thought to be liberated as the consequence of platelet adhesion and activation. Others are thought to be expressed as constitutive elements of the arterial wall. The final effects of the growth factors are similar to those of the inflammatory cellular infiltration: the genesis of the myofibroblasts and the production of extracellular matrix resulting in hyperplastic lesions.

One characteristic of hyperplastic lesions is the apparent loss of normal regulation of cellular growth. In this regard, hyperplastic lesions resemble low-grade malignant lesions: the loss of contact inhibition, uncontrolled proliferation, and unregulated production of cellular materials. Based on these observations, another etiologic theory suggests that intimal hyperplasia is the result of loss of inhibition of the normal growth of the cells of the arterial wall. In this theory, loss of inhibition of growth afforded by the intact arterial wall results in the loss of differentiation and uncontrolled proliferation of medial smooth muscle cells. Cell culture experiments have demonstrated that there is interaction between the endothelium and the medial myofibroblasts. There is evidence that the endothelial cells exert an inhibitory effect and thus stabilize the growth of the medial cells. When the endothelium is denuded, then the medial cells migrate, replicate, and elaborate matrix.

Hemodynamic theories of recurrent stenosis suggest that the hyperplastic lesions form as a response to the turbulence and shear stress exerted by the bloodstream at the carotid bifurcation.[18] Specific hemodynamic factors that have been implicated include the volume of blood flow, the shear stress generated by such flow, the exposure of local baroreceptors to altered tension, and the turbulence generated at the bifurcation of the carotid. On a cellular level, there is evidence that endothelial cells respond to a variety of physical stimuli, and that these stimuli will alter their growth pattern as well as the phenotypic characteristics of the cells themselves. According to the hemodynamic theory of recurrent stenosis, the recurrence is the consequence of alterations in such factors as shear stress and tangential pressure on the cellular constituents of the arterial wall. This in turn accelerates the division, growth, and proliferation of cellular components in order to restore the more stable, less compliant environment of the intact arterial wall. One appealing feature of this theory is its ability to explain both the predilection of the primary atherosclerotic plaque and the recurrent hyperplastic lesion for the carotid bifurcation.

Regardless of which etiologic theory is invoked, several events are common to both hyperplastic as well as atherosclerotic lesions: proliferation of undifferentiated cells, migration of the myofibroblasts into the subintima, and elaboration and deposition of a fibrous matrix material. In the atherosclerotic variant, the matrix becomes calcified over the course of time. It has been proposed that hyperplastic lesions are accelerated precursors of atherosclerotic lesions, and that the latter derive from the former as a consequence of time and calcification. Whether these two distinctive lesions are related in such a manner remains unclear. Ultimately, they differ significantly with respect to several characteristics. Of particular importance, their long-term growth and symptomatic potential separates both lesions into two distinct clinical entities.

NATURAL HISTORY

The natural history of a recurrent carotid lesion is the clinical expression of the morphologic and pathologic changes to which it is subjected over the course of time. These changes are determined, in large part, by the lesion's constituent elements as well as the interplay between these elements and their host environment. Intimal hyperplastic lesions and recurrent atherosclerotic lesions display remarkably different natural histories. This is thought to reflect the differences in the constitution of these two lesions. Additionally, these differences in composition lead to dif-

TABLE 1.

Incident of Recurrent Stenosis, and Symptomatic Recurrence in Selected Cases Reported Over the Past Decade

Authors	Year	No. of Cases	Mean Follow-up (mos)	Recurrent Stenosis* (%)	Symptomatic Recurrence* (%)
Baker et al.[30]	1983	133	20	11.0	2.0
Salvian et al.[31]	1983	105	28	7.0	5.0
O'Donnell et al.[1]	1985	276	38	11.0	2.0
Das et al.[21]	1985	1,726	42	1.8	1.8
Nichols et al.[19]	1985	145	18	17.0	2.0
Hertzer et al.[23]	1987	917	21	31.0	—
Sanders et al.[2]	1987	109	24	8.0	—
Eikelboom et al.[24]	1988	129	12	11.0	—
Healey et al.[20]	1989	301	48	21.0	—
Bertin et al.[32]	1989	155	18	8.3.0	—
Clagett et al.[15]	1989	152	22	12.9	—
Salenius et al.[25]	1989	257	77	13.0	—
Reilly et al.[12]	1990	131	15	18.0	—
Mattos et al.[16]	1993	409	42	10.8	2.4
Hansen et al.[10]	1993	232	6	9.2	0.9
Gelabert et al.[11]	1994	268	18	11.0	0

*Note that recurrences include hemodynamically significant recurrences (whenever possible).

ferent interactions between the lesions and their host environment, the blood (Table 1).

INTIMAL HYPERPLASIA

Hyperplastic lesions are principally composed of fibrous tissue: myofibroblasts and their collagenous extracellular matrix. These elements are remarkably stable. The lesions are surfaced by an intact endothelium which effectively separates the lesion from the overlying blood. Phenotypically, the endothelial surface appears to maintain the critical antithrombotic properties of normal endothelium and thus does not appear to be as thrombogenic as the exposed arterial media would be. A remarkable property of the hyperplastic lesion appears to be its ability to sustain near-occlusive growth without exceeding its nutrient supply. Additionally, the tensile strength of hyperplastic lesions appears to be more uniform and homogeneous than is the case in an atherosclerotic plaque. Thus hyperplastic lesions do not present with evidence of intralesion necrosis, infarction, or intraplaque hemorrhage. While these lesions are thought to occasionally regress with time, the mechanism of this regression is not well understood. It would appear that the lesions do not regress by mechanisms such as liquefaction or excavation, but rather by a gradual reduction of the substance of the lesion. It is not known whether the lost mass represents cellular or matrix material, or both.

Because of their progressive growth, hyperplastic lesions may cause arterial stenosis. Eventually, they may generate symptoms on the basis of either restriction of carotid blood flow or carotid occlusion with thrombosis of the distal vessel. The growth of hyperplastic carotid plaques appears to be initiated by arterial injury. It is then thought to be sustained by hemodynamic forces acting on the arterial wall. Clinical evidence suggests that the growth of these lesions is limited. Most will not occlude an arterial lumen, although some may. What factors govern the duration and rate of growth of the hyperplastic lesions remains unclear.

Mattos and associates[7] reported a series of 380 patients who underwent 409 endarterectomies. These patients were serially examined with duplex scans over a 16-year period. Among these patients, 44 recurrent stenoses were identified (10.8% crude incidence). Analysis by the life table method suggested that 70% of the recurrent lesions occurred within the first 2 years following surgery. One of these patients became symptomatic within the first 2 years following surgery. At the end of 10 years only 2 of the 44 recurrences had become symptomatic. The authors concluded that the lesions were remarkably stable and had a low likelihood of either transient ischemic attacks (TIAs) or stroke. This finding was echoed in a recent report from UCLA.[11] Investigators were able to distinguish true recurrences and residual lesions by the use of completion arteriography and early postoperative duplex scanning. The crude incidence of true recurrent lesions was noted to be only 4.3%. By life table analysis, the 3-year incidence of recurrent stenosis was 11%. The clinical fate of these lesions was benign. None of the recurrent carotid stenoses were associated with new neurologic symptoms.[11]

A benign prognosis for recurrent stenosis has also been reported by

Strandness and his colleagues in two separate papers. In 1985 Nicholls et al.[19] reported a series of 134 patients who had undergone a total of 145 endarterectomies and were followed with duplex scans for an average of 4 years. The authors noted that most of the recurrences were identified within 24 months of surgery. They further noted that, of the six strokes recorded in the overall group, one occurred in association with arterial occlusion. The others were in unobstructed arteries. Of the six TIAs recorded in the follow-up period, only two were associated with recurrent stenosis. In a later paper, Healey et al.[20] reported the clinical outcome of 301 patients who had undergone endarterectomy and had been followed by the same group of surgeons. They noted that while TIAs occurred in 12% of the patients with recurrent stenosis and stroke occurred in 3% of this group, the incidence of these events was not statistically different from that observed in the postoperative patients without recurrence.

The ability to regress is a unique feature of hyperplastic lesions. Evidence of regression has been derived on the basis of serial duplex scans of patients with early recurrent stenosis. While the initial reports were subject to skepticism, this phenomenon has been identified in several papers from different institutions. Accordingly, regression of the early hyperplastic recurrent stenosis is now thought to occur in as many as one fourth to one third of instances. One of the first reports of the regression of hyperplastic lesions was that of Nicholls et al. who reported in 1985 that approximately 22% of patients developed recurrent stenosis generally within 24 months of surgery.[19] Also noted was the regression of almost one fourth of these lesions so that the persistence of recurrent stenosis was 17% at the end of the study. In 1987 Sanders et al.[2] reported 14 instances of regression of postoperative restenosis, and suggested that it occurred more commonly in arteries with low-grade restenosis. This observation was reaffirmed by Healey and associates[26] in a publication in 1989. They reported that a 7-year actuarial analysis recorded the occurrence of restenosis in 31% of patients. About one third of these regressed during the observation period, so that the prevalence of recurrent stenosis at the end of the study period was 21%. More recently, in 1990, Reilly and colleagues[12] reported that 16% of lesions regressed in their study. The impression which these reports yield is that some early lesions may be very active biologically and as the stimulus for their development abates, they may regress.

ATHEROSCLEROSIS

The biologic behavior of recurrent atherosclerotic lesions is considerably different from that of myointimal hyperplasia. In contrast to the hyperplastic lesions, atherosclerotic lesions are known to progress through a series of stages characterized by gradual plaque growth and subsequent degeneration. The mature and degenerating plaque is characterized by a propensity toward symptomatic presentation. In these later stages of growth, the lesions display several pathologic interactions with the endothelium blood which generate thromboembolic symptoms. This is due to pathologic processes of surface thrombosis, thromboembolization, intraplaque hemorrhage, and ulceration with plaque embolization. In contrast, hyperplastic lesions are relatively quiescent. They do not demonstrate surface thrombosis, ulceration, or intralesion hemorrhage. Accordingly, they do not generate embolic lesions and are less frequently symptomatic.

Atherosclerotic plaques generate cerebrovascular symptoms by means of a combination of arterial occlusive disease and intraarterial embolization. Progressive stenosis may produce symptoms in some patients on the basis of arterial insufficiency. More commonly, severe stenosis leads to occlusion and subsequent acute ischemic symptoms. Those patients who are able to tolerate the loss of perfusion from one carotid still face the potential of secondary events, such as propagation and embolization of thrombus within the internal carotid trunk above the occlusion. Perhaps more significant are the embolic symptoms of recurrent atherosclerotic plaques. Like primary atherosclerosis, these recurrent atherosclerotic plaques are deficient in both endothelial surfacing and plaque consistency. Thus both atheroemboli and thromboemboli are seen more frequently with recurrent atherosclerotic lesions than with recurrent hyperplastic lesions. It follows that recurrent atherosclerotic plaques are more likely to require surgical intervention.

Stoney and String[4] reported a sharp bimodal distribution in the presentation of recurrent carotid lesions. They further noted that those lesions which presented after 2 years were atherosclerotic, whereas those which presented before 2 years were hyperplastic. Das and colleagues[21] noted that 8 (27%) of the 29 late (>2 years) restenoses in their series were symptomatic at the time of reoperation. In 1992, Ricotta and associates[9] reported a series of 35 patients who were identified as having severe (>80%) recurrent stenosis. Of the 5 patients who developed neurologic symptoms, all but 1 presented 2 years after endarterectomy. In their discussion, these authors were impressed by the benign and stable nature of the early recurrent lesions despite their severity. It appears from this report that symptoms were more common in older lesions. Thus, the late carotid stenosis, which is more likely to be atherosclerotic, is also more likely to become symptomatic.

More recently, Gagne and colleagues[22] reported a 19-year experience with reoperation for carotid restenosis. The indication for reoperation was the development of cerebrovascular symptoms in 23 patients (80%), and progression toward preocclusive lesions in 6 patients (20%). Almost 60% of all lesions were caused by recurrent atherosclerosis. This report emphasizes the significant difference between hyperplastic and atherosclerotic lesions. It also serves to indicate the durability of carotid endarterectomy; their reoperative cohort represented only 1.6% of their patients who had undergone carotid endarterectomy. It would thus appear that symptomatic presentations are more common with recurrent atherosclerotic lesions.

PRESENTATIONS

The presentation of recurrent carotid lesions fall into four principal categories: (1) asymptomatic stenosis, (2) asymptomatic occlusion, (3) symptomatic stenosis, and (4) symptomatic occlusions. Because of the ability of duplex scanners to monitor changes in carotid blood hemodynamic variables, and to image changes in the arterial wall, it has become relatively easy to follow patients after carotid endarterectomy and identify the presence of recurrent lesions regardless of the presence of symptoms.

Most vascular surgeons have incorporated routine duplex scanning into their practice so that their patients undergo several duplex scans in the years following endarterectomy. Because of this, most recurrent carotid stenoses are identified at a relatively early and asymptomatic stage. Using the same method, it is possible to characterize the composition of plaques and differentiate the recurrent hyperplastic lesions from the recurrent calcific or atherosclerotic lesions.

While most recurrent lesions remain asymptomatic, between 1% and 15% of hyperplastic lesions may generate symptoms. Of these, between 15% and 25% of symptomatic presentations represent strokes.[2, 17, 24–26, 28] Symptomatic presentations appear to be more commonly associated with recurrent atherosclerotic lesions. Because of the selective nature of reports which focus on recurrent atherosclerosis, it is difficult to assess the incidence of symptoms associated with recurrent atherosclerosis. It is thought to be significantly higher than the incidence of symptoms associated with hyperplastic recurrences.

Progression of a recurrent carotid stenosis to occlusion is a relatively rare event. Most lesions remain asymptomatic and quiescent for years. The incidence of occlusion following endarterectomy appears to be about 1% to 2%.[10, 12, 24, 25] As many as one third of acute occlusions

TABLE 2.

Incidence of Recurrent Stenosis, Carotid Occlusion, and Occlusion-Related Symptoms in Selected Cases

Authors	Year	No. of Cases	Recurrent Stenosis (%)	No. of Late Occlusions	No. of Symptomatic Occlusions*	
					CVA	TIA
Nicholls et al.[19]	1985	145		1	1	—
Hertzer et al.[23]	1987	917	31	4	—	—
Sanders et al.[2]	1987	109	8	1	—	—
Eikelboom et al.[24]	1988	129	11	3	—	—
Healey et al.[20]	1989	301	21	2	—	
Clagett et al.[15]	1989	152	12.9	11	4	—
Salenius et al.[25]	1989	257	13	5	—	—
Reilly et al.[12]	1990	131	18	8	—	—
Mattos et al.[16]	1993	409	10.8	7	1	1
Hansen et al.[10]	1993	232	9.2	4	—	—
Gelabert et al.[11]	1994	268	11	0	—	—

*Note that CVA indicates cerebrovascular accident (stroke) and TIA indicates a transient ischemic attack. Symptomatic occlusions refer to late occlusions which presented with symptoms.

may present with stroke symptoms (Table 2). Even at the time of the occlusion, the development of symptoms appears to be dependent principally upon cerebral collateral circulation. If the hemodynamic alteration imposed by a carotid occlusion is tolerated without event, the probability of a late stroke appears to be very low, although some patients may experience late embolic events following asymptomatic carotid occlusion.

SCREENING

Since most recurrent carotid stenoses discovered in the course of routine postoperative duplex scanning are asymptomatic, the value of these routine scans have been called into question. Studies in the early postoperative period serve to document the patency of the artery operated on. Another important application in the early postoperative period is to identify any significant residual lesions, thus certifying the completeness of the endarterectomy. Later, duplex scans are often obtained for two reasons: to identify progression of plaque stenosis on the contralateral side, and to survey for recurrent stenosis on the postendarterectomy side.

The debate regarding the value of routine postoperative duplex scanning focuses on a cost-benefit assessment. While it is clear that 10% to 20% of patients may develop some form of recurrent stenosis following carotid endarterectomy, the number of patients who progress to hemodynamically significant stenosis is remarkably smaller. As few as 0.5% of all patients may require reoperation for recurrence. Additionally, even fewer patients sustain recurrent symptoms in the first 5 years following endarterectomy. About 0.01% of all patients will have recurrent symptoms related to a recurrent stenosis and require surgical correction. Furthermore, the probability that a completed stroke would be the first presentation of recurrent stenosis is exceedingly low (0.0001%). Finally, the probability of suffering a stroke upon complete occlusion of a recurrent carotid stenosis is undefined. In addressing this issue, Mattos and colleagues posed a question regarding the clinical impact of routine carotid duplex scanning.[17] They reviewed their experience with routine postoperative duplex scanning and concluded that recurrent carotid stenosis is an early postoperative event that is typically benign and generally remains stable over long periods of time. Accordingly, clinical evaluation is of prime importance, and routine postoperative duplex scanning is not necessary. This conclusion is similar to that reached by Ricotta et al.[7] and Cook et al.[29] in two different publications. Cook and colleagues noted that the incidence of symptomatic events in the postoperative period is low. Because of this, periodic postoperative scans to assess the development and progression of a recurrent stenosis are not merited. Follow-up duplex studies are warranted for evaluation of contralateral carotid disease and should be based on the status of the noninvolved artery.[29] Ricotta et al.[9] arrived at a similar conclusion: routine periodic postoperative duplex scanning is not justified simply for the documentation of recurrent stenosis and prevention of postoperative occlusion.

MEDICAL THERAPY

Current therapy for recurrent carotid stenosis consists of one of several elements: first is risk factors management; second, specific pharmacotherapy for prevention or inhibition of recurrent stenosis; finally, surgical approaches for prevention and reconstruction following recurrent carotid stenosis.

The most elemental approach to the problem of recurrent carotid stenosis is the management of risk factors for atherosclerotic arterial disease. Once risk factors such as smoking, hyperlipidemia, or diabetes are identified they should be modified or eliminated. This represents an attempt to control both progression of generalized atherosclerosis as well as a nonspecific means of reducing the risk of recurrent atherosclerotic carotid stenosis. The adoption of risk factor–controlling protocols is based on the assumption that the risk factors may contribute to the progression of recurrent stenosis, be it hyperplastic or atherosclerotic. It should be recognized that the evidence implicating these risk factors is tenuous and not based on clear prospective data.

Pharmacotherapy for recurrent carotid stenosis is directed toward either preventing restenosis or restricting the progression of an established lesion in the early postoperative period. Several agents have been used in this effort: aspirin, dipyridamole, angiotensin-converting enzyme (ACE) inhibitors and corticosteroids. All have been considered potentially to be beneficial with regard to the goal of inhibiting neointimal hyperplasia. None of these agents have proved of benefit in controlled clinical situations. Experimental evidence supports the possible role of ACE inhibitors as well as dexamethasone. Both these agents have been reported to inhibit the development of intimal hyperplasia in animal subjects. Anecdotal clinical experience with these last two groups of agents suggests that their clinical use may present significant problems. Certain patients may be unable to tolerate the effect of these medications and thus the clinical application may be limited. Accordingly, use of these agents for inhibition of intimal hyperplasia should be avoided outside the context of a controlled trial.

SURGICAL APPROACHES

The two principal surgical approaches to the problem of recurrent carotid stenosis involve either an attempt to prevent the problem from occurring, or the correction of the recurrence once it has occurred. Preventive measures are meant to mitigate the effect of a possible recurrent lesion. Corrective surgical measures may be necessary if a severe recurrent stenosis has been identified.

PREVENTION OF RECURRENCE

The principal surgical maneuvers employed to reduce the risk of recurrent stenosis involve meticulous and complete endarterectomy, and patch closure of the arteriotomy. Residual carotid plaque is thought to be a significant risk factor for the development of postendarterectomy carotid stenosis.[8, 30] While many authors would argue that this represents an inadequacy of the original operation, residual lesions predisposed to the reaccumulation of plaque and are associated with development of symptoms. Accordingly, the first principle of prevention of recurrence is to perform a meticulous endarterectomy.

The plane of the endarterectomy may bear a significant impact on the risk of recurrence. If the plane is too shallow, a large residual plaque may remain. If the plane is too deep, there may be a problem in ending the endarterectomy smoothly and an abrupt transition may result at the endpoint. Such an abrupt endpoint transition may result in an intimal flap, which in turn may predispose to an early stenosis or occlusion.

Carotid patch angioplasty closure has been suggested as a means of reducing the risk of restenosis. Patch closure is thought to work by means of several mechanisms. First, it enlarges the arterial diameter. The larger vessel diameter may reduce the impact of a recurrent lesion. A given volume of hyperplastic lesion in a small artery may cause significant stenosis; in a larger artery the same volume of lesion may not be significant. Since many lesions seem to grow to a given size and then become quiescent, patching may prevent many recurrences from resulting in a significant degree of stenosis. Another manner in which patch closure may decrease the risk of recurrent stenosis is by improving the hemodynamic configuration of the endarterectomy. Severe turbulent blood flow is among several hemodynamic factors which are thought to be associated with recurrent lesions. Patch angioplasty has been advocated as a means of reducing such turbulent flow. Finally, patch closure may help stabilize the distal endpoint. This in turn may result in a decreased possibility of an intimal flap occurring.

Despite these proposed benefits regarding the use of patch closure, the clinical experience as reported in medical literature suggests that the actual results are mixed. In a prospective randomized study of carotid patching presented in 1993, Meyers et al.[28] reported no significant difference in the incidence of recurrent stenosis or of cerebrovascular symptoms. A total of 136 patients underwent 163 endarterectomies over a period of 46 months. They were randomized to one of three groups (patch, no patch, obligatory patch), prospectively enrolled, and followed for about 5 years. The result was that recurrence of stenosis as well as stroke-free survival rates were similar among study groups. It should be noted that this report represents a dramatic change in data from an earlier report (1989) by the same authors in which they suggested that patch closure resulted in significantly increased recurrence rates.[15]

Hertzer and associates[23] reported a study favoring vein patch angioplasty in which 801 patients underwent 917 carotid endarterectomies. The use of patch closure was at the discretion of the surgeons. Patients were followed on a routine basis. After a mean follow-up period of 21 months, a significant difference was noted in the incidence of recurrent stenosis between the patch angioplasty (9%) and primary closure groups (31%). While not a randomized study, this report strongly suggests a benefit of routine patch closure. Further supporting the use of patch angioplasty is a report by Eikelboom and colleagues presented in 1988.[24] This report describes a prospective randomized study in which patients were divided between patch closure and primary closure. After 1 year of follow-up, the patch closure group had a significantly lower rate of significant restenosis than the primary closure group (3.5% vs. 21%).

CORRECTION OF RESTENOSIS

The decision to repair recurrent carotid stenosis is based on two general indications: development of recurrent neurologic symptoms, and progression of the recurrence to a preocclusive stage. If recurrent stenosis is the source of neurologic symptoms such as TIAs or mild stroke, then repair is merited to prevent a major stroke. If the lesion has progressed to a preocclusive stage, then repair is considered to be indicated as an effort to prevent occlusion of the internal carotid artery (and to reduce the risk of subsequent stroke).

Several assumptions underlie the decision to operate on a carotid restenosis. The principal assumption is that a recurrent carotid lesion presents a significant risk of stroke and that the risk of the reoperative surgical procedure is low. An estimation of the risk of carotid reoperations may be obtained in the results presented by Gagne and associates.[14] They reported a series of patients operated on at New York University. In all, 29 patients underwent reoperation for recurrent stenosis over a period of 19 years. A total of three postoperative TIAs and one hypoglossal nerve injury occurred in this series. No other perioperative neurologic events or deaths occurred. This report stands in contrast to that of Piepgras and colleagues[29] who reported a 10% reoperative complication rate. This rate was four times greater than the risk of surgery for primary atherosclerosis. Specifically noted in their report were four major strokes, and two minor strokes and two TIAs. At the Cleveland Clinic, Das and colleagues[21] noted an overall reoperative complication rate of 13.8%. Of these, 9.2% represented transient cranial nerve dysfunction. The nonfatal stroke rate was 1.5%, and the mortality rate was 3.1%.

Surgical mortality for primary or reoperative carotid surgery generally has been reported to be in the range of 0.2% to 2.0%. In a report from University of California, San Francisco, in 1976, Stoney and String[4] reported a mortality rate of 3.2%. Piepgras and associates[29] reported no deaths, although two of their patients sustained myocardial infarctions. In general, most surgeons seem to agree that the risk of cranial nerve injury or other complications in the course of reoperative carotid surgery is increased when compared to the original operation.

Because of the significant difference in the pathologic potential of hyperplastic and atherosclerotic lesions, asymptomatic hyperplastic lesions are thought to represent relatively little risk. Given the technical difficulties associated with carotid reoperations and their potentially increased risk, most surgeons are willing to observe recurrent stenosis for either the development of symptoms or signs of progression toward occlusion before reoperation is considered.

Operations designed to correct recurrent carotid stenosis employ one of three approaches: (1) the lesion is resected, (2) a repeat endarterectomy is accomplished, or (3) patch angioplasty is performed to relieve the stenosis. The choice of which procedure applies to the situation at hand is decided by the characteristics of the lesion and the condition of the artery.

The surgical alternatives for repair of a recurrent hyperplastic lesion include either replacement of the arterial segment or patch angioplasty. Patch angioplasty is the standard technique used for repairing recurrent stenosis due to hyperplastic lesions. This is because the fibrous hyperplastic lesion frequently is not amenable to repeat endarterectomy. The plane in the medial layer of the arterial wall is frequently obliterated by the hyperplastic lesion. The drawback of patch angioplasty in this setting is that the hyperplasia remains in place. Some concern exists that the lesion still may subsequently progress to reocclude the arterial lumen. On the other hand, patch angioplasty is less complex than arterial resection and reconstruction, and thus it is more appealing in some circumstances.

Arterial resection and reconstruction have commonly been reserved for those instances where the possibility of further recurrence is very high, or where the artery appears so damaged by either disease or dissection that replacement is advisable. Tertiary recurrences (a recurrence following reoperation for recurrent stenosis) may be an indication for resection of the arterial segment and graft reconstruction. The surgical technique in these instances involves replacement of the arterial segment with a short segment of saphenous vein or prosthetic material. If the diseased segment involves the internal carotid, the graft is tailored to replace the internal segment only. If the recurrence involves both the internal and common carotid, the graft is used to replace the diseased segment, and the external carotid is either reimplanted or ligated. Ligation of the external carotid is performed when the artery has been so damaged or diseased that it cannot be readily reattached to the common carotid trunk. An additional reason to ligate the external carotid may be a concern with the prolongation of cerebral ischemia during the reoperation. The consequences of ligating this artery are usually minimal, since collateral circulation from the contralateral carotid provides abundant vascular supply to the face. The most important consequence of external carotid ligation is loss of an important cerebral collateral pathway.

The choice of material for graft replacement of the carotid artery generally is limited to saphenous vein, Dacron graft, or polytetrafluoroethylene (PTFE). Given that carotid replacement usually is performed in a reoperative field, a benefit may be derived from the preferential use of saphenous vein because of its resistance to infection. It should be recognized, however, that the risk of infection following carotid surgery is very low. Accordingly, prosthetic material appears to be well tolerated. There seems to be little evidence that either vein or prosthetic graft is superior with respect to recurrent stenosis, so the choice of prosthetic material is based largely on the preference of the surgeon.

Repeat endarterectomy may be quite appropriate when recurrent carotid stenosis is atherosclerotic. Preoperative factors which might suggest this cause include the presence of calcification on duplex scanning, as well as the interval from the original operation to the date of reoperation. If the recurrent plaque appears to be heavily calcified or contains heterogeneous material on a duplex scan, then a repeat endarterectomy may be possible. If the interval from the original endarterectomy to the reoperation is more than 36 months, it also is more likely that an atherosclerotic recurrence is present. The surgical approach to these lesions is based on the principles of reoperative carotid surgery: meticulous dissection of all vascular structures, careful preservation of adjacent nerves, and patch closure of the arteriotomy. Of particular importance, patch closure is recommended in order to reduce the risk of further recurrent (tertiary) stenosis.

Tertiary stenosis is an unusual event, and the optimal management of this lesion is not well established. The principal alternatives include patch angioplasty or resection and reconstruction of the artery. If patch angioplasty has previously been performed, then consideration should be given to resecting the artery and replacing the segment with the interposition of a saphenous vein or prosthetic graft. In many instances, the question is moot since the third operation on a previously patched carotid may result in an artery so damaged that replacement clearly is necessary.

CONCLUSION

The discovery of a recurrent carotid stenosis frequently occurs as a consequence of routine postoperative surveillance following carotid endarterectomy. Serial duplex scans may reveal the development and progression of hyperplastic lesions. Most of these reach a given size and then remain fixed, without further growth or regression. A small number may progress to the point of occlusion, and a few others may regress. While several risk factors have been associated with the development of carotid restenosis, their relative importance remains largely unexplained. Female sex, small arterial diameter, tobacco exposure, and hyperlipidemia all have been associated with recurrent stenosis, and its prevention may best be afforded by patch closure during the original carotid arteriotomy. It is evident that most of these lesions are benign. The incidence of symptoms from an early recurrent stenosis is very low. For this reason, aside from an early postoperative duplex scan to establish patency of the artery operated on, serial duplex studies are not recommended for observation of a recurrent lesion. However, late scans may be warranted for evaluation of the contralateral carotid.

Another important question regards the correct management of patients with recurrent stenosis. Again, since the symptomatic presentation of these lesions is unusual, most early recurrences will not require reoperation. Surgery is clearly indicated for symptomatic lesions, and perhaps for a preocclusive hyperplastic lesion. Atherosclerotic recurrences are probably best managed in a manner similar to the primary carotid lesion: symptomatic stenoses of greater than 70% and asymptomatic stenoses greater than 80% should be surgically repaired.

Successful management requires an understanding of the nature of the lesion as well as the risk that it represents. The role of surgery in restenosis centers on the prevention of stroke in patients with recurrent symptoms and the prevention of occlusion in those who appear to be at increased risk. Perhaps most important is the recognition that many recurrences may be preempted by the judicious use of patch reconstruction as part of the original operation.

REFERENCES

1. O'Donnell TF, Callow AD, Scott G, et al: Ultrasound characteristics of recurrent carotid disease: Hypothesis explaining the low incidence of symptomatic recurrence. *J Vasc Surg* 1985; 2:26–41.
2. Sanders E, Hoeneveld H, Eikelboom B, et al: Residual lesions and early restenosis after carotid endarterectomy. *J Vasc Surg* 1987; 5:731–737.
3. Sterpetti A, Schultz R, Feldhaus R, et al: Natural history of recurrent carotid artery stenosis. *Surg Gynecol Obstet* 1989; 168:217–223.
4. Stoney RJ, String ST: Recurrent carotid stenosis. *Surgery* 1976; 80:705–710.
5. Bodily K, Zierler R, Marinelli M, et al: Flow disturbances following carotid endarterectomy. *Surg Gynecol Obstet* 1980; 151:77–80.
6. Turnipseed WD, Berkoff HA, Crummy A: Postoperative occlusion after carotid endarterectomy. *Arch Surg* 1980; 115:573–574.
7. Baker JD: Recurrent stenosis of the carotid artery: Incidence, diagnosis, prognosis, and management. In Moore WS (ed): *Surgery for Cerebrovascular Disease*. New York, Churchill Livingstone, 1987, pp 703–713.
8. Bandyk D, Kabenick H, Adams M, et al: Turbulence occurring after carotid bifurcation endarterectomy: A harbinger of residual and recurrent carotid stenosis. *J Vasc Surg* 1988; 7:261–274.
9. Ricotta J, O'Brien M, DeWeese J: Natural history of recurrent and residual stenosis after carotid endarterectomy: Implications for postoperative surveillance and surgical management. *Surgery* 1992; 112:656–663.
10. Hansen F, Linbald B, Persson N, et al: Can recurrent stenosis after carotid endarterectomy be prevented by low-dose acetylsalicylic acid? A double-blind, randomized, and placebo-controlled study. *Eur J Vasc Surg* 1993; 7:380–385.
11. Gelabert H, El-Marrsy S, Moore W: Carotid endarterectomy with primary closure does not adversely affect the rate of recurrent stenosis. *Arch Surg* 1994, in press.
12. Reilly LM, Okuhn SP, Rapp JH, et al: Recurrent carotid stenosis: a consequence of local or systemic factors? The influence of unrepaired technical defects. *J Vasc Surg* 1990; 11:448–459.
13. Blaisdell F, Lim RJ, Hall A: Technical result of carotid endarterectomy. Arteriographic assessment. *Am J Surg* 1967; 114:239–246.
14. Clagett G, Rich N, McDonald R, et al: Etiologic factors for recurrent carotid artery stenosis. *Surgery* 1983; 93:313–318.
15. Clagett G, Patterson C, Fisher D, et al: Vein patch versus primary closure for carotid endarterectomy. *J Vasc Surg* 1989; 9:213–223.
16. Mattos M, van Bemmelen P, Barkmeire L, et al: Routine surveillance after carotid endarterectomy: Does it affect clinical management? *J Vasc Surg* 1993; 17:819–831.
17. Colburn MD, Moore WS: Myointimal hyperplasia, in Moore WS (ed): *Vascular Surgery: A Comprehensive Review*, ed 4. Philadelphia, WB Saunders, 1993, pp 673–693.
18. Zarins CK, Zatina MA, Giddens DP, et al: Shear stress regulation of artery lumen diameter in experimental atherogenesis. *J Vasc Surg* 1987; 5:413–420.
19. Nicholls S, Phillips D, Bergelin R, et al: Carotid endarterectomy. Relationship of outcome to early restenosis. *J Vasc Surg* 1985; 2:375–381.
20. Healy DA, Zierler RE, Nicholls SC, et al: Long-term follow-up and clinical outcome of carotid restenosis. *J Vasc Surg* 1989; 10:662–669.

21. Das M, Hertzer N, Ratliff N, et al: Recurrent stenosis. A five year series of 65 reoperations. *Ann Surg* 1985; 202:28–35.
22. Gagne P, Riles T, Imparato A, et al: Redo endarterectomy for recurrent carotid artery stenosis. *Eur J Vasc Surg* 1991; 5:135–140.
23. Hertzer N, Beven E, O'Hara P, et al: A prospective study of vein patch angioplasty during carotid endarterectomy. *Ann Surg* 1987; 206:628–35.
24. Eikelboom B, Ackerstaff R, Hoeneveld H, et al: Benefit of carotid patching: A randomized study. *J Vasc Surg* 1988; 7:240–247.
25. Salenius JP, Haapanen A, Harju E, et al: Late carotid restenosis: aetiologic factors for recurrent carotid artery stenosis during long-term follow-up. *Eur J Vasc Surg* 1989; 3:271–277.
26. Cook J, Thompson B, Barnes R: Is routine duplex examination after carotid endarterectomy justified? *J Vasc Surg* 1989; 12:334–340.
27. Green R, McNamara J, Ouriel K, et al: The clinical course for residual carotid arterial disease. *J Vasc Surg* 1991; 13:112–120.
28. Myers S, Valentine J, Chervu A, et al: Saphenous vein patch versus primary closure for carotid endarterectomy: Long term assessment of a randomized prospective study. *J Vasc Surg* 1994; 19:15–22.
29. Piepgras D, Marsh W, Mussman L, et al: Recurrent carotid stenosis: Results and complications of 57 operations. *Ann Surg* 1986; 203:205–213.
30. Baker WH, Hayes AC, Mahler D, et al: Durability of carotid endarterectomy. *Surgery* 1983; 94:112–115.
31. Salvian A, Baker J, Machleder H, et al: Cause and noninvasive detection of restenosis after carotid endarterectomy. *Am J Surg* 1983; 146:29–35.
32. Bertin V, Plecha F, Rodgers G, et al: Recurrent stenosis by duplex scanfollowing carotid endarterectomy. *Arch Surg* 1989; 124:866–869.

Aortic Graft Infections

Hazim J. Safi, M.D.

Associate Professor of Surgery, Baylor College of Medicine, Houston, Texas

Stefano Bartoli, M.D.

Visiting Assistant Professor, Baylor College of Medicine, Houston, Texas

I nfection of aortic grafts is a rare but dreadful complication of vascular surgery. Although the incidence of graft infections has declined since the advent of prophylactic antibiotics administered during vascular procedures, they remain a serious problem and carry a high rate of morbidity and mortality.[1, 2]

Unfortunately, the classic treatment for graft infection—excision and extraanatomic bypass—has not produced uniformly good results, and the search continues for better methods. In our experience, graft excision and in situ replacement, reinforced with omentum or muscle flap coverage, with up to 6 weeks' intravenous (IV) antibiotic therapy, followed by lifelong oral antibiotics, give the most promising results. Occasionally, an extraanatomic graft is called for. Clinical manifestation, virulence of bacteria, extensiveness of the infection in the graft, and location of the graft in the patient will ultimately dictate surgical decisions.

This review of aortic graft infections explores surgical techniques, weighing the pros and cons of solutions for the situation at hand. We begin with an outline of the epidemiology, the clinical presentation, and the diagnostic tools.

INCIDENCE, MORBIDITY, MORTALITY

Despite the actual increase in the number of patients for aortic graft implant surgery, we believe we have seen a decline in the percentage of infected grafts. Correct cumulative numbers for the incidence of vascular graft infections are difficult to determine owing to the variable intervals between graft implantation and clinical manifestation of infection (from 4 weeks to more than 10 years) and also because patients have sometimes been treated at separate hospitals for graft implantation and graft infection. The overall incidence of vascular graft infections lies between 0.5% and 6.0% (Tables 1 and 2).

Antibiotic therapy and assiduous surgical procedures provide protection against many graft infection-causing bacteria. We advocate timing angiography within 24 hours before surgery, antiseptic preoperative bathing, and shaving the skin just before the time of surgery. We prepare the skin with povidone-iodine (Betadine) and apply adhesive skin drapes. During the operation, tissues are handled gently, good hemostasis is se-

TABLE 1.
Incidence of Prosthetic Graft Infection*

Author	Period	No. of Grafts	No. of Infections	Incidence (%)
Szilgayi	1952–1971	2,145	41	1.9
Goldstone	1959–1973	566	14	2.5
Casali	1967–1979	652	20	3.1
Yashar	1966–1977	590	15	2.5
O'Hara	1961–1985	3,652	51	0.6

*Modified from Simon GL, Parenti DM, Trout HH III: Arterial and vascular graft infections, in Giordano JM (ed). *The Basic Science of Vascular Surgery.* Mount Kisco, NY, Futura, 1988, 723–745.

TABLE 2.
Results of Aortic Graft Infection*

Author	Year	No. of Infections	Mortality (%)	Amputations (%)
Liekweg	1977	84	49	8
Turnipseed	1983	20	40	15
O'Hara	1986	84	28	29
Reilly	1987	101	16	23
Yeager	1990	38	26	21

*Modified from Ricotta JJ, Faggioli GL, Stella A, et al: *Am J Surg* 1991; 162:145–149.

cured, and wounds are closed accurately. In all cases, we prescribe perioperative antibiotic prophylaxis (see below).

ONSET OF INFECTION

Unfortunately, despite meticulous surgical techniques, infection can begin in a number of ways at the time of graft implantation. If this occurs, morbidity, primarily from lower limb amputations, and mortality remain high. Identifying different causal factors is important.

Most frequently, infections arise from graft contamination. The organism contacts and lodges in the graft because of inadequate sterilization, a breakdown in sterile technique, contact with skin or intraabdominal organs, or from bacteria residing within the native artery. Bacteria from anatomic structures unrelated to the operation may also reach the graft via blood.[3, 4] Postoperatively, hematoma, lymphatic damage, or development of thrombus creates a potential habitat for infection. Another possible cause, still debated, is simultaneous nonvascular procedures.[5, 6] The highest percentage of infected grafts occurs in femoropopliteal grafts (2.5%), followed by aortofemoral (2.0%), axillobifemoral (1.0%), and aortoiliac (<0.5%). Aortic infection mortality rates have actually decreased from 50% to 20% during the last 10 years. With femoral graft infection, the mortality rate is generally lower, at 10% to 20%, but the amputation rate approaches 80%.[2, 7]

BACTERIOLOGY

Staphylococcus aureus was previously the most commonly identified bacterium, responsible for up to 50% of graft infections. *Staphylococcus epidermidis*, a low-virulence organism, is now responsible for a growing number, if not the majority, of clinically observed cases.[8] The identification of this bacterium is important because it reinforces our decision to perform in situ surgery or selective preservation of a graft. Because of the low virulence of *S. epidermidis*, antibiotic therapy is effective in suppressing the infection.

Graft infection is usually bacterial, although other reported causes are fungi, mycoplasmas, and mycobacteria. The incidence of gram-negative organisms and mixed infections is also rising.[9] Prophylactic antibiotics administered against *S. aureus* as well as a greater number of gram-negative organisms found within hospital environments may be the cause of this shift. This increase may also reflect improved culture techniques.

An important feature of *S. epidermidis* is its ability to produce slime, enabling it to adhere to biomaterials, and to encase itself in a protective biofilm, thereby protecting it from antibiotics. Penetration of this protective armor, releasing the bacterium into the blood, can happen at any time, causing early or late infection.[10]

When clinical signs of infection are present, culture of graft material in broth media without surface biofilm disruption will, in most cases, recover the infection microorganism. When signs of infection are absent, the documentation of graft colonization requires the addition of surface biofilm disruption, important to the culture technique.[11] More important than the infected graft culture is the culture of the adjacent arterial wall because, as claimed by Malone et al.,[12] the morbidity and mortality of graft infection treatment are linearly and directly related to arterial culture. Positive arterial wall cultures have been significantly correlated with disruption of suture lines and hemorrhage following repair of infected grafts.

Preoperatively, for vascular surgery, we administer cefamandol as a prophylactic against any staphylococcus infection: 2 g IV at the induction of anesthesia, then 2 g every 4 hours, for 24 hours.

With a graft infection and positive culture, the choice of antibiotics is determined by culture sensitivity. Our course is IV antibiotics for 6 weeks followed by lifelong oral antibiotics. Patients are instructed to report any subsequent intolerance to antibiotics; hence the importance of keeping records of the bacteria and their sensitivity if the original antibiotic must be replaced.

In a minority of cases, a culture is negative and it is difficult to choose the appropriate antibiotics. In these cases, in order to guarantee protection against *S. epidermidis,* we administer both vancomycin and a broad-spectrum antibiotic, e.g., ceftazidime IV for 6 weeks, followed by lifelong oral antibiotics. Our choice here is minocycline.

TABLE 3.
Antibiotic Therapy of Graft Infection

Bacterial/Fungal Infection	Administration		
	Preoperative	Six Weeks (IV)	Lifelong (Oral)
Prophylactic	Cefamandole		
Bacterial culture			
Positive		Antibiotic depends on culture sensitivity	Antibiotic depends on culture sensitivity
Negative		Vancomycin and ceftazidine (empiric)	Minocycline (empiric)
Candida		Amphotericin B	Fluconazole

In the event of a fungal infection *(Candida)* our antibiotic therapy is first, amphotericin B IV, followed by lifelong therapy with fluconazole (Table 3).

CLINICAL PRESENTATION

We know that much of the damage has already taken place when clinical symptom of an infected graft make their appearance. Symptoms may range from fever, leukocytosis, and recurrent nonspecific pain to the deceptively vague symptoms of weight loss or malaise. The most telling sign, a palpable mass, may not emerge at all since the location of symptoms is not necessarily that of the infection. Negative blood cultures will not always mean absence of infection, as noted in our discussion about *S. epidermidis*. Obviously, no single tool exists for the diagnosis of graft infection and the clinician must rely on history, physical examination, a high index of suspicion, and findings of various radiologic and isotopic studies to confirm the diagnosis.

We most frequently use angiography, combined with computed tomography (CT) scanning, as a diagnostic tool. Angiography is useful in determining the patency of graft segments as well as leakage from the suture line, both of significant importance in treatment decisions. Anastomotic false aneurysms and graft occlusions can be visualized by angiography, but not perigraft fluid or gas, for which CT scanning is important.

Another useful tool is ultrasound. Ultrasound can identify perigraft fluid and gas in some cases, and is optimal for revealing false aneurysms or abscesses, especially in the groin. Ultrasound, however, does not produce a good image in the lower abdomen and pelvis.[13]

Nuclear medicine studies like indium 111-labeled white blood cell scans have significant false-positive and false-negative rates. A new technique, ^{111}In-labeled immunoglobulin G, shows both improved sensitivity and specificity for infection.[14] Another process, technetium 99m hexametazime, reportedly has 100% sensitivity, and 94.4% specificity for detecting aortic graft infection.[15] Magnetic resonance imaging (MRI) provides excellent fat-fluid contrast, but cannot separate postoperative changes from inflammation, and has poor muscle-fluid contrast.[16] New

TABLE 4.
Testing Sensitivity and Specificity for Prosthetic Graft Infection*

Test	Sensitivity (%)	Specificity (%)
CT scan	57	100
[111]In WBC scan	96	85
[111]In IgM scan	91	100
[99m]Tc scan	100	94
MRI	85	100

*Modified from LaMuraglia GM, Fischman AJ, Strauss HW, et al: *J Vasc Surg* 1989; 10:20–28; and Fiorani P, Speziale F, Rizzo L, et al: *J Vasc Surg* 1993; 17:87–96.

MRI applications continue to develop methods with high sensitivity (85%) and specificity (100%).[15]

In summary, we use angiography to detect the presence of occlusion and false aneurysms and CT scanning for detection of perigraft fluid. MRI may be as good as the CT scan, but it is limited by cost and often the patient's claustrophobia (Table 4).

SURGICAL TECHNIQUES

In general, surgeons agree that in the case of anastomotic disruption, systemic sepsis, or occlusion, all infected graft material must be removed and systemic antibiotics administered. There is less agreement regarding the ideal replacement conduit.

Problems of operative management center around four critical questions: (1) in situ or extraanatomic reconstruction; (2) selective, synchronous, or staged arterial reconstruction; (3) total vs. partial excision; and (4) selection of allograft, homograft, or prosthetic material for revascularization.

Some authors believe the infected graft to be an absolute indication for extraanatomic bypass, continuing to give credence to the principle that prosthetic material should not be permanently placed in an infected field.[17-20] Despite the use of staged procedures, however, late morbidity remains high with this approach, in addition to the potential for fatal blowout of the aortic stump. Retrograde thrombosis, caused by proximal propagation of an intraluminal thrombosis, is another complication of the remaining aortic stump that can result in renal failure.

The most common complication of extraanatomic bypass is occlusion of the bypassed graft. Revascularization with new grafts before infected graft excision may avoid the obligatory ischemic time to the

TABLE 5.

Sequence and Staging of Extraanatomic Bypass and Aortic Graft Excision*

	Surgical Results		
Timing	Mortality	Amputation	Extraanatomic Graft Sepsis
Sequential or staged			
Extraanatomic bypass followed by graft excision	25%	11%	20%
Traditional			
Graft excision followed by extraanatomic bypass	43%	46%	23%

*Modified from Reilly LM, Stoney RJ, Goldstone J, et al: *J Vasc Surg* 1987; 5:421–431.

lower extremities and lead to fewer amputations. There is, however, the theoretical risk of bacteremic seeding of the new graft material if it is placed before removal of the infected prosthesis. Clinical results indicate that this type of revascularization is satisfactory if staged with an interval of no more than 1 week for chronic aortic graft infections. Whether revascularization is performed before or after infected aortic graft excision, however, does not appear to alter the eventual outcome. In the end, we agree that neither schedule provides a reduction in the return of infection, and decreased surgical stress is the only advantage of staging[21] (Table 5).

The solution to the problem of maintaining extraanatomic graft patency continues to be explored through new bypass routes and improved prosthetic material. An interesting report is the use of the descending thoracic aorta to the iliofemoral or femorofemoral artery bypass. The first such operation was performed by Lester R. Sauvage in 1956, and reported in 1961 with a 20-month graft patency. Theoretically, this method provides an inflow source superior to other extraanatomic reconstructions, but still does not require aortic cross-clamping, and avoids the abdominal cavity[22] (Fig 1).

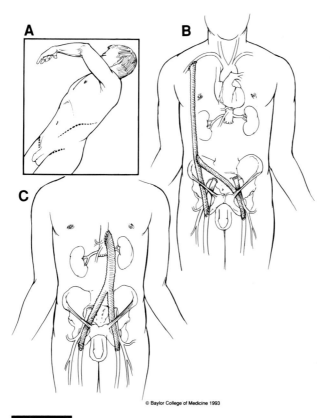

© Baylor College of Medicine 1993

FIGURE 1.

To improve the patency rate of the axillobifemoral graft, replacement with a descending thoracic aortobifemoral bypass graft was used. **A,** incisions for descending bifemoral bypass graft. **B,** axillobifemoral graft. **C,** descending bifemoral bypass graft.

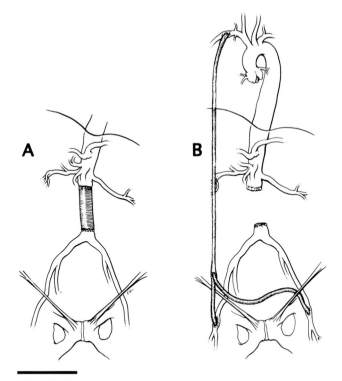

FIGURE 2.

A, infected graft, infrarenal abdominal aorta. **B,** axillobifemoral graft replacement of **A.**

INFRARENAL AORTIC GRAFT

In 1961, Blaisdell et al. reported the first clinical use of axillary–femoral artery bypass to revascularize the lower limbs after removal of an infected aortic prosthetic graft.[23] This new bypass was tunneled through a noninfected clean field. This method, however, is associated with a significant risk of operative death as well as frequent late complications.

Nonetheless, some papers evaluating this procedure found fairly good results and specified the indications as patients with gross, frank retroperitoneal pus surrounding the anastomosis of the graft to the artery. Treatment was specified as complete excision of infected prosthetic ma-

TABLE 6.

Revascularization With Excision*

	Surgical Results	
	Mortality	**Graft Sepsis**
In situ	32%	11%
Extraanatomic replacement	38%	15%

*Modified from Yeager RA, Porter JM: *Ann Vasc Surg* 1992; 6:485–491.

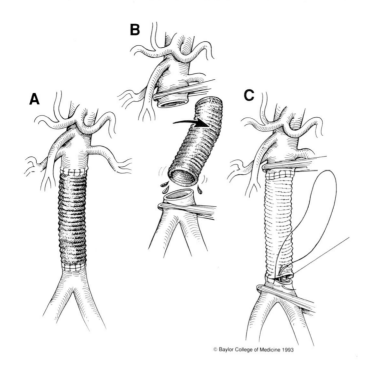

© Baylor College of Medicine 1993

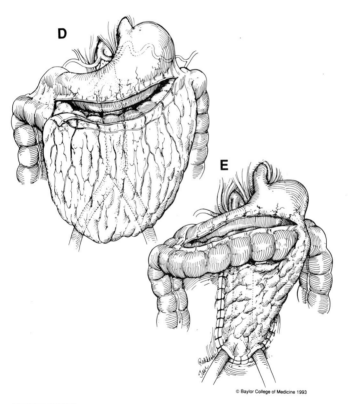

© Baylor College of Medicine 1993

FIGURE 3.

A, infected Dacron graft, infrarenal abdominal aorta. **B,** infected graft excised. **C,** new Dacron graft replacement. **D,** mobilized omentum. **E,** graft wrapped with omentum.

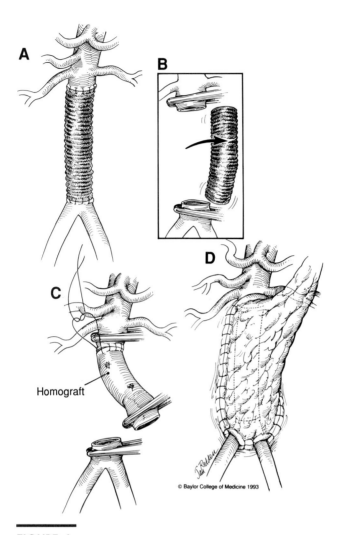

FIGURE 4.

A, infected graft, infrarenal abdominal aorta. **B,** infected graft excised. **C,** new in situ homograft replacement. **D,** homograft wrapped with omentum.

terial; complete debridement of all infected retroperitoneal tissues, including the aorta; aortic ligation; omental coverage of the aortic stump; and extraanatomic bypass accompanied by high-dose culture-directed antibiotic therapy.

In our opinion, extraanatomic bypass replacement is best suited for the infrarenal-abdominal graft when, on physical examination, infection is rampant, bacteria are virulent, and there is no violation of the groins. In this case we advise oversewing the aortic stump and prefer the sequence of extraanatomic bypass surgery before graft removal (Fig 2).

Aortic stump dehiscence is a significant late cause of death in patients surviving extraanatomic surgical treatment of aortic vascular graft infections. Two factors in the pathogenesis of late aortic stump dehiscence are persistent periaortic infection and bacterial virulence.[23] To avoid this deadly complication, we and other surgeons began to experiment with in situ graft replacement.[24–26]

For the infrarenal abdominal aortic graft with infection of one or both groins, bacteria of low virulence, and a relatively small amount of pus, we prefer in situ abdominal aortic graft replacement wrapped with omentum, followed by lifelong antibiotic therapy. This treatment obviates the aortic stump problem related to virulence of bacteria, the problem of poor graft flow, and that of poor patency (Table 6).

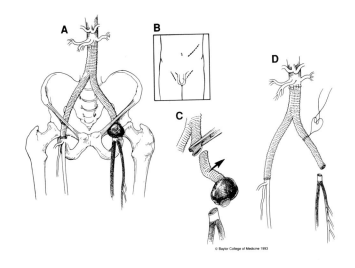

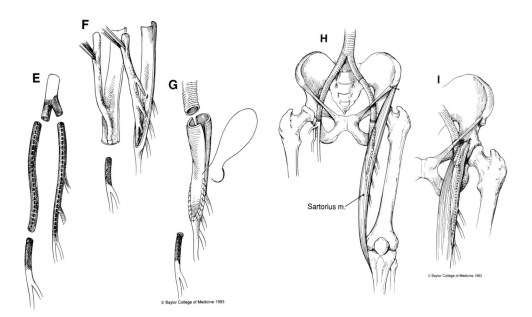

FIGURE 5.

A, local infection and false aneurysm of left distal anastomosis of aortobifemoral graft, and occlusion of deep femoral and superficial femoral arteries. **B,** incisions for partial removal of aortobifemoral graft. **C,** partial excision of graft. **D,** sutured partial graft replacement. **E,** endarterectomy of left deep femoral and superficial femoral arteries. **F** and **G,** profundaplasty of left deep femoral artery using autologous superficial artery. **H** and **I,** sartorius muscle mobilized and wrapped around arterial reconstruction.

TABLE 7.
Muscle Flaps for Regional Coverage*

Region	Muscles
Neck to supraclavicular fossa	Sternocleidomastoid
	Pectoralis major
	Latissimus dorsi
Mediastinum	Pectoralis major
	Omentum
	Rectus abdominis
	Latissimus dorsi (rarely)
Trunk–lateral chest	External oblique/serratus anterior
	Rectus abdominis
	Latissimus dorsi
	Pectoralis major
	Omentum
Groin to upper thigh	Rectus femoris
	Rectus abdominis
	Tensor fascia lata
	Sartorius

*Modified from Mixter RC, Turnipseed WD, Smith DJ, et al: *J Vasc Surg* 1989; 9:472–478.

We prefer in situ treatment for localized or circumscribed and chronic aortic sepsis and also for patients with aortoduodenal fistula.[27, 28] After complete excision of all prosthetic graft material, the patient must be treated with radical debridement of all inflammatory retroperitoneal tissue, including the aorta. The in situ aorta is then reconstructed to restore distal perfusion and the graft is separated from the overlying gastrointestinal tract by interposition of viable tissue such as omentum or prevertebral fascia.[29] In our opinion this is best followed by long-term antibiotics, 6 weeks IV, and lifelong oral therapy (Fig 3).

We also believe that an infected infrarenal aortic graft is best replaced with a homograft. The homograft is an excellent temporary measure for 2 or 3 years, after which it is replaced with a prosthetic graft. Homografts provide optimal resistance to infection, permitting a patient to fully recover from infection before the prosthetic implant. They are not a permanent solution, especially when dealing with highly virulent organisms and incompletely debrided infected tissues. Homograft antigenicity, causing late deterioration, probably due to an immunologic reaction, must be considered. Kieffer et al.[30] suggests careful debridement, coverage of homograft with viable tissue, administration of appropriate antibiotics, and close clinical and ultrasonic surveillance after in situ replacement. Unfortunately, we do not yet have confirmation of the benefit of homografts provided by long-term results (Fig 4).

A further problem with the homograft is storage. Possibly this problem could be solved with an organization of homograft arterial cryopreservation banks.

With aortofemoral grafts it is also important to avoid wound infection of the groin, as this has resulted in an increasing incidence of late anastomotic false aneurysms or overt graft infection.[31, 32] Most infected groin problems may be managed conservatively, with radical graft excision necessary for only a few intractable cases. Therefore we propose different surgical solutions, depending on the circumstances.[33-36] If the graft is patent, intact prosthetic graft surgery can wait and the patient is treated solely with antibiotic therapy. If the graft is occluded, we perform partial removal of the graft. If there is anastomotic false aneurysm or bleeding, we conduct graft removal. In all cases we employ radical debridement and IV antibiotics, with muscle flaps to cover the infected groin wound (Fig 5).

In the selection of a muscle flap, certain technical criteria must be considered. In the island flap design, there must be enough leverage at the rotation point to cover the wound totally. The vascular supply of the muscle must be preserved, since the success of the procedure depends on the viability of the muscle and there must be only limited functional loss from the donor site.[37] The muscles we use most frequently for groin infection are the sartorius and rectus abdominis (Table 7).

ASCENDING AND TRANSVERSE AORTIC ARCH GRAFT

As ascending and transverse aortic arch graft infection is not an area in which the choice of graft excision and extraanatomic bypass is applicable. With an infected ascending arch graft, we check the graft for patency, the infection's resistance to antibiotics, and aortic valve insufficiency or aortocardiac fistula. Occasionally, in cases of less obvious pus or when removal of a graft is hazardous owing to severe adhesions, or when disruption between the graft and arterial wall would also be hazardous, we treat this portion of a graft with antibiotic therapy alone. Otherwise, the graft is excised and replaced. The perigraft inflammation, mediastinum, and chest wall are debrided to remove all existing infection, and the sternum is wrapped with omentum (Fig 6).

THORACOABDOMINAL AORTIC GRAFT

The few known cases of infected thoracoabdominal aortic prostheses suggest that most of the infections are fatal and therefore go unreported. This portion of the aorta is also not feasible for extraanatomic bypass. For the infected graft of the thoracoabdominal aorta, our guidelines for treatment are prompt reoperation with complete debridement of the infection area and necrotic tissue. The infected prosthetic material is removed and replaced in situ, and blood flow is restored through clean operative fields. Dead space around the prosthesis is filled with healthy, well-vascularized tissue. The tissue used around the prosthesis may be available locally from thymus gland, mediastinal pleura, or may be a pedicle flap of omentum or pectoral muscle. A perigraft catheter is inserted for antibiotics administration for 6 weeks.[38] This is followed by lifelong oral antibiotics (Fig 7).

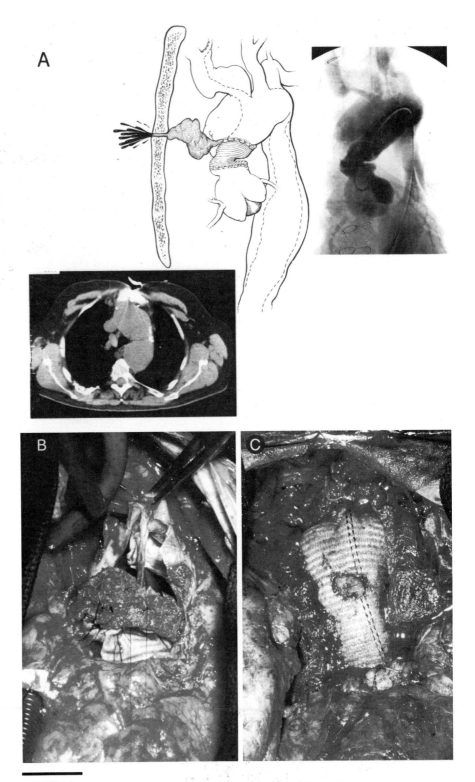

FIGURE 6.
A, CT scan *(lower left inset)* showing infection of ascending aorta, transverse arch, and descending aorta. *Line drawing* shows ascending aortocutaneous fistula. *Upper right inset:* Aortogram. **B,** the previous aortic graft in place with felt, and with false and true lumina of dissected aorta. **C,** the new Dacron graft; ascending and transverse aorta. **B,** the previous aortic graft in place with felt, and with false and true lumina of dissected aorta. **C,** the new Dacron graft; ascending and transverse aorta.

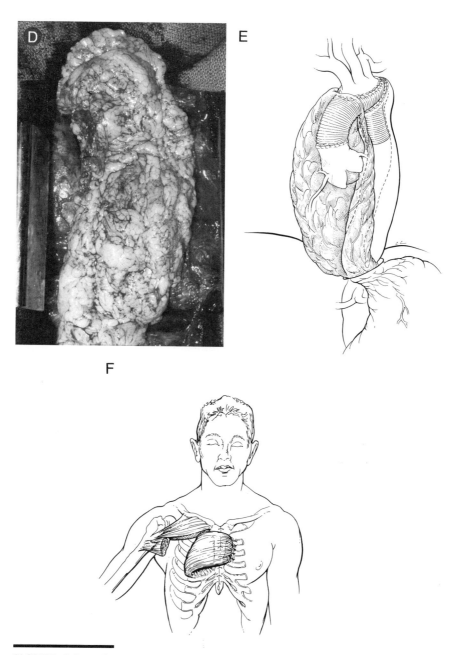

FIGURE 6 (cont.).

D, the greater omentum wrapped around the ascending aorta and mediastinal structure. **E,** replacement of graft, ascending aorta, transverse arch, and descending aorta using elephant trunk technique, wrapped with greater omentum. **F,** sternum wrapped with right pectoral muscle.

MULTIPLE GRAFT INFECTIONS

Recently, we were met with the challenge of a patient with a history of multiple aortic bypass graft operations and graft infections. His preoperative diagnosis was descending thoracic aortic bifemoral bypass graft infection. We removed the descending bifemoral bypass graft, replacing

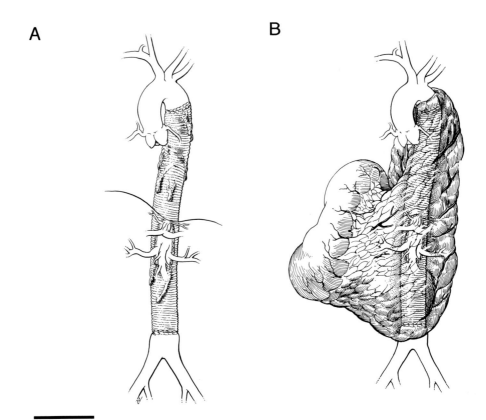

FIGURE 7.

A, infected graft, thoracoabdominal aorta. **B,** graft replacement with greater omentum wrap.

it with a polytetrafluoroethylene (PTFE) bifurcation graft via thoracoabdominal exploration (Fig 8).

GRAFT MATERIAL

Currently, we see no greater value in Dacron or PTFE for initial graft placement. Persistent high rates of mortality and morbidity demand development of better methods for prevention of primary or secondary aortic graft infection.

Either Dacron or PTFE can be used for in situ graft replacement, but there remains in either the probability of new graft infection. Some experimental studies have suggested that PTFE resists infection better than Dacron. However, no randomized clinical study concludes that Dacron is more vulnerable to infection than PTFE. Thus, at present, there is no firm principle favoring the choice of one of these replacement graft types over the other.

Research continues on the still controversial methods of graft endothelial seeding and antibiotic-bonded grafts. Grafts seeded with autologous endothelial cells[39] and antibiotic-bonded grafts (with a collagen matrix release system) may resist late bacteremic challenge. So far, studies

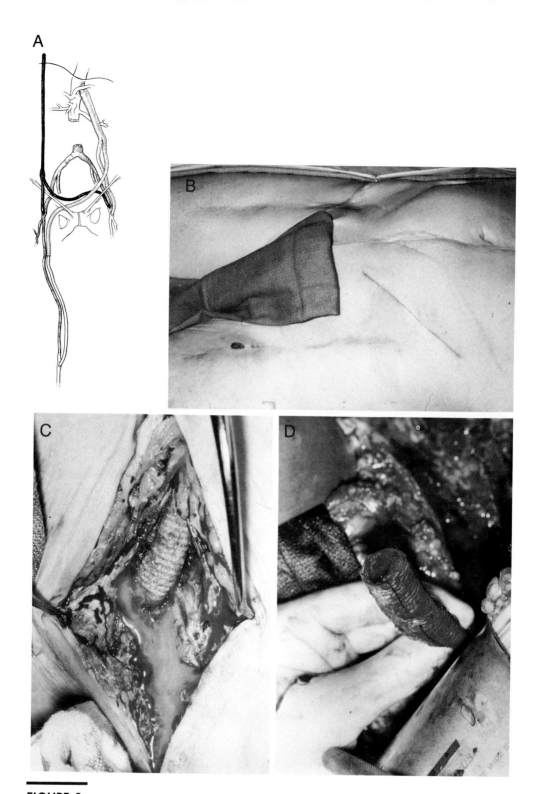

FIGURE 8.

A. occluded axillobifemoral Dacron graft and infected abdominal aortobifemoral popliteal Dacron graft, replaced with descending bifemoral bypass graft with poly-tetrafluoroethylene (PTFE) femoropopliteal graft. **B.** multiple scars and draining pus on left thigh. **C,** left groin incision showing infected graft and pus. **D,** removal of infected descending thoracoabdominal aortic graft through thoracoabdominal approach.

(Continued.)

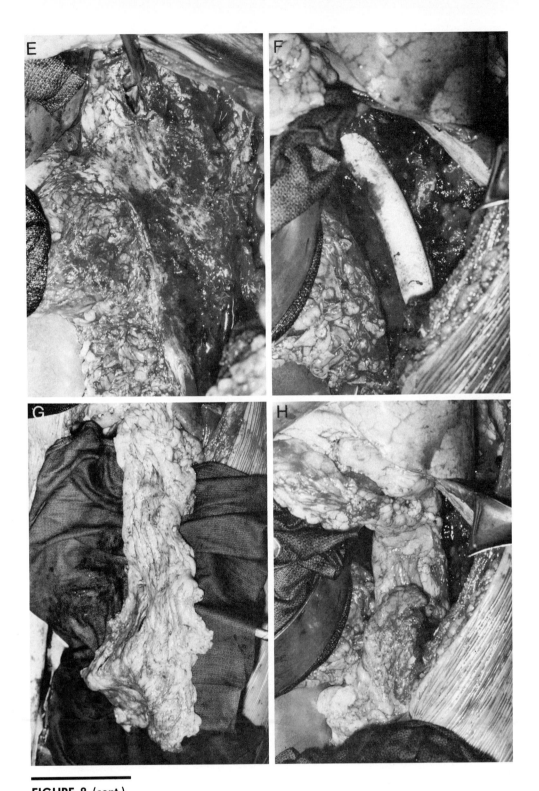

FIGURE 8 (cont.).

E, descending thoracoabdominal aortic graft removed. **F,** descending aortobifemoral PTFE graft in place. **G,** mobilized greater omentum. **H,** greater omentum wrapped around PTFE graft.

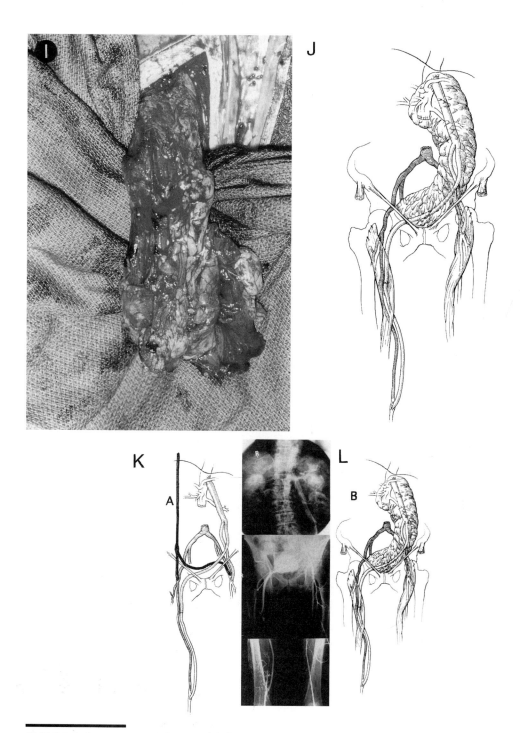

FIGURE 8 (cont.).

I, mobilized sartorius muscle. **J,** new graft with omentum, wrapped and sutured. **K,** aortogram and artist's illustration of descending thoracic aortic graft in place as well as occluded previous axillobifemoral graft. **L,** illustration of descending thoracic aortobifemoral graft in situ replacement and greater omental wrap; sartorius muscle wrap for groin.

of antibiotic bonding conclude that antibiotic effectiveness persists for at least 1 week, and can serve as a prophylactic tool against perioperative vascular graft infection, but require additional supplemental antibiotics in the presence of preexisting infection.[40-43]

SUMMARY

Aortic graft infection is a rare, but very serious complication of vascular surgery. The ideal treatment for graft infection is yet to be found. We believe that in situ replacement of infected grafts in the ascending aorta, transverse arch, thoracoabdominal aorta, and infrarenal abdominal aorta to be the most practical. The new graft is wrapped with viable pedicle tissue, and IV antibiotics are administered for 6 weeks followed by lifelong oral antibiotics. In our practice, the role of extraanatomic replacement is reserved for infrarenal aortic graft infection with no groin involvement. The homograft is a temporary alternative for borrowing time in the hope that infection can first be irradicated before ultimate, prosthetic graft in situ replacement. In the future, new techniques, such as graft pretreatment with antibiotics, or endothelial seeding, may substantially reduce graft infection. For the time being, we believe that treatment for graft infection based on careful consideration of clinical presentation, location of the infected graft, and appropriate surgery, with equal attention to appropriate antibiotics, will give the most acceptable results.

ACKNOWLEDGMENT

We gratefully acknowledge Amy Wirtz Newland's editorial assistance.

REFERENCES

1. O'Brien T, Collin J: Prosthetic vascular graft infection. Br J Surg 1992; 79:1262–1267.
2. Yeager RA, Porter JM: Arterial and prosthetic graft infection. Ann Vasc Surg 1992; 6:485–491.
3. Herbst A, Kamme C, Norgen L, et al: Infections and antibiotic prophylaxis in reconstructive vascular surgery. Eur J Vasc Surg 1989; 3:303–307.
4. Earnshaw JJ, Slack RCB, Hopkinson B, et al: Risk factors in vascular surgical sepsis. Ann R Coll Surg Engl 1988; 70:139–143.
5. Bickerstaff LK, Hollier LH, Van Peenan HS, et al: Abdominal aortic aneurysm repair combined with a second procedure—morbidity and mortality. Surgery 1984; 95:487–491.
6. Thomas JH, McCroskey BL, Iliopoulos JI, et al: Aorto-iliac reconstruction combined with non-vascular operations. Am J Surg 1983; 146:784–787.
7. Ricotta JJ, Faggioli GL, Stella A, et al: Total excision and extra-anatomic by-pass for aortic graft infection. Am J Surg 1991; 162:145–149.
8. Bandyk DF, Berni GA, Thiele BL, et al: Aortofemoral graft infection due to Staphylococcus epidermidis. Arch Surg 1984; 119:102–108.
9. Bunt TJ: Synthetic vascular graft infections. Surgery 1983; 93:733–746.
10. Martin LF, Harris JM, Fehr DM, et al: Vascular prosthetic infection with Staphylococcus epidermidis: Experimental study of pathogenesis and therapy. J Vasc Surg 1989; 9:464–471.

11. Bergamini TM, Bandyk DF, Govostis D, et al: Infection of vascular prostheses caused by bacterial biofilms. *J Vasc Surg* 1988; 7:21–30.

12. Malone JM, Lalka SG, McIntyre KE, et al: The necessity for long-term antibiotic therapy with positive arterial wall cultures. *J Vasc Surg* 1988; 8:262–267.

13. Hansen ME, Yucel EK, Waltman AC: STIR imaging of synthetic vascular graft infection. *Cardiovasc Intervent Radiol* 1993; 16:30–36.

14. LaMuraglia GM, Fischman AJ, Strauss HW, et al: Utility of the indium 111-labeled human immunoglobulin G scan for the detection of focal vascular graft infection. *J Vasc Surg* 1989; 10:20–28.

15. Fiorani P, Speziale F, Rizzo L, et al: Detection of aortic graft infection with leukocytes labeled with technetium 99m-hexametazime. *J Vasc Surg* 1993; 17:87–96.

16. Olofsson PA, Auffermann W, Higgins CB, et al: Diagnosis of prosthetic aortic graft infection by magnetic resonance imaging. *J Vasc Surg* 1988; 8:99–105.

17. O'Hara PJ, Hertzer NR, Beven EG, et al: Surgical management of infected abdominal grafts: Review of a 25-year experience. *J Vasc Surg* 1986; 3:725–731.

18. Rutherford RB, Patt A, Pearce WH: Extra-anatomic bypass: A closer view. *J Vasc Surg* 1987; 6:437–446.

19. Yeager RA, Moneta GL, Taylor LM, et al: Improving survival and limb salvage in patients with aortic graft infection. *Am J Surg* 1990; 159:466–469.

20. Porter JM, Harris EJ, Taylor LM, et al: Extra-anatomic bypass: A new look (supporting view). *Adv Surg* 1993; 26:133–149.

21. Reilly LM, Stoney RJ, Goldstone J, et al: Improved management of aortic graft infection: The influence of operation sequence and staging. *J Vasc Surg* 1987; 5:421–431.

22. Stoney RJ, Quigley TM: Extra-anatomic bypass: A new look (opposing view). *Adv Surg* 1993; 26:151–162.

23. Blaisdell FW, Hass AD: Axillary-femoral artery bypass for lower extremity ischemia. *Surgery* 1963; 54:563–568.

24. Bandyk DF: Diagnosis and treatment of biomaterial-associated vascular infections. *Infect Dis Clin North Am* 1992; 6:719–729.

25. Bandyk DF, Bergamini TM, Kinney EV, et al: In situ replacement of vascular prostheses infected by bacterial biofilms. *J Vasc Surg* 1991; 13:575–583.

26. Robinson AJ, Johansen K: Aortic sepsis: Is there a role for in situ graft reconstruction? *J Vasc Surg* 1991; 13:677–684.

27. Walker WE, Cooley DA, Duncan JM, et al: The management of aortoduodenal fistula by *in situ* replacement of the infected abdominal aortic graft. *Ann Surg* 1987; 205:727–732.

28. Higgins RSD, Steed DL, Julian TB, et al: The management of aortoenteric and paraprosthetic fistulae. *J Cardiovasc Surg* 1990; 31:81–86.

29. Mehran RJ, Graham AM, Ricci MA, et al: Evaluation of muscle flaps in the treatment of infected aortic grafts. *J Vasc Surg* 1992; 15:487–494.

30. Kieffer E, Bahnini A, Koskas F, et al: In situ homograft replacement of infected infrarenal aortic prosthetic grafts: Results in forty-three patients. *J Vasc Surg* 1993; 17:349–356.

31. Newington DP, Houghton PW, Baird RN, et al: Groin wound infection after arterial surgery. *Br J Surg* 1991; 78:617–619.

32. Taylor SM, Mills JL, Fujitani RM, et al: The influence of groin sepsis on extraanatomic bypass patency in patients with prosthetic graft infection. *Ann Vasc Surg* 1992; 6:80–84.

33. Samson RH, Veith FJ, Janko GS, et al: A modified classification and approach to the management of infections involving peripheral arterial prosthetic grafts. *J Vasc Surg* 1988; 8:147–158.

34. Calligaro KD, Westcott CJ, Buckley RM, et al: Infrainguinal anastomotic arterial graft infections treated by selective graft preservation. *Ann Surg* 1992; 216:74–79.
35. Calligaro KD, Veith FJ, Schwartz ML, et al: Are gram-negative bacteria a contraindication to selective preservation of infected prosthetic arterial grafts? *J Vasc Surg* 1992; 16:337–346.
36. Cherry KJ, Roland CF, Pairolero PC, et al: Infected femorodistal bypass: Is graft removal mandatory? *J Vasc Surg* 1992; 15:295–305.
37. Mixter RC, Turnipseed WD, Smith DJ, et al: Rotational muscle flaps: A new technique for covering infected vascular grafts. *J Vasc Surg* 1989; 9:472–478.
38. Hargrove WC, Edmunds LH: Management of infected thoracic aortic prosthetic graft. *Ann Thorac Surg* 1984; 37:72–77.
39. Keller JD, Falk J, Bjornson S, et al: Bacterial infectibility of chronically implanted endothelial cell-seeded expanded polytetrafluoroethylene vascular grafts. *J Vasc Surg* 1988; 7:524–530.
40. Chervu A, Moore WS, Gelabert HA, et al: Prevention of graft infection by use of prostheses bonded with rifampin/collagen release system. *J Vasc Surg* 1991; 14:521–525.
41. Chervu A, Moore WS, Chvapil M, et al: Efficacy and duration of antistaphylococcal activity comparing three antibiotics bonded to Dacron vascular grafts with a collagen release system. *J Vasc Surg* 1991; 13:897–901.
42. Colburn MD, Moore WS, Chvapil M, et al: Use of an antibiotic-bonded graft for in situ reconstruction after prosthetic graft infections. *J Vasc Surg* 1992; 16:651–660.
43. Haverich A, Hirt S, Karck M, et al: Prevention of graft infection by bonding of gentamycin to Dacron prostheses. *J Vasc Surg* 1992; 15:187–193.

Advances in the Noninvasive Diagnosis and Surgical Management of Chronic Venous Insufficiency

Agustin A. Rodriguez, M.D.
Vascular Surgery Fellow, Tufts University School of Medicine, New England
Medical Center Hospitals, Boston, Massachusetts

Thomas F. O'Donnell, Jr., M.D.
Chief, Vascular Surgery Section, Professor of Surgery and Chair, Department of
Surgery, Tufts University School of Medicine, New England Medical Center
Hospitals, Boston, Massachusetts

V enous surgery preceded arterial surgery, yet progress in venous reconstruction has lagged significantly behind advances in arterial reconstruction. The precise reason for this developmental difference is not
known, although two factors have likely played major roles: (1) lack of
accurate tests to establish the presence of venous insufficiency and to
gauge its severity, and (2) the equivocal efficacy of surgery for reflux disease.

The conventional management of advanced chronic venous insufficiency (Society for Vascular Surgery/International Society for Cardiovascular Surgery [SVS/ISCVS] stage II or III)[1] has entailed the use of a pano-
ply of lotions and creams for skin care as well as compressive bandages,
none of which has been shown to be superior to the original compressive
bandage developed by Unna over 100 years ago.[2] Frustration over the inability of some ulcers to heal with conservative therapy, and, more important, the frequent recurrence of ulcers, led to the development of a
variety of surgical procedures. Most of these procedures were carried out
on the superficial system, without regard for abnormalities in the deep
system. The interruption of perforating veins, as well as the stripping and
ligation of the saphenous vein, carried a recurrence rate of anywhere from
20% to 30%.[3] The birth of modern venous surgery based on anatomic and
physiologic criteria had to await refinements in venography and the development of novel noninvasive techniques.

It is the purpose of this chapter to review recent advances in both
noninvasive diagnosis and surgical management of chronic venous insufficiency (CVI).

Advances in Vascular Surgery, vol. 2
© 1994, Mosby–Year Book, Inc.

PATIENT EVALUATION

Several questions must be answered during the evaluation of patients with CVI:

1. Is CVI present?
2. How severe is it?
3. What is the pathologic process—obstruction, valvular incompetence, or both?
4. What are the levels (proximal, distal, proximal and distal) and systems (deep, perforator, superficial, individually or in combination) involved?

Currently available noninvasive methods for assessing CVI can be divided into *hemodynamic*, e.g., photoplethysmography (PPG), air plethysmography (APG) and *anatomic*, e.g., duplex scan (DS), methods. This division is not rigid, since physiologic information can also be gained from the DS by calculation of the valve closure time. By utilizing these various tests, the precise level and degree of involvement can be determined and surgical therapy instituted when appropriate.

QUANTITATIVE PHOTOPLETHYSMOGRAPHY

Rationale

Photoplethysmography is a simple, inexpensive and operator-independent technique for evaluating patients with CVI. We prefer quantitative photoplethysmography (QPG) by light reflection rheography (LRR) over PPG because it provides quantitative information on both venous emptying and venous refill times. The LRR contains three light-emitting diodes (LEDs) and a thermistor probe. Light emitted through the skin is reflected back from red blood cells in direct proportion to the blood content of the subdermal venous plexus. Reflected light is translated into an electric signal which allows quantification of venous blood volume.

Technique

The probe is taped 10 cm above the medial malleolus. A baseline measurement is taken with the patient seated and the foot placed flat on the floor. The patient is then instructed to perform ten tiptoe exercises over a 15-second period. The examination is repeated three to five times with a 3-minute rest period in between exercises, to prevent effects mediated by reactive hyperemia. In order to avoid temperature artifacts, only patients with skin temperatures in the range of 28° to 32° C should be studied. The probe should not be placed over areas of active infection or inflammation.

Normally, there will be a decrease in blood volume following exercise, which will return to baseline after 25 seconds. If there is no normalization of flow after 25 seconds, tourniquets are applied above the ankle and above and below the knee and the test is repeated with sequential removal of these tourniquets. If there is complete normalization, the patient has isolated superficial system incompetency. If the time interval is shortened by more than 5 seconds, the patient has combined superficial and deep system incompetency. The location of the tourniquet(s) respon-

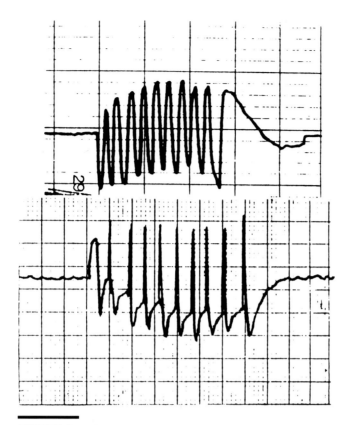

FIGURE 1.

Comparison between light reflection rheography *(top)* and invasive venous pressure measurements *(bottom).* This patient was shown to have deep valvular incompetency on descending phlebography. Both studies show a shortened venous refill time (<5 seconds) and a failure of the ambulatory venous pressure to decrease with exercise, resulting in venous hypertension. (From O'Donnell TF: The surgical management of deep venous valvular incompetence, in Rutherford RB (ed): *Vascular Surgery,* ed 3. Philadelphia, WB Saunders, 1989, pp 1612–1626. Used by permission.)

sible for the normalization or improvement points to the level of involvement. LRR was compared with invasive pressure measurements in our laboratory[4] and significant correlation was established (r = .93, P < .05). Excellent correlation was also observed between the drop in venous pressure with exercise and the concomitant change in light reflection (Fig 1).

AIR PLETHYSMOGRAPHY

Rationale

Christopoulos et al.[5] described a plethysmographic technique which provides several important parameters of venous physiology. APG is used to evaluate both reflux (by measurement of venous refill time, VRT) as well as the integrity of the calf muscle pump (by calculation of the venous ejection fraction, EF). APG also provides an indirect estimation of ambulatory venous pressure. APG assesses volume changes within the entire limb.

Technique

A tubular polyvinyl sleeve is placed over the calf and is connected to a pressure transducer which has been calibrated with a known volume of saline (Fig 2). The air-filled cuff is then applied to the calf and the leg is elevated 45 degrees. This provides a baseline reading of the empty leg. Volume changes are derived from pressure changes in the sensing cuff. The patient quickly stands while holding onto a walker so that the body weight is supported by the contralateral leg. Venous filling of the leg is then recorded continuously, until a plateau is reached, which is the functional venous volume (VV). By convention, 90% of VV is used in calculating the venous filling index (VFI). The time to reach 90% VV is defined as venous filling time 90% (VFT 90) while the venous filling index, a measure of reflux, is calculated from 90% VV/VFT 90 (in mL/sec). The VFI relates directly to the degree of venous reflux present and is independent of the venous volume reservoir. Normal VFI is usually less than

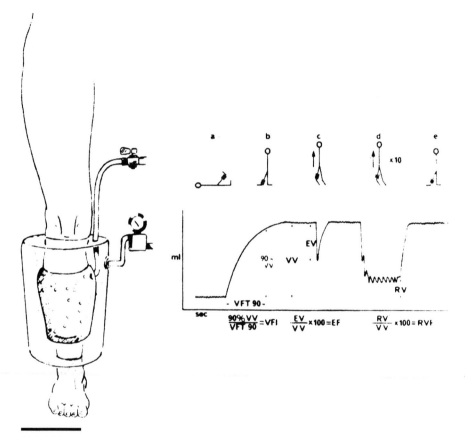

FIGURE 2.

Diagram of the technique of air plethysmography as described by Christopoulos et al.[5] Representative volume changes with patient supine (a), with weight on contralateral leg (b and e), with one tiptoe exercise (c), and with ten tiptoe exercises (d). VFT = venous filling time; VFI = venous filling index; RVF = residual volume fraction; EF = ejection fraction; RV = residual volume; EV = ejected volume; VV = functional venous volume. (From O'Donnell TF Jr, McEnroe CS, Heggerick P: Surg Clin North Am 1990; 70:176. Used by permission.)

2 seconds, while in patients with popliteal venous reflux, the range is 7 to 28 seconds. Tourniquets are applied to the leg to assess the contribution of the superficial venous system. The patient then performs a tiptoe movement with both legs and shifts weight off the test leg. The amount of volume decrease in the APG is the ejection volume (EV). The EF is then calculated as EF = EV/VV × 100. EF represents the degree of fitness of the calf muscle pump. When a steady plateau is again reached, the patient performs ten rapid tiptoe exercises. The residual volume is then the difference between volume at the end of the tiptoe exercises and the baseline. The residual volume fraction (RVF), which has been shown to correlate with the ambulatory venous pressure (AVP), is then calculated as RVF = RV/VV × 100. In summary, APG determines the degree of reflux, the capability of the calf muscle pump, and the AVP.

DUPLEX SCAN

Rationale
Duplex scanning provides the following information: (1) the cause of deep venous reflux, i.e., postthrombotic syndrome (PTS) vs. primary valvular incompetency; (2) the levels involved, i.e., superficial, communicating veins, or deep; and (3) the magnitude of reflux. This technique has been used for at least 10 years, and while it is the most sensitive examination available, it is highly operator- and interpreter-dependent. Duplex imaging permits examination of the superficial venous system, including the greater and lesser saphenous veins as well as the perforating veins.[6] The deep venous system—femoral, superficial femoral popliteal, and calf veins—can also be scrutinized.

Technique
All patients are examined supine and prone on a standard tilt table in 45-degree reverse Trendelenburg's position. This allows for maximal filling of the venous tree and is essential for evaluation of the perforating veins. All evaluations are done with an 8-MHz probe which allows for a 4.0-cm depth of penetration, with axial and lateral resolutions of 0.3 mm and 0.7 mm respectively.

APPLICATION OF NONINVASIVE TECHNIQUES

Evaluation of the Superficial and Deep Systems
The superficial and deep venous systems are evaluated first for the presence or absence of acute or chronic thrombus, as described by Karkow et al.[7] The internal diameter of all vessels is noted, documenting the extent of superficial varicosities and deep venomegaly, when present. Doppler signals are obtained at the common femoral level with attention to the normal spontaneous and phasic signals. The iliac veins are indirectly evaluated using the integrated pulsed Doppler signal at the level of the common femoral vein (CFV). A spontaneous and phasic signal is indirect evidence of proximal patency. Gross distention of the CFV and difficulty compressing vessel walls in the absence of intraluminal thrombus is indirect evidence of proximal venous outflow obstruction. Valvular competency is also determined using the integrated pulsed Doppler sig-

nal. The Valsalva maneuver, proximal and distal manual compression, automatic pneumatic tourniquets, as well as having a patient blow into a rubber glove, can all be used in an attempt to elicit reflux. Final determination of the integrity of each valve is made by reviewing the audible Doppler as well as the recorded spectrum for signs of unidirectional or bidirectional flow.

Evaluation of the Communicating System
Evaluation of the perforating veins begins at midthigh, followed by the calf and ankle regions.[8] Perforating veins are those that penetrate the fascia and which can be seen to connect the superficial and deep systems. Attention is directed to evaluating their anatomic and functional characteristics, as was done for the superficial and deep veins. Venous flow characteristics were evaluated by directing the integrated pulsed Doppler signal into the perforator lumen and having the patient perform a Valsalva maneuver, or through manual compression. Valvular integrity is determined by documenting unidirectional (competent) or bidirectional (incompetent) flow. The precise location of these incompetent perforating veins can be marked on the skin with an indelible marker.

Anatomic B-Mode
Changes in the superficial venous system consistent with varicose involvement are indicated by an increased saphenous vein diameter and variation in wall thickness, as well as similar changes in the saphenous tributaries. Chronic deep venous involvement usually presents with recanalization changes: the vein demonstrates an irregular lumen with highly echoic and thickened walls. Venous occlusion reveals echoic homogeneous material in the vessel lumen. The echo characteristics of the thrombus are dependent on the collagen content, and generally, older occlusions are hyperechoic. The vein wall is noncompressible and there is no flow in the vein. Occasionally, collaterals are visualized proximal and distal to the occlusion, especially when it has been a longstanding occlusion.

Valvular incompetency resulting from postthrombotic changes is characterized by either absent or markedly thickened valves. Motionless, scarred valves that fail to coapt are observed on dynamic scanning. Primary valvular incompetency, on the other hand, appears as redundant and multifolded valve structures.

DUPLEX QUANTITATION OF VALVE CLOSURE TIME

Rationale
Recent studies by van Bemmelen et al.[9] have shown that the Valsalva maneuver may not be sufficient to provoke reflux in a significant percentage of patients, and thus may underestimate the degree of reflux.

Technique
van Bemmelen et al.[9] have standardized an alternative method which produces uniform reflux. Patients are examined in the upright position while holding onto a walker and supporting their weight on the contralateral leg. A pressure cuff is placed around the limb and inflated to occlude venous flow, then rapidly deflated. The duration of venous flow proxi-

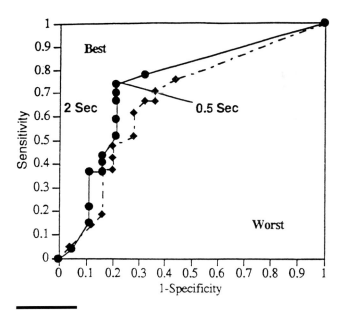

FIGURE 3.

Receiver operator characteristic curve for popliteal valve closure time by duplex ultrasound using (-●-) normal to mild (SVS/ISCVS stages 0 and I) chronic venous insufficiency (CVI) vs. moderate to severe CVI (stages II and III) as the outcome measure and (-♦-) using ulcerated (stage III) vs. nonulcerated (stages 0, I and II). (From Iafrati MD, Welch H, O'Donnell TF, et al: Correlation of venous noninvasive tests with the SVS/ISCVS clinical classification of chronic venous insufficiency. Presented at the New England Society for Vascular Surgery Meeting, Cambridge, Mass, Oct 28, 1993.

mal to the area of rapid pneumatic cuff deflation is recorded using Doppler spectral analysis. For the superficial femoral vein, a 24-cm-wide cuff is used, and is inflated to 80 mm Hg. For the evaluation of the popliteal vein, a 12-cm-wide cuff is applied around the calf and inflated to 100 mm Hg. The distance between the cuff and the transducer was always less than 5 cm. Examination of the tibial veins is done with a foot cuff inflated to 120 mm Hg. Both color Doppler and spectral analysis are recorded and the latter is used to quantify the degree of reflux. Normal reflux time using this technique is less than 0.5 second (Fig 3). Masuda and Kistner[10] have compared this technique to descending venography and found that competency of the valve correlated best with reflux times shorter than 1 second.

AMBULATORY STRAIN-GAUGE PLETHYSMOGRAPHY

Rationale

The noninvasive "cousin" of ambulatory venous pressure measurements, ambulatory strain-gauge plethysmography attempts to correlate changes in calf volume following exercise with the degree of venous insufficiency present.

Technique

Silastic strain gauges are placed circumferentially around the calf at its widest portion. Compression cuffs similar to those used for measurement of duplex valve closure time are placed around the thigh. Venous occlusion is produced by rapid inflation of the thigh cuffs to a pressure of 60 mm Hg, while subsequent changes in calf volume are continuously recorded (Fig 4). These measurements are performed at rest with the leg elevated approximately 30 cm above the level of the heart. After obtaining baseline measurements, exercise tests are then performed.[11] The strain gauges are taped securely in place to avoid movement during exercise. The treadmill is set at an angle of 10 degrees and a speed of 7 km/hr, and the patient is required to walk for a period of at least 3 minutes during which calf volumes are continuously recorded. Volume curves for the plethysmographic recordings are measured at 5, 10, 15, 20, 30, 60, 100, 120, 140, and 180 seconds following the initiation of exercise. At each of these intervals the changes in the calf volume are measured, and each value is compared to the resting baseline.

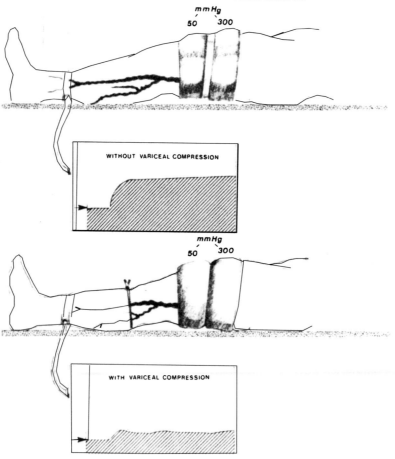

FIGURE 4.

Schematic of the technique for strain-gauge plethysmography. Changes in calf volume following inflation of proximal, then distal cuffs can be correlated with grade of venous reflux *(top)*. The contribution of the superficial venous system can be assessed by the placement of a superficial tourniquet prior to cuff inflation *(bottom)*. (From O'Donnell TF Jr, McEnroe CS, Heggerick P: *Surg Clin North Am* 1990; 70:175). Used by permission.)

A RATIONAL APPROACH TO DIAGNOSIS

We now examine how these various tests can help in establishing if CVI is present. Since many patients present with leg swelling, without other stigmata of CVI, it is important to rule out lymphedema and other systemic causes.

IS CVI PRESENT?

Quantitative photoplethysmography can be used reliably to establish the presence of CVI. Sarin et al.[12] have compared PPG to DS (using the latter as the gold standard), and have found PPG to have reliable sensitivity and better specificity with 15 seconds as the optimal discriminant value.

SEVERITY OF CVI

In our laboratory,[13] we evaluated 770 limbs by QPG and showed good correlation between VRT and the clinical severity of CVI.[4] These results are similar to earlier studies employing AVP measurements.[5] Eighty percent of patients with stage III disease had VRTs of less than 15 seconds, and a mean VRT of 9 seconds. EF by APG failed to correlate with clinical grade of disease. RVF, VFI, VRT, and valve closure time all demonstrated trends toward progressive deterioration of venous hemodynamics as the clinical severity of CVI worsened.

WHAT SYSTEMS ARE INVOLVED

The precise level of involvement has important therapeutic implications. Patients with advanced stage II or III disease and only superficial system involvement will benefit from simple saphenous vein stripping, with interruption of incompetent perforating veins (ICPVs), if present. With the use of tourniquets, PPG usually will distinguish between patients with superficial and deep venous incompetency in patients with *competent* perforating veins. DS with identification of ICPVs allows a more selective surgical approach by the use of limited incisions over the ICPV[8] or by laparoscopic methods.[14]

Recent efforts at selective preservation of the greater saphenous vein (GSV) mandates preoperative assessment of superficial valve competency. If the saphenous vein is dilated, tortuous, and grossly incompetent, it should be removed. In contrast, preservation of the GSV is associated with lower morbidity and subsequent availability of an essential conduit. Valve closure time within the saphenous system assessed by DS, as described by van Bemmelen,[9] is quite satisfactory at making this determination. A recent study in our own laboratory of 65 limbs referred with varicose veins showed that 70% had an abnormal GSV as defined by reflux greater than 0.6 second, while incompetency was limited to branch veins in the remainder of the superficial system.[15] DS, therefore, allows preservation of the GSV in nearly one third of patients who require only ligation and excision of tributaries.

WHAT IS THE PATHOLOGIC PROCESS—OUTFLOW OBSTRUCTION, VALVULAR INCOMPETENCY, OR BOTH?

Air plethysmography and DS have unique attributes and should be regarded as complementary in the evaluation of the deep venous system.

APG provides a global hemodynamic assessment of venous function and sorts out the various hemodynamic components (e.g., valvular reflux by VFI; residual venous volume [RVV], which correlates with AVP; and the integrity of the calf muscle pump by EF). DS provides both anatomic as well as precise hemodynamic information regarding the function of a specific segment. More than 70% of patients with stage II or III disease have deep venous system involvement, and valvular incompetency is the major underlying pathologic feature in more than 90% of them.[11]

ASSESSMENT OF OUTFLOW OBSTRUCTION

Raju and Fredericks[16] have emphasized the need to establish the functional (hemodynamic) rather than the anatomic significance of phlebographically proven ileofemoral obstruction in deciding the need for surgery. They recommend measuring arm-foot pressure differences both at rest and following reactive hyperemia, where normal limbs will exhibit less than a 5-mm Hg pressure difference. In contrast, patients with mild to moderate outflow obstruction will have a resting pressure difference of greater than 5 mm Hg, which will increase to the range of 10 to 15 mm Hg following reactive hyperemia. In limbs with severe venous outflow obstruction, the resting pressure difference is in the 15 to 20-mm Hg range, and it does not increase following reactive hyperemia. APG can also be used to estimate the degree of outflow obstruction. Christopoulos et al.[5] have shown that normal limbs will expel approximately 40% of their total venous volume within the first second. In mild to moderate obstruction there is a reduction ranging from 30% to 40%. Patients with severe venous claudication expel less than 30% of their total venous volume during the first second. Recently, Baumgartner et al.[11] employed dynamic strain-gauge plethysmography to determine the degree of venous outflow obstruction. The baseline calf volume of a normal limb decreases during the initial 30 seconds of exercise then increases to 0.01 mL during 3 minutes of exercise, at which time a plateau is reached. Patients with mild to moderate venous obstruction demonstrate a greater increase in leg volume with exercise and a longer time to reach a plateau. In contrast, patients with significant outflow obstruction and venous claudication have a marked rise in limb volume within the first 1.5 minutes of exercise and never establish a plateau before exercise is curtailed by the onset of pain. At this point, the transport capacity of the collateral veins is insufficient for the exercise-induced increase in arterial flow. These last two techniques, APG and strain-gauge plethysmography, represent reliable noninvasive methods for determining the degree of outflow obstruction.

ASSESSMENT OF PERFORATOR INCOMPETENCY

Color-flow DS will not only visualize ICPVs but will also establish their location with sufficient precision to allow site-specific selective incisions (Fig 5).

ASSESSMENT OF DEEP VENOUS VALVULAR INCOMPETENCY

Total valve closure time provides the best balance between sensitivity and specificity for the determination of reflux. Only patients deemed to have

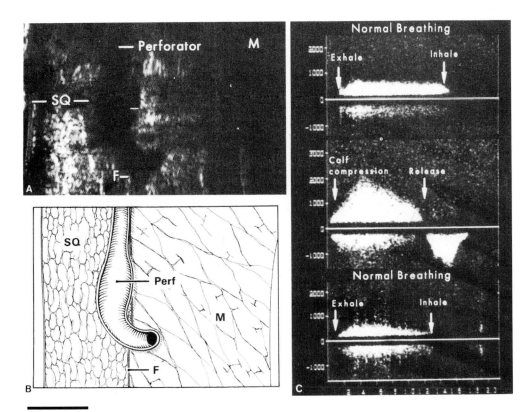

FIGURE 5.

Duplex image of incompetent perforator. Duplex scan image **(A)** and artist's rendering of incompetent perforating vein **(B)**. SQ = subcutaneous tissue; F = fascia; M = muscle; Perf = perforator. **(C)** Venous flow characteristics *(top to bottom)*: phasic venous flow variation with respiration; bidirectional venous flow following calf compression; and return of normal venous flow signal. x = *axis*, time (seconds); *y-axis*, frequency shift (Hz). (From Hanrahan LM, Araki CT, Fischer JB, et al: *J Cardiovasc Surg* 1991; 32:87–97. Used by permission.)

grade 3 or 4 reflux as described by van Bemmelen[9] should undergo descending phlebography in preparation for surgery.

IS THERE POSTOPERATIVE IMPROVEMENT?

Hemodynamic function should be routinely assessed with quantitative PPG, APG, and DS quantitation of valve closure time in patients following popliteal vein valve transplantation or valvuloplasty. Anatomic patency is best determined by duplex B-mode scan. Patients undergo ascending and descending phlebography within 2 weeks of surgery to determine the immediate postoperative patency rate.

SURGICAL THERAPY

The various surgical management options are outlined in Table 1.

SUPERFICIAL VENOUS INSUFFICIENCY

Patients with superficial venous insufficiency (SVI) should undergo superficial vein stripping and ligation with subfascial ligation of incompe-

TABLE 1.
Surgical Management of Chronic Venous Insufficiency

I. Superficial venous insufficiency
   A. Ligation and stripping
      1. Greater saphenous/tributaries
      2. Lesser saphenous/tributaries
   B. Interruption of perforating veins
II. Valvular reflux
   A. Primary valvular insufficiency
      1. Valvuloplasty
         a. Open
         b. Closed (angioscopic)
      2. External venous support
         a. Diameter reduction of vein by interrupted sutures
         b. Psathakis external sling
         c. Dacron "cuff"
   B. Postthrombotic syndrome
      1. Valve autotransplantation
      2. Vein segment transposition
III. Venous outflow obstruction
   A. Iliac vein obstruction
      1. Autogenous femorofemoral crossover graft
      2. Prosthetic femorofemoral crossover graft
   B. Femoral vein obstruction
      1. Autogenous saphenopopliteal bypass
      2. Prosthetic saphenopopliteal bypass

tent perforating veins when present. While ligation can be done through the traditional medial subfascial approach,[17] or through a more cosmetic posterior "stocking-seam" incision,[18] selective small incisions over the ICPV usually heal with the least noticeable scarring. DS can identify the specific site of ICPVs allowing ligation through small incisions directly over the perforator. Alternatively, the laparoscopic superficial approach can be applied.[14] Both techniques significantly reduce the morbidity associated with conventional approaches.

VALVULAR REFLUX
Patients with valvular reflux can be further classified based upon primary valvular insufficiency (PVI), PTS, or a combination of both.

PRIMARY VALVULAR INCOMPETENCY
Patients with isolated PVI are the best candidates for valvuloplasty. The valve most accessible for surgery is located in the proximal superficial femoral vein (SFV) near its junction with the profunda femoris vein (PFV). The CFV, SFV, PFV, and GSV are approached through a longitudinal incision placed over the CFV. Raju and Fredericks[16] prefer to carry out the dissection with a scalpel rather than with cautery to minimize veno-

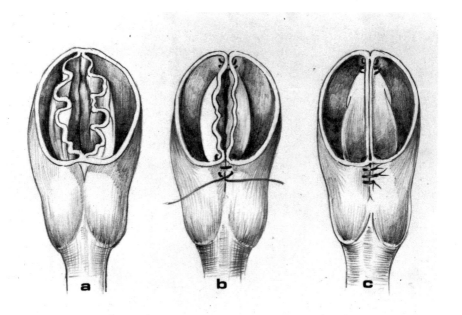

FIGURE 6.

Valvuloplasty by the open technique. A venotomy has been made above the valve, the valve is seen to be incompetent and floppy (a); one suture has been placed at either side (b); the valve cusps have been reefed with three interrupted 7-0 nonabsorbable (Prolene) sutures and competency has been achieved (c).

spasm. Unlike those veins that have had prior thrombophlebitis, there is no perivenous scarring surrounding the veins of patients with PVI. Approximately 4 cm of SFV is isolated. The proximal valve is recognized by its characteristic bulge in the proximal SFV. Following heparinization, soft, noncrushing vascular clamps are placed on the CFV, PFV, and SFV below the valve.

Three open approaches for exposure of the valve have been advocated. Kistner[19] prefers a longitudinal venotomy made at the valve commissure, whereas Raju and Fredericks[20] advocate a transverse venotomy placed above the valve. Sottiurai[21] uses a combination of transverse and longitudinal venotomy. The transverse venotomy is placed proximal to the valve structure at the level of the junction of the PFV and CFV. Extreme care should be exercised to avoid damage to the commissure. Kistner recommends that the longitudinal venotomy be started inferior to the valve, so that lengthening of the venotomy can be made while visualizing the valve commissure and cusps.[19]

We prefer to place 7-0 monofilament sutures through the vein wall for retraction in order to visualize the valve structures. The redundant wall cusp can then be "reefed" to the valve commissure by placing a 7-0 monofilament mattress suture at each commissure. Rather than passing the same suture through the valve structure to shorten it, we prefer interrupted mattress sutures (Fig 6). Raju and Frederick[16] recommend shortening the valve cusp length by about 20% at each commissure. This suture advances the valve cusp cephalad and thereby shortens the valve cusp. The double-armed stay sutures placed previously in the vein as stay sutures are then used to repair the venotomy using interrupted technique to minimize further reduction of the vessel lumen. Valve competency is then tested by the "strip test."

Alternatively, valvuloplasty can be carried out using the closed approach described by Kistner[19] or under angioscopic guidance as described and preferred by our group.[22]

When this last technique is employed, the angioscope is inserted through either a large tributary of the proximal GSV (which is invariably absent), or via a branch of the femoral vein and passed distally into the SFV (Fig 7). Saline solution is then infused through the angioscope to assess valvular competency. Once the diagnosis is confirmed, valve repair is then performed. Monofilament sutures are placed across the commissure of the valve leaflets from the outside, while the angioscope is used within the lumen to observe and guide suture placement. After placing two or three sutures on each side of the valve, it is again tested for competency by saline infusion under direct angioscopic visualization. Incompetent perforating veins should be interrupted when present. If superficial venous stripping is performed, it should not be done concomitantly with this procedure in order to avoid bleeding due to perioperative heparinization. Pneumatic compression boots and heparinization are used in the immediate postoperative period, and patients are maintained on Coumadin (warfarin sodium) for a period of 6 months, during which elastic compression stockings are worn.

Seven recently published series attempts to define the indication, role efficacy, and long-term outcome of direct valvular reconstruction for PVI.

Kistner and his group, who pioneered the development of direct valvular reconstruction, examined their results following venous valve re-

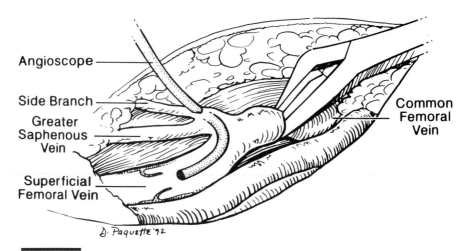

FIGURE 7.

Technique of angioscopic valvuloplasty. The angioscope is inserted through the tributary or stump of the previously ligated greater saphenous vein into the superficial femoral vein. Diagnosis of valvular incompetency is made, the valve is repaired, and competency of repair is assessed under direct visualization with the angioscope. (From Welch HJ, McLaughlin RL, O'Donnell TF: *J Vasc Surg* 1992; 16:694–700.)

construction in 51 limbs (48 patients).[10] Main indications for operation were severe stasis with ulceration (57%) or severe pain and edema (43%). The patients were also subdivided into three anatomic groups: PVI (47%), PTS (29%), and mixed (PVI-PTS, 24%).

All of these patients clinically had stage II or III disease as defined by SVS/ISCVS criteria,[1] and all had grade 3 or 4 venous reflux on descending phlebography. Twenty-two of these patients had preoperative APG and all were severely abnormal. Open direct valvular repair with ligation of ICPVs was performed on all patients. Clinical outcome was graded 0 to 3 as follows:

Class

0	Excellent result: asymptomatic extremity without need for elastic support
1	Good result: mild symptoms of swelling, pain, or indurative change
2	Fair result: moderate symptoms of swelling, pain, or skin changes; no ulcer
3	Poor result: ulceration or disabling pain or edema

Fifty-nine percent of patients had dramatic improvement from class 3 or 2 to 1 or 0, with 33% of patients restored to full activity without elastic support. The 10-year cumulative success rate by life table analysis was 60%.

DS or descending phlebography documented competent valves (or mild reflux) in 86% of class 1 or 0 patients compared to 47% of class 3 or 2 patients ($P = .0011$). This difference suggests that the prevention of recurrence of disabling symptoms or ulcers is highly dependent on achieving structural valvular competency at the time of surgery. The ulcer recurrence rate seemed to be lower when incompetent perforators were divided or no incompetent perforators were present (36%) compared to when left untreated (69%), although this difference did not attain statistical significance. It would seem logical from these data, however, that incompetent perforators should be divided when present. Of significance, Kistner[19] noted that most failures usually occurred within 4 years in the majority of cases (12/15).

The next large series was reported by Raju and Fredericks[20] who studied 107 venous valve reconstructions followed over a period of 2 to 8 years. The most common cause of insufficiency in this series was PVI. Arm-foot venous pressure differences and changes in venous pressure in response to reactive hyperemia were used to rule out and grade the degree of venous obstruction. Valsalva foot venous pressure was employed as an index of reflux. The primary indication for surgery was venous stasis ulceration in 71% of patients. No patient with venous outflow obstruction was operated on. Patients underwent direct open valvular repair through a transverse venotomy as well as ligation of the saphenofemoral junction. If the previously incompetent vein was found to become competent from "venospasm," an external Dacron "jacket" was performed instead of direct valvuloplasty. This was done in order to maintain the "competent luminal dimension."[20]

Sixty-nine percent of patients in this series experienced either healing of the ulcer or marked symptomatic improvement. Eleven patients (10%) required a secondary procedure for recurrent ulcer or symptoms. Interestingly, recurrence in two instances was due to recanalization of the saphenous vein. In these two cases, saphenofemoral disconnection resulted in long-term healing. The authors further point out that the presence of abnormal lymphangiographic findings did not adversely affect the results of valvular reconstruction for the relief of edema. The most consistent test to assess reflux in this series was the Valsalva foot venous pressure measurement rather than the ambulatory venous pressure.[20]

Cheatle and Perrin[23] studied 52 limbs in 42 patients who underwent SFV valvuloplasty for recurrent venous ulceration or severe stasis. Forty-four of these limbs had adjunctive surgery of the superficial or perforating veins. Twenty-one limbs had intractable venous ulceration, while 31 limbs had pain, swelling, and lipodermatosclerosis. All had grade 3 or 4 reflux on descending phlebography. Hypercoagulability was a specific exclusion criterion. Patients underwent direct valvuloplasty using Sottiurai's technique,[21] and 94% had simultaneous interruption of the perforating veins.

Patients were followed with DS and PPG. At 1-year follow-up, 85% were free of reflux on DS, and 68% had normalization of their venous refill times. At 1-year follow-up, there was one instance of ulcer recurrence (9%).

The next series was reported by Eriksson[24] and his group from Sweden who have summarized their experience with direct valvuloplasty in 22 limbs (20 patients) with severe deep venous insufficiency (DVI, class 3 or 2), and who had undergone multiple previous procedures on their superficial system. All patients with SVI underwent perforator ligation prior to valve reconstruction.

All patients underwent ascending and descending venography prior to surgery and had grade 3 or 4 reflux. Only patients with PVI were operated on. The valve most commonly chosen for repair was the most proximal SFV valve utilizing the technique originally described by Kistner.[19] All patients were systemically heparinized at the time of their operation and received postoperative dextran for a period of 3 days.

Follow-up ranged from 6 to 84 months, with 53% of limbs showing improvement after 84 months. Doppler examination documented competent valves in all limbs at 6 months' follow-up and all seven clinical failures subsequently demonstrated incompetency of the repaired valve on descending venography. These investigators were the first to call attention to the importance of the status of the PFV following this repair. Improvement in physiologic parameters following surgery only occurred when this vein was documented to be competent.

Sottiurai[21] described his experience on 20 patients with recurrent ulcers (class 3) at a mean follow-up of 37 months. Sixteen patients (80%) had their ulcers healed.

Simkin and his group[25] have reported their experience with seven patients, three of whom underwent Kistner valvuloplasty and four, intraluminal femoral and popliteal valvuloplasty. The latter technique, as described by the author, diminishes the caliber of the vein throughout its length by placing multiple U-shaped polypropylene sutures. In the authors' experience, 50% of patients had healed ulcers at long-term follow-up, the duration of which was unspecified.

Our group[22] has recently reported results for superficial vein valvuloplasty in nine limbs (six patients), all of which were clinically stage III with grade 4 or 3 reflux on descending venography. In addition to valvuloplasty, interruption of incompetent perforators was performed in five limbs, and three limbs underwent stripping and ligation of superficial varicose veins. Two patients had external expanded polytetrafluoroethylene (PTFE) "wraps." The last five limbs had angioscopic evaluation of the repair, and two of these had closed, angioscopically guided repairs. After a mean follow-up period of 20 months, all patients had healed ulcers and there were no recurrences. The two patients who had the expanded PTFE wraps and no postoperative anticoagulation had deep venous thrombosis (DVT). Duplex quantitation of venous reflux was normalized postoperatively in those patients who had angioscopically guided repairs. It should be noted that in this subgroup, two patients required an additional suture to render the valve competent, a necessity

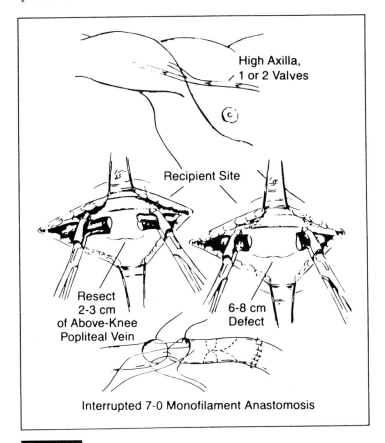

FIGURE 8.

Axillary vein-to-popliteal vein transplantation. The surgical steps involved in axillary vein-to-popliteal vein transplantation are shown schematically. (From O'Donnell TF, Mackey WC, Shepard AD, et al: *Arch Surg* 1987; 122:475. Used by permission.)

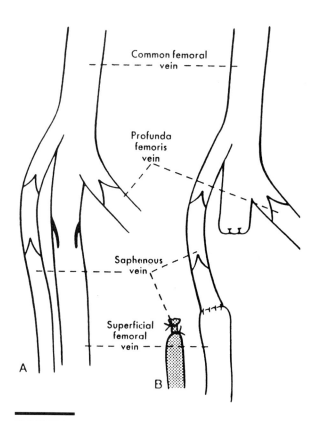

FIGURE 9.

Venous segment transposition. The proximal valve of the superficial femoral vein (SFV) is incompetent (a). The distal SFV is transposed to the greater saphenous vein to provide the latter's competent valves (b). Alternatively, the SFV may be anastomosed end to side, thus utilizing the competent valves of the profunda femoris vein. (From O'Donnell TF Jr, Shepard AD: Chronic venous insufficiency, in Jarrett F, Hirsch SA (eds): *Vascular Surgery of the Lower Extremity*. St Louis, Mosby–Year Book, 1985).

which would not have been appreciated without the benefit of angioscopy. The valvuloplasties evaluated angioscopically also demonstrated much shorter valve closure times for both the SFV and popliteal vein.

The combined experience of well over 170 patients who underwent open valvuloplasty for recurrent venous stasis ulceration shows that, on average, greater than 70% of ulcers can be expected to heal with no mortality and minimal morbidity. Angioscopic evaluation of vein valve repair appears to improve hemodynamic and functional results in this preliminary experience.

Perforating veins should be ligated if found to be incompetent as is true in most patients with advanced venous stasis. Failure to ligate incompetent perforating veins has been associated with a higher rate of ulcer recurrence.[19, 26]

We believe that the ideal candidate for valvuloplasty has primary valvular insufficiency characterized by stage II or III clinical disease with grade 3 or 4 reflux on descending venography. Angioscopy and ligation of incompetent perforators in conjunction with the judicious use of anticoagulation and support hose all lead to improved results.

Other options for these patients include the Psathakis external sling[27] and the Dacron cuff.[28] The use of these procedures is limited to valves which become competent as a result of venospasm with prior documentation of incompetency on preoperative descending phlebogram. Results so far have not been as satisfactory as with the direct approach.

POSTTHROMBOTIC SYNDROME

Patients with the PTS are candidates for vein valve transplant as described by Taheri et al.[29] They recommended that a valve-bearing segment of the brachial vein be interposed into the incompetent SFV (Fig 8). We have long advocated that the popliteal vein is the logical site for interposition since it is invariably incompetent in patients with advanced

TABLE 2.

Surgical Therapy for Chronic Venous Insufficiency*

Series	No. of Limbs	Ulcer (%)†	Ulcer Healing (%)‡	
			(Short)	(Long)
Valvuloplasty				
Masuda & Kistner[10]	51	57	NA	57
Raju & Fredericks[16]	107	78	85	63
Cheatle & Perrin[23]	52	40	NA	NA
Eriksson[24]	22	NA	64	62
Sottiurai[21]	20	100	NA	80
Simkin et al.[25]	7	100	NA	50
Welch et al.[22]	9	100	100	100
Venous transposition				
Ferris & Kistner[30]	14	NA	80	NA
Johnson et al.[26]	12	33	100	67
O'Donnell et al.[32]	9	100	100	78
Vein valve transplant				
Taheri et al.[29]	43	40	NA	94
Raju & Fredericks[16]	24	80	79	42
O'Donnell et al.[32]	12	100	100	92
External venous support				
Psathakis[27]	44	23	100	100

*NA = not available.
†The percentage of limbs studied preoperatively whose indication for surgery was intractable ulcer.
‡The percentage of limbs that underwent complete healing following short (6 months) or long (>2 years) follow-up.

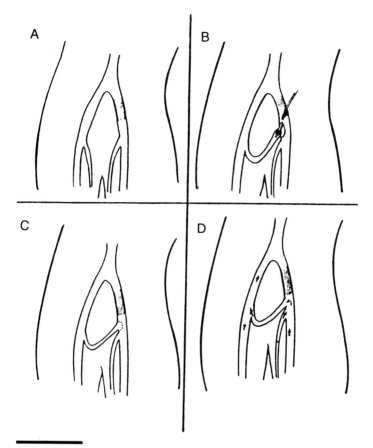

FIGURE 10.

Saphenofemoral crossover graft. **A,** obstructed left ileofemoral segment. **B,** the contralateral saphenous vein is tunneled subcutaneously across the pubis to the left groin. **C,** end-to-side anastomosis. **D,** venous return from the left leg now flows through the graft to the right iliac system. (Modified from Dale WA: Surgery 1966; 59:117.)

CVI and serves as the "gatekeeper" above the calf venous pump mechanism. In addition, we prefer the larger axillary vein because of its greater caliber and more appropriate size match with the popliteal vein.

Another option for these patients is Kistner's venous segment transfer (transposition).[30] The incompetent SFV is divided close to its junction with the PFV and anastomosed to the GSV below a competent venous valve (Fig 9). When the GSV is absent, the SFV is anastomosed end to side to the PFV.

The long-term results reported so far for segment transfer performed for PTS have not been as encouraging as those reported for valvuloplasty performed in patients with PVI (Table 2). Ferris and Kistner[30] have suggested that this difference may actually be due to differences in the pathologic processes between these two entities.

PATIENTS WITH VENOUS OUTFLOW OBSTRUCTION

A variety of operations have been devised in an attempt to help patients with venous outflow obstruction (VOO). The first such operation was the femorofemoral cross-pubic graft devised by Palma and Esperon[31] for unilateral iliac vein obstruction (Fig 10). Other operations include: saphenopopliteal bypass, saphenofemoral bypass, and direct reconstruction of obstructed segments. Both autogenous and prosthetic materials have been used, with some advocating the use of a distal arteriovenous fistula to increase flow through the graft and theoretically improve long-term patency. The best results have thus far been achieved when the obstruction is due to extraluminal compression with concomitant sparing of the intrinsic venous architecture.[32] Dale[33] and Bergan and Yao[18] have reported long-term patency rates of 72% to 75%, while Husni[17] suggests that extirpation of secondary varicose veins as well as ligation of ICPVs appears to improve results.

FOLLOW-UP EVALUATION

All patients should be carefully monitored following direct venous reconstruction. DS or ascending phlebography (segment transfer) or both ascending and descending phlebography followed by serial duplex examinations (valve transplant or valvuloplasty groups) should be performed. Consideration should be given to APG, and if the patient had an ulcer preoperatively, its size should be measured at each office visit with the aid of a clear plastic tracing. The goal of venous surgery should be the prevention of ulcer recurrence and the amelioration of stasis symp-

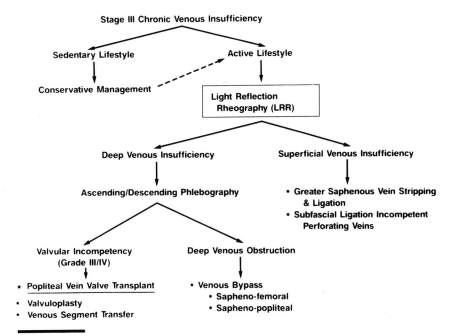

FIGURE 11.

Algorithm for management of stage III chronic venous insufficiency (CVI). Patients with active lifestyles and disabling CVI should undergo initial assessment by noninvasive means (e.g., duplex scan, air plethysmography). Subsequent management is dictated by phlebography. We prefer angioscopically guided valvuloplasty for grade III and IV primary valvular incompetency, and popliteal vein valve transplantation for postthrombotic syndrome; venous segment transfer or bypass is dictated by the nature of the obstructed segment.

toms to allow the patient to return to regular activity. The accomplishment of these goals can only be ascertained after a long period of careful follow-up. Thorough preoperative evaluation, careful planning of surgery (Fig 11), and meticulous follow-up should reward both patient and surgeon with excellent and lasting results.

REFERENCES

1. Porter JM, Rutherford RB, Clagett GP, et al: Reporting standards in venous disease. *J Vasc Surg* 1988; 8:172–181.
2. Cordts PR, Hanrahan LM, Rodriguez AA, et al: A prospective randomized trial of Unna's boot versus Duoderm CGF hydroactive dressing plus compression in the management of venous leg ulcers. *J Vasc Surg* 1992; 15:480–486.
3. Burnand KG, Lea T, O'Donnell TF Jr, et al: Relationship between post-phlebitic changes in the deep veins and results of surgical treatment of venous ulcers. *Lancet* 1976; 1:936–938.
4. McEnroe CS, O'Donnell TF, Mackey WC: Correlation of clinical findings with venous hemodynamics in 386 patients with chronic venous insufficiency. *Am J Surg* 1988; 156:148–152.
5. Christopoulos DG, Nicolaides AN, Szendro G, et al: Air plethysmography and the effect of elastic compression on venous hemodynamics of the leg. *J Vasc Surg* 1987; 5:148–159.
6. Hanrahan LM, Araki CT, Rodriguez AA, et al: Distribution of valvular incompetence in patients with venous stasis ulceration. *J Vasc Surg* 1991; 13:805–812.
7. Karkow WS, Ruoff BA, Cranley JJ: B-mode venous imaging, in Kempczinski RF, Yao JST (eds): *Practical Noninvasive Vascular Diagnosis*, ed 2. St Louis, Mosby–Year Book, 1987, pp 464–485.
8. Hanrahan LM, Araki CT, Fisher JB, et al: Evaluation of the perforating veins of the lower extremity using high resolution duplex imaging. *J Cardiovasc Surg* 1991; 32:87–97.
9. van Bemmelen PS, Bedford G, Beach K, et al: Quantitative segmental evaluation of venous valvular reflux with ultrasonic duplex scanning. *J Vasc Surg* 1989; 10:425–431.
10. Masuda EM, Kistner RL: Long-term results of venous valve reconstruction: a 4- to 21-year follow-up. Presented at the 46th Annual Meeting of the Society for Vascular Surgery, Chicago, June 8–9, 1992.
11. Baumgartner I, Franzeck UK, Bollinger A: Venous claudication evaluated by ambulatory plethysmography. *Phlebology* 1992; 7:2–6.
12. Sarin S, Shields DA, Scurr JH, et al: Photoplethysmography: A valuable tool in the assessment of venous dysfunction. *J Vasc Surg* 1992; 15:154–162.
13. O'Donnell TF Jr, Welch H: Value of non-invasive techniques in assessing chronic venous insufficiency and guiding surgical management. Unpublished data, 1993.
14. O'Donnell TF: The surgical management of deep venous valvular incompetence, in Rutherford RB (ed): *Vascular Surgery*, ed 3. Philadelphia, WB Saunders, 1989, pp 1612–1626.
15. Iafrati MD, O'Donnell TF, McLaughlin R, et al: Comparative trial of clinical examination and photoplethysmography in the management of varicose veins. Presented at the fifth Annual Meeting of the American Venous Forum, Orlando, Fla, Feb 25, 1993.
16. Raju S, Fredericks R: Venous obstruction: An analysis of 137 cases with he-

modynamic, venographic and clinical correlations. *J Vasc Surg* 1991; 14:305–313.

17. Husni EA: Reconstruction of veins: The need for objectivity. *J Cardiovasc Surg* 1983; 24:525–528.

18. Bergan JJ, Yao JST (eds): *Surgery of the Veins.* Orlando, Fla, Grune & Stratton, 1985.

19. Kistner RL: Surgical repair of the incompetent femoral vein valve. *Arch Surg* 1975; 110:1336–1342.

20. Raju S, Fredericks R: Valve reconstruction procedures for non-obstructive venous insufficiency: Rationale, techniques, and results in 107 procedures with two- to eight-year follow-up. *J Vasc Surg* 1988; 7:301–310.

21. Sottiurai VS: Technique in direct venous valvuloplasty. *J Vasc Surg* 1988; 8:646–649.

22. Welch HJ, McLaughlin RL, O'Donnell TF: Femoral vein valvuloplasty: Intra-operative angioscopic evaluation and hemodynamic improvement. *J Vasc Surg* 1992; 16:694–700.

23. Cheatle TR, Perrin M: Venous valve repair: A report of 52 cases. *J Vasc Surg* 1994; 19:404–413.

24. Eriksson I: Vein valve surgery for deep valvular incompetence, in Eklöf B, Gjöres JF, Thulesius O, et al (eds): *Controversies in the Management of Venous Disorders.* London, Butterworths, 1989, pp. 267–279.

25. Simkin R, Estebam JC, Bulloj R: By-pass veno-venosos y valvuloplastias en el tratamiento quirurgico del sindrome post-trombotico. *Angiologia* 1988; 1:30–34.

26. Johnson ND, Queral LA, Flinn WR, et al: Late objective assessment of venous valve surgery. *Arch Surg* 1981; 116:1461–1468.

27. Psathakis ND: The substitute "valve" operation by technique II in patients with post-thrombotic syndrome. *Surgery* 1984; 95:542–548.

28. Jessup G, Lane RJ: Repair of incompetent venous valves: A new technique. *J Vasc Surg* 1988; 8:569–575.

29. Taheri SA, Lazar E, Elias SM, et al: Vein valve transplantation. *Surgery* 1982; 91:28–33.

30. Ferris EB, Kistner RL: Femoral vein reconstruction in the management of chronic venous insufficiency. *Arch Surg* 1982; 117:1571–1579.

31. Palma EC, Esperon R: Vein transplants and grafts in the surgical treatment of the post-phlebitic syndrome. *J Cardiovasc Surg* 1960; 1:94–107.

32. O'Donnell TF, Mackey WC, Shepard AD, et al: Clinical, hemodynamic and anatomic follow-up of direct venous reconstruction. *Arch Surg* 1987; 122:474–482.

33. Dale WA: Crossover vein grafts for iliac and femoral venous occlusion. *Res Staff Phys* 1983; 58–64.

PART V

Issues in Basic Science

Raynaud's Phenomenon: Vasospastic Disease and Current Therapy

Marie D. Gerhard, M.D.
Vascular Medicine and Atherosclerosis Unit of the Cardiovascular Division of
Brigham and Women's Hospital, Boston, Massachusetts

Mark A. Creager, M.D.
Vascular Medicine and Atherosclerosis Unit of the Cardiovascular Division of
Brigham and Women's Hospital, Boston, Massachusetts

E pisodic vasospastic digital ischemia, or Raynaud's phenomenon, was first described by Maurice Raynaud in 1862. It consists of episodes of well-demarcated digital pallor or cyanosis following environmental or local cold exposure (Fig 1). Raynaud's phenomenon can be provoked by low environmental temperatures, by touching a cold object, and occasionally by emotional distress. Usually color changes are confined to the fingers and toes; less often the ear lobes, tip of the nose, and tip of the tongue are affected. Pallor is caused by vasospasm eliminating blood flow to the digit. The arterioles, venules, and capillaries of the digit then dilate as ischemia progresses. Deoxygenated blood collects in these vessels, resulting in cyanosis. These color changes may be accompanied by feelings of cold, numbness, and paresthesias. Digital vasospasm resolves with rewarming. The resulting hyperemia often causes a throbbing sensation, and imparts a bright-red color to the affected digit. The color of the digit usually returns to normal following such an episode. The classic triphasic color response is not experienced by all patients. Some patients experience only pallor *and* cyanosis and others note only pallor *or* cyanosis. The clinical severity of Raynaud's phenomenon varies markedly from individual to individual. Symptom patterns range from mild infrequent attacks to prolonged episodes of digital ischemia.

The diagnosis of Raynaud's phenomenon is based on the patient's historical account, since patients do not often present to their physician during an acute episode. Environmental conditions that decrease whole-body temperature can cause digital vasospasm. Daily activities such as removing items from a refrigerator freezer or gripping a cold steering wheel may also induce an episode of digital ischemia. Unfortunately, simple office maneuvers such as placing the patient's hand in ice water do not reliably induce Raynaud's phenomenon. Physical findings in subjects range from a normal examination to overt digital ischemia, digital ulcers, gangrene, and autoamputation.

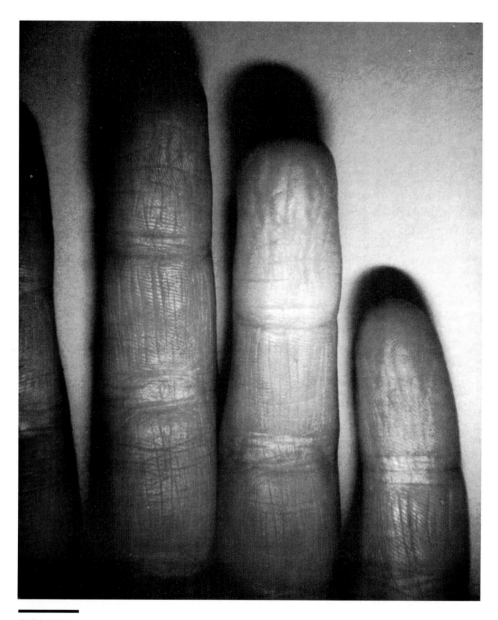

FIGURE 1.

Well-demarcated pallor occurring in a single finger as a result of Raynaud's phenomenon. (From Creager MA: Vasospastic diseases in Loscalzo J, Creager MA, Dzau V (eds): *Vascular Medicine*. Boston, Little, Brown, 1992, p 984. Used by permission.)

PRIMARY RAYNAUD'S PHENOMENON

The classification of Raynaud's phenomenon is separated into primary, i.e., unassociated with any other disease process, or secondary, i.e., occurring as a consequence of another disease or treatment. Allen and Brown[1] established five minimal requisites for the diagnosis of primary Raynaud's phenomenon based on data from 150 patients: (1) a history of vasospastic attacks precipitated by cold or emotional stimuli, (2) bilat-

TABLE 1.
Classification of Primary Raynaud's Phenomenon*

Bilateral episodic attacks of acral cyanosis or pallor
Strong and symmetric peripheral pulses
No digital pitting, ulcerations, or gangrene
No signs or symptoms of systemic disease associated with Raynaud's
  phenomenon
Symptoms >2 yr
Normal nail-fold capillaries
Negative antinuclear antibody test
Normal erythrocyte sedimentation rate

*Modified from Allen EV, Brown GE: *Am J Med Sci* 1932; 183:187–200; and LeRoy EC, Medsger TA Jr: *Clin Exp Rheumatol* 1991; 10:485–488.

eral involvement of the extremities, (3) the absence of gangrene, or gangrene that is confined to the fingertips, (4) the absence of evidence of underlying disease that could be responsible for the vasospastic episodes, and (5) a history of symptoms for at least two years (Table 1).

More recently, LeRoy and Medsger[2] have modified these criteria for the diagnosis of primary Raynaud's phenomenon based on a retrospective study of 240 patients. The history includes episodes of acral pallor or cyanosis, and physical findings include the presence of strong symmetric peripheral pulses without evidence of digital pitting, ulcerations, or gangrene. Laboratory criteria have been added and include normal nail-fold capillaroscopy, antinuclear antibody test with titer less than 100 for all patterns and epitopes, and erythrocyte sedimentation rate less than 20 mm/hr (see Table 1).

PREVALENCE

The prevalence of Raynaud's phenomenon depends on the means of data collection, the definition utilized, and the climate. A small number of studies have used questionnaires to examine the prevalence of Raynaud's phenomenon in the selected populations. In one of the earliest of these studies, 122 medical students and nurses aged 19 to 45 years were questioned about whether they had episodes of digital pallor and cyanosis during cold exposure.[3] Nineteen (31%) of the 62 women and 15 (25%) of the 60 men reported such episodes. Sixty-seven female physical therapists in Denmark were evaluated for Raynaud's phenomenon by questionnaire and measurement of digital blood flow during local cooling.[4] Eight subjects (22%) had both a history of white, numb fingers with cold exposure and abnormal finger blood flows during digital cooling. Among 520 subjects queried in England, 8.3% of men and 17.6% of women aged 20 to 59 years were estimated to have Raynaud's phenomenon.[5] In South Carolina, 4.6% of 1,752 randomly selected subjects reported episodes of digital pallor or cyanosis in response to cold temperatures.[6] The prevalence rate in South Carolina is much lower than those found in the earlier studies. In most of these studies a distinction was not made between primary and secondary Raynaud's phenomenon.

Geographic variation in the prevalence of Raynaud's phenomenon was confirmed in a study involving the general population in Charleston, South Carolina, and Tarentaise, Savoie, France.[7] In Tarentaise, the temperatures throughout the year average 10° C lower than those in Charleston. Initially, subjects interviewed by phone gave a higher prevalence of digital pallor and cyanosis in response to cold in Tarentaise (31.1%) than in Charleston (17.9%). Subsequently, medical teams confirmed the diagnosis of Raynaud's phenomenon based on four components: (1) cold sensitivity, (2) reported color change, (3) identification of pallor or cyanosis from a color scale, and (4) identification of pallor or cyanosis from hand photographs which included attacks of Raynaud's phenomenon. Prevalence of the diagnosis was three times higher in Tarentaise (16.8%) than in Charleston (5.0%). The prevalence was higher in women (20.1% and 13.5%) than in men (5.7% and 4.3%) in Tarentaise and Charleston, respectively. Also, the mean age of women with Raynaud's phenomenon in Tarentaise was 10 years lower than in Charleston.

PROGNOSIS

Patients with primary Raynaud's phenomenon generally have a favorable prognosis. This clinical impression was substantiated by Gifford and Hines[8] who followed 307 medically treated patients with primary Raynaud's phenomenon for an average of 12 years. The average duration of symptoms was 17 years. Symptoms disappeared in 10%, improved in 36%, and worsened in 16% of patients. Ulcers and digital skin changes developed in 13%, but only 0.4% had digital amputations. Alleviation of symptoms occurred in 50% of the subgroup of patients who moved to a warmer climate. It is important to note that the diagnosis of connective tissue disorders had not reached its current level of sophistication when this study was reported in 1957. More recently, Clavijo and Krahenbuhl[9] studied 136 patients with primary (18%) and secondary (82%) Raynaud's phenomenon and found very similar results. Symptoms improved in 36%, were unchanged in 48%, and worsened in 16% of these subjects followed for an average of 3.9 years. Of those with primary Raynaud's phenomenon, symptoms improved in 25% and worsened in 12%. Predictors for poor prognosis in these subjects included digital skin necrosis, an abnormal Allen's test, and age greater than 60 years; these findings are typical of secondary Raynaud's phenomenon. Age of onset and presence of sclerodactyly did not appear to predict poor prognosis. Gerbracht et al.[10] followed 87 subjects with at least a 2-year history of primary Raynaud's phenomenon. After a follow-up period of at least 5 years, 4 (5%) of these subjects developed scleroderma and 15 (17%) developed positive antinuclear antibodies.

PATHOPHYSIOLOGY

There are some unique features of the digital circulation to consider in understanding the pathophysiology of Raynaud's phenomenon. The cutaneous vessels of the fingers and toes are supplied only by sympathetic adrenergic vasoconstrictor fibers, unlike other regional circulations which are supplied by sympathetic vasodilator and vasoconstrictors fibers. Cold exposure can result in digital vasoconstriction due to reflex activation of the sympathetic nervous system. Raynaud's phenomenon occurs only in skin areas with arteriovenous anastomoses proximal to the capillary circulation. The arteriovenous anastomoses directly connect the arterial and venous circulation via richly innervated coiled vessels with thick muscular walls. Fingertip blood flow can vary from 1 to 180 mL/100 mL/min tissue when these arteriovenous shunts close in cold environments and open in warm environments. The arteriovenous anastomoses are largely under sympathetic nervous system control.

Digital artery patency results from the balance between vascular smooth muscle contractile forces and the intravascular pressure. In Raynaud's phenomenon, normal physiologic vasoconstriction is replaced by digital artery vasospasm. *Vasospasm* is defined as an excessive vasoconstrictor response to stimuli which results in obliteration of the vascular lumen rather than the expected modest reduction of the luminal diameter. A number of mechanisms have been proposed to explain Raynaud's phenomenon. These include: (1) increased efferent sympathetic stimulation to the digital artery, (2) a local digital fault resulting in increased activity to vasoconstrictor stimuli, (3) decreased intraluminal pressure, and (4) excessive vasoconstrictor stimuli (Table 2).

INCREASED SYMPATHETIC NERVOUS SYSTEM ACTIVITY

Maurice Raynaud first suspected that excessive sympathetic nervous system activity might be the cause of the episodic digital ischemia, because of the bilateral nature of the vasospastic attacks that he observed. The idea is intuitively appealing, but support for this hypothesis has not been convincing. Peacock[11] found that norepinephrine and epinephrine concentrations were higher in the wrist veins of subjects with primary Raynaud's phenomenon than in control subjects, and were highest in the subjects with the most clinically severe Raynaud's phenomenon. Kontos and Wasserman,[12] however, found normal levels of norepinephrine in the brachial arterial and venous blood of subjects with Raynaud's phenomenon. Also, both normal subjects and persons with Raynaud's phenomenon had simi-

TABLE 2.
Mechanisms Proposed to Explain the Pathophysiology of Raynaud's Phenomenon

---

Excessive sympathetic efferent activity results in vasoconstriction of
  digital vessels
A local vascular fault of digital vessels allows them to overreact to
  normal vasoconstrictor stimuli
Decreased intravascular pressure allows the vessel to collapse when
  vasoconstrictor tone increases
Increased amounts of circulating or local vasoconstrictor substances
  results in vasospasm in response to vasoconstrictor stimuli

lar responses to the administration of intraarterial tyramine. Reflex sympathetic vasoconstriction was similar in both patients with Raynaud's phenomenon and control subjects.[13] Fagius and Blumberg[14] measured skin nerve sympathetic activity from the right median nerve in seven patients with primary Raynaud's phenomenon and in ten healthy subjects both at rest and with immersion of the left hand in cold water. Sympathetic outflow increased comparably in subjects of both populations. These data suggest that increased sympathetic nervous system activity proximal to the digits is not the cause of episodic digital ischemia in patients with Raynaud's phenomenon.

LOCAL VASCULAR FAULT

Increased sensitivity of digital vessels to normal levels of sympathetic stimuli was first proposed by Sir Thomas Lewis[15] as an explanation for digital vasospasm during cold exposure, and he used the phrase "local vascular fault." He was able to produce digital vasospastic attacks in response to cold despite nerve blockade or sympathectomy. However, many of these subjects had secondary Raynaud's phenomenon and possibly structurally abnormal vessels. Jamieson et al.[16] also found evidence for local vascular hyperreactivity. They studied patients with primary Raynaud's phenomenon and control subjects. The temperature of one hand was maintained at 36° C while the other was kept at 26° C. When ice was applied to the patient's neck, the magnitude of reflex vasoconstriction was similar in both populations in the warm hand but exaggerated in the cold hand of patients with Raynaud's phenomenon.[16] Freedman et al.,[17] in 1989, reported that vasospastic attacks could be induced in response to environmental plus local cooling in patients with primary and secondary Raynaud's phenomenon both before and after digital nerve block. Vasospastic attacks were precipitated in 80% of the subjects with primary Raynaud's phenomenon before digital nerve block and in 66% following digital nerve block. In the subjects with scleroderma, 80% demonstrated vasospastic attacks before digital nerve block and 60% after nerve block. Therefore, in the majority of patients, vasospastic attacks occurred despite the absence of efferent digital nerve activity. Taken together, these data suggest that there is indeed a "local vascular fault" which promotes vasospastic attacks during stimuli that would typically result in modest vasoconstriction.

The precise nature of the local fault is not known, but cold-induced changes in vascular reactivity may be relevant. The intracellular concentration of high-energy phosphates and influx of calcium needed for the contractile machinery of the vessel wall is decreased with cooling.[18, 19] This would normally limit vasoconstriction during cooling. In contrast, adrenergic-mediated vasoconstriction is augmented by cooling. This occurs despite decreased release of norepinephrine from sympathetic nerve endings in the vessels.[20, 21] This suggests that α-adrenergic receptor sensitivity is altered by cooling. Of these, α_2-adrenoreceptors are more sensitive to changes in temperature than α_1-adrenoreceptors.[22] α_2-Adrenoreceptor-mediated responses are augmented with cooling and depressed with warming, while the converse is true for α_1-adrenoreceptor responses.[22, 23] Coffman and Cohen[24] administered α_1- and α_2-adrenoreceptor antagonists to subjects with primary Raynaud's phenomenon during reflex sympathetic vasoconstriction. Finger blood flow and vascular resistance increased significantly in those who received the α_2-adrenoreceptor antagonist yohimbine, but not in those who received the α_1-antagonist prazosin. This study suggests that α_2-adrenoreceptors in human digits are important in producing digital vasoconstriction during cooling. These investigators also administered α-adrenoreceptor agonists and found that subjects with Raynaud's phenomenon had augmented responses to the α_2-adrenoreceptor agonist clonidine and not to the α_1-adrenoreceptor agonist phenylephrine. These data suggest that increased activity or number of postjunctional α_2-adrenoreceptors could contribute to episodic digital vasospasm. Flavahan and colleagues[25] examined the distribution of α-adrenoreceptors in the arteries of human limbs amputated from patients without vascular disease. They found that α_2-adrenoreceptors were more numerous than α_1-adrenoreceptors in the digital arteries. Cooke et al.[26] studied finger blood flow responses to yohimbine and prazosin in control subjects and patients with Raynaud's phenomenon. They found that postjunctional α_1-adrenoreceptors appear to predominate in the control of digital vasoconstriction in normal subjects. In patients with Raynaud's phenomenon, postjunctional α_1-1 and α_2-adrenoreceptors appear equally important in regulation of finger blood flow. Keenan and Porter[27] observed that the density of platelet α_2-adrenoreceptors is increased in patients with Raynaud's phenomenon. Together, these studies suggest that increased activity of postjunctional α_2-adrenoreceptors could result in episodic digital vasospasm in patients with Raynaud's phenomenon.

DECREASED INTRAVASCULAR PRESSURE

Blood vessel patency requires a favorable balance between intravascular distending pressure and constricting tension in the arterial wall. This is illustrated in a study by Landis[28] who measured intravascular pressure in patients with primary Raynaud's phenomenon by micropipette introduced into a large digital capillary. Capillary pressure fell during cyanosis, consistent with proximal vessel closure. It has been reported[29] that brachial artery blood pressure is lower in patients with primary Raynaud's phenomenon than in control subjects, suggesting that in these subjects less external pressure is required to stop blood flow. Furthermore, brachial and digital blood pressures are lower in primary Raynaud's patients than in control subjects during reflex sympathetic vasoconstriction induced by body cooling.[30] Not all subjects with low pressures have Raynaud's phenomenon, suggesting that this is only a partial explanation of the pathophysiology. Nonetheless, many disorders associated with secondary Raynaud's phenomenon cause low digital artery pressures, e.g., atherosclerosis and thromboangiitis obliterans (see below).

INCREASED VASOCONSTRICTOR SUBSTANCES

Increased concentrations of endogenously produced vasoconstrictor substances may contribute to digital vasospasm. These include serotonin, angiotensin II, thromboxane A_2, and endothelin. Plasma and platelet serotonin levels are occasionally elevated in patients with Raynaud's phenomenon.[31] Serotonin levels are highest in those with secondary Raynaud's phenomenon.[32] Serotonin acts directly on smooth muscle to cause vasoconstriction, and also augments the constrictor responses to other neurohumoral mediators such as catecholamines, histamine, and angiotensin II. Both platelet release of serotonin and infusion of serotonin have been shown to result in digital constriction and cyanosis.[33-35] The contribution of serotonin to Raynaud's phenomenon is unclear. Both digital pulse volume and fingertip temperature increased in patients with primary and secondary Raynaud's phenomenon who received intravenous ketanserin.[36] However, intravenous ketanserin does not improve digital blood flow if given to patients with Raynaud's phenomenon before a cold challenge.[37] A serotonin antagonist, ketanserin facilitates recovery of digital temperature following provoked vasospastic attacks.[38] Thus serotonin may contribute to digital vasospasm. However, chronic administration of ketanserin has had inconsistent effects on the symptoms of Raynaud's patients, making serotonin's contribution to vasospastic attacks less clear.[36, 39-42]

Levels of the vasoconstrictor angiotensin II are not elevated in most patients with Raynaud's phenomenon, but may be if a patient has coexistent renal artery stenosis or renal parenchymal disease. Captopril, an angiotensin-converting enzyme inhibitor, improved Raynaud's phenomenon in two patients with scleroderma being treated for malignant hypertension.[43] In this unusual situation, high levels of angiotensin II may have exacerbated digital vasospasm in patients with known Raynaud's phenomenon.

Patients with Raynaud's phenomenon secondary to systemic sclerosis have been found to have increased urinary excretion of the metabolite thromboxane B_2. This suggested a possible role for vasoconstrictors released during platelet aggregation in Raynaud's phenomenon. The thromboxane synthetase inhibitor dazoxiben did not affect fingertip blood flow in patients with Raynaud's phenomenon studied in warm and in cool environments.[44] Administration of a thromboxane receptor antagonist and a thromboxane synthase inhibitor did not change responses to local cold challenge in either patients or controls[45] despite a 95% reduction in thromboxane B_2 levels. These data do not support a significant role for this platelet-derived vasoconstrictor in Raynaud's phenomenon.

The endothelium produces many potent vasoactive substances. An alteration in the balance of these vasoconstrictive and vasodilative substances could potentially result in vasospasm. Levels of endothelin-1 are elevated in patients with Raynaud's phenomenon and increase further in response to a cold stimulus,[46, 47] suggesting a possible role for this potent vasoconstrictor in the development of Raynaud's phenomenon. Malondialdehyde levels indicative of free radical activity are elevated in patients with primary and secondary Raynaud's phenomenon.[48] Increased levels of free radicals could potentially impair endothelial vasodilator function and tip the balance toward vasoconstriction. However, a recent study found no difference in agonist-stimulated release of endothelium-derived relaxing factor in patients with Raynaud's phenomenon compared to control subjects.[49] In one study of 22 patients,[50] plasma levels of the endothelial product factor VIII correlated with disease activity. These data raise the possibility that endothelial damage and dysfunction may contribute to the development of Raynaud's phenomenon.

SECONDARY CAUSES OF RAYNAUD'S PHENOMENON

Table 3 lists the secondary causes of Raynaud's phenomenon.

CONNECTIVE TISSUE DISORDERS

The most frequent secondary cause of Raynaud's phenomenon in tertiary referral centers is a connective tissue disorder. These account for 35% to 72% of cases of secondary Raynaud's phenomenon.[51–53] In one such series, scleroderma accounted for 90% of the connective tissue disorders.[54]

Raynaud's phenomenon occurs in 90% of patients with *scleroderma*.[55] In the early stages of diffuse scleroderma, Raynaud's phenomenon may be the only manifestation, and physical examination and laboratory tests may be normal. From 33% to 50% of scleroderma patients initially

TABLE 3.
Secondary Causes of Raynaud's Phenomenon

Connective tissue diseases	Neurologic disorders
Scleroderma	Stroke
Systemic lupus erythematosus	Syringomyelia
Rheumatoid arthritis	Poliomyelitis
Dermatomyositis and	Carpal tunnel syndrome
polymyositis	Drugs
Vascultis	Bromocriptine
Arterial occlusive disease	β-Adrenergic blocking agents
Atherosclerosis	Dopamine
Thromboangiitis obliterans	Ergot derivatives
Thromboembolic disease	Toxins
Thoracic outlet syndrome	Vinyl chloride
Thermal or vibration injury	Ergot
Vibration white finger	Chemotherapeutic agents
Mechanical percussive injury	Vinblastine
Hypothenar hammer syndrome	Bleomycin
Electric shock injury	
Frostbite	
Blood dyscrasias	
Hyperviscosity syndromes	
Polycythemia vera	
Thrombocytosis	
Myeloproliferative disorders	
Cold agglutinin disease	
Cryglobulinemia	
Cryofibrinogenemia	

present with Raynaud's phenomenon. The CREST syndrome is a specific form of diffuse scleroderma, consisting of subcutaneous calcifications, Raynaud's phenomenon, esophageal dysmotility, sclerodactyly, and telangiectasia. In contrast to diffuse scleroderma, localized scleroderma is limited to the skin and subcutaneous tissues and is not accompanied by Raynaud's phenomenon.[56] Scleroderma, like Raynaud's phenomenon, is more likely to occur in females than in males. Vasospastic attacks are often more frequent and more severe in patients with scleroderma than in patients with primary Raynaud's phenomenon.

The most sensitive and specific indicator of diffuse scleroderma is the presence of proximal scleroderma.[57] *Proximal scleroderma* is defined as "tightness, thickening and non-pitting induration of the skin proximal to the metacarpophalangeal or metatarsophalangeal joints, affecting other parts of the extremities, face, neck or trunk usually in a bilateral symmetrical pattern and almost always including sclerodactyly."[57] The shiny skin appears to be tightly drawn and bound to its underlying structures; this is most prominent in the sclerodactyly seen in the fingers and toes. As the skin tightens and the tendons fibrose, the fingers become retracted in the flexed position. Because of tightening of the facial skin, there is recession of the lips with diminution of mouth size (Fig 2). The gums are often visible. Other skin manifestations include Raynaud's phenomenon, sausagelike swelling of the fingers, telangiectasia, abnormal skin pigmentation, and digital pitting scars (Fig 3). Arthritis and acral osteolysis can occur. Visceral manifestations include renal failure, myocardial involvement, basilar pulmonary fibrosis, esophageal dysmotility, and colonic sacculations.

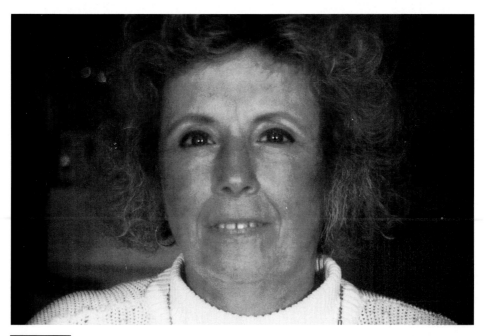

FIGURE 2.
Tightening of facial skin and diminution of mouth size are evident in this patient with scleroderma.

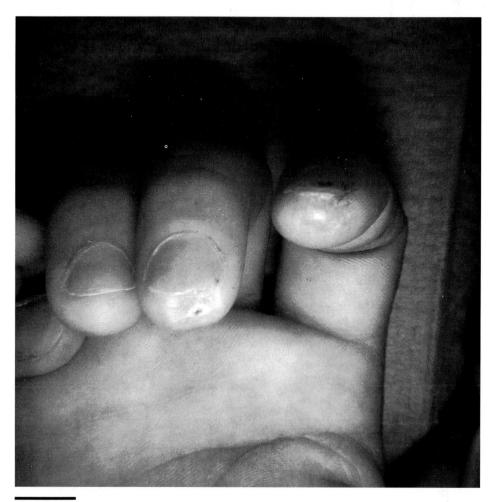

FIGURE 3.
Digital pitting and ulcerations in a patient with scleroderma. (From Creager MA: Vasospastic disease, in Loscalzo J, Creager MA, Dzau V (eds): *Vascular Medicine.* Boston, Little, Brown, 1992, p 985. Used by permission.)

Antinuclear antibodies using HEp-2 cell lines are found in approximately 95% of scleroderma patients.[58] Antibodies to the Scl-70 antigen, centromere, and nucleolus are specific for scleroderma.[59] Mild hypergammaglobulinemia, elevated sedimentation rate, and rheumatoid factor can also be present in scleroderma. Nail-fold capillaroscopy is often abnormal early in the course of scleroderma. Digital vascular obstructive lesions are suggested by flattened pulse volume recordings and decreased digital systolic pressures (see Diagnosis). Angiography often demonstrates digital vascular occlusions. Pathologically, there is an increase in collagen bundles in the dermis and subcutaneous tissues cause calcification and loss of skin appendages in the involved skin. Intimal and medial fibrosis and thickening in the walls of the arteries and arterioles narrow the vascular lumen.

The course of diffuse scleroderma is variable, but usually progressive. Involvement of the viscera predicts a poor prognosis. Development of gangrene in the terminal phalanges may lead to autoamputation or surgical amputation. A cumulative survival rate of 45% at 7 years after diagnosis was documented in a group of 309 patients with diffuse scleroderma.[60] Both surgical and medical therapy in scleroderma are supportive and dependent upon the systems affected. There is no specific treatment for scleroderma.

Raynaud's phenomenon is present in 20% to 25% of patients with *systemic lupus erythematosus (SLE)*[57, 61, 62] and usually occurs after other manifestations of this autoimmune disease. Endarteritis of the small digital vessels causes persistent ischemia that often results in gangrene. SLE is a multisystem disorder which occurs predominantly in 20- to 40-year-old women, and is more prevalent in African Americans than in other races. Skin findings with SLE include malar rash, photosensitivity, discoid rash, and oral ulcers. Other findings include nonerosive arthritis, pleuritis or pericarditis, and seizures or unexplained psychosis. Many of the clinical manifestations are due to vasculitis affecting the arterioles and venules. Laboratory findings can include proteinuria and hemolytic anemia with leukopenia or lymphopenia or thrombocytopenia. Antibodies to double-stranded DNA and Sm nuclear antigen are common, as is false-positive syphilis serology. Immune complex deposition produces an inflammatory response. In one small series, corticosteroid treatment improved Raynaud's phenomenon secondary to SLE.[63]

Dermatomyositis and *polymyositis* are inflammatory diseases of skeletal muscle characterized by weakness of the girdle muscles. Raynaud's phenomenon occurs in 25% to 30% of these patients.[57, 64] In dermatomyositis, skeletal muscle abnormalities are accompanied by characteristic skin findings. Gottron's papules are violaceous-to-erythematous patches over the extensor surfaces of the hand which are pathognomonic for dermatomyositis. In addition to the characteristic heliotrope rash on the upper eyelids and around the nail beds, patients may have the more nonspecific findings of erythema, maculopapular rash, and eczematoid dermatitis. One third develop myocarditis and others develop esophageal dysmotility. Non-necrotizing lymphocytic vasculitis and gastrointestinal tract ulcers are more common in childhood dermatomyositis.

Laboratory tests used to diagnose dermatomyositis and polymyositis include elevated serum levels of creatine kinase, aldolase, lactate dehydrogenase, and myoglobinuria. There is often nonspecific elevation of the erythrocyte sedimentation rate and antinuclear antibodies may be present. Nail-fold capillaroscopy demonstrates dilated disorganized capillaries associated with avascular areas and hemorrhages.[65, 66] An electromyogram will detect myopathy. Prednisone is the treatment of choice for acute exacerbations of dermatomyositis and polymyositis.

Patients with *rheumatoid arthritis* may have vasculitis of medium-sized vessels as well as obliterative endarteritis of the small vessels.[67, 68] Focal ischemia and infarction appear as small brown periungual areas. Angiograms reveal digital artery occlusions in many patients with rheumatoid arthritis.[69] Studies of finger blood flow in patients provide evidence that provokable vasospasm is evident early in rheumatoid arthritis; later, vascular occlusions predominate as immune complexes are deposited on the vessel wall.[70] Findings in rheumatoid arthritis include morning joint stiffness, joint pain or tenderness on motion, joint swelling, and subcutaneous nodules. Bone erosions are often evident on radiologic examination. Synovial fluid in acute rheumatoid arthritis may have leukocyte counts greater than 20,000/mm^3 with predominance of polymorphonuclear leukocytes. The presence of rheumatoid factor and elevated erythrocyte sedimentation rate are often noted. Therapeutic management begins with salicylates and rest, but often progresses to more complicated immunosuppressive regimens.

ARTERIAL OCCLUSIVE DISEASE

Occlusive disease of medium and small arteries is present in 10% to 20% of all patients presenting to tertiary referrals centers with Raynaud's phenomenon.[54] These disorders include atherosclerosis, thromboangiitis obliterans, and extrinsic compression of the subclavian artery.

Atherosclerosis may contribute to Raynaud's phenomenon by reducing perfusion pressure proximal to the digital artery. Proximal arterial occlusions may decrease distal intravascular distending pressure, making the distal vessel more prone to vasospasm in response to sympathetic stimuli. Atherosclerosis may also affect the digital arteries. The incidence of occlusive digital arterial lesions in unselected patients increases with age,[69] as does the incidence of atherosclerosis. Peripheral atherosclerosis is most common in men in their sixth decade and women in their seventh decade. In a group of 26 patients with digital artery atherosclerosis, 8 reported lower extremity claudication and 8 died from ischemic heart disease.[71] In one series, all patients with Raynaud's phenomenon attributed to atherosclerosis had evidence of lower extremity or coronary atherosclerosis.[54] Symptoms of atherosclerosis elsewhere such as claudication, angina, and transient ischemic attacks often suggest the diagnosis. Raynaud's phenomenon secondary to atherosclerosis tends to be unilateral and related to the affected extremity. Physical examination often reveals decreased or absent pulses in the involved extremity. Decreased perfusion pressures are evident on noninvasive vascular testing. Digital arterial occlusive disease can cause severe and prolonged ischemia, which is quite distinct from the episodic digital vasospasm seen in Raynaud's phenomenon.

Thromboangiitis obliterans (Buerger's disease) is a segmental inflammatory occlusive vascular disorder which involves small and medium-sized arteries and veins.[72, 73] Allen and Brown[74] suggested that Raynaud's phenomenon may occur in as many as 30% of patients with thromboangiitis obliterans during the course of the disease. It is estimated to be present in 2% to 5% of all patients presenting with Raynaud's phenomenon.[51, 53, 74] Thromboangiitis obliterans is most prevalent in males under 40 years of age of Asian or Eastern European descent. It occurs almost exclusively among cigarette smokers. The cause of thromboangiitis obliterans is unknown. An increased incidence of HLA-B5 and -A9 antigens and an increased cellular immune response to collagen types I and III have been found in these patients.[75] The first symptoms of thromboangiitis obliterans are often apparent following local trauma.[76, 77] The distal vessels of both the upper and lower extremities are most often affected.[78]

Common clinical presentations include: Raynaud's phenomenon with digital ulceration, intermittent claudication affecting the calf and the arch of the foot, and migratory thrombophlebitis. Symptoms of cerebral, visceral, or coronary involvement are less common.[79-81] Physical examination is notable for normal proximal pulses and diminished or absent distal pulses. Segmental, smooth, tapering distal lesions may be evident on arteriography. Occluded vessels often have abundant collaterals in a tree root pattern.

A definitive diagnosis of thromboangiitis obliterans is made from biopsy of an acute arterial lesion. Pathologic examination of acute lesions demonstrates polymorphonuclear leukocyte infiltration of all arterial layers, an intact internal elastic lamina, and the absence of medial necrosis.[76] The vessel lumen is frequently occluded by thrombus. Perivascular fibrosis and recanalization are often evident in the chronic arterial lesions, but these contain no specific morphologic features. Lesions of different ages can be seen in any one vessel. Medical therapy with corticosteroids, anticoagulants, and immunosuppressive agents is not useful. Smoking cessation is the one therapy which clearly improves the prognosis in patients with thromboangiitis obliterans.

Thoracic outlet syndrome is the most frequently encountered disorder in cases of unilateral Raynaud's phenomenon.[82] The mechanism of Raynaud's phenomenon is probably multifactorial, involving decreased perfusion pressure secondary to subclavian artery compression and altered sympathetic efferent activity caused by irritation of the brachial plexus. Neurovascular compression of the thoracic outlet is usually accompanied by claudication, weakness, numbness, and paresthesias, which are most pronounced in the inner arm and fourth and fifth fingers. Compression of the subclavian vein results in swelling of the upper extremity. Cervical ribs, abnormal insertion of the scalenus anticus muscle, abnormalities of the first thoracic rib or clavicle, and abnormal insertion of the pectoralis minor muscle can each act to compress the subclavian artery and brachial plexus in certain positions.

Subclavian bruits may be audible on physical examination. Arterial pulses are often normal on routine examination unless provocative maneuvers are performed. The costoclavicular, scalenus, and hyperabduction maneuvers can also suggest the location of the abnormality and are diagnostic of thoracic outlet syndrome if they reproduce the signs and symptoms of decreased radial pulse, pallor, and numbness in the hand. Chest radiography is useful to detect the presence of cervical ribs or apical lung masses. Nerve conduction velocities may be abnormal if the brachial plexus is involved. Arteriography is indicated only if emboli occur, suggesting the presence of a poststenotic aneurysm.

Conservative management may be effective in up to 70% of patients with thoracic outlet syndrome.[83] This includes avoiding positions that aggravate the symptoms, and exercises to strengthen the shoulder girdle and to improve posture. Maintaining the shoulder in an abducted and slightly elevated position during sleep can help relieve compression of the neurovascular bundle. Patients with significant vascular compromise and patients with cervical ribs compressing the thoracic outlet do appear to benefit from surgery.[84]

TRAUMATIC VASOSPASTIC DISEASE

Traumatic vasospastic disease can result from vibration injury, mechanical percussive injury, frostbite, thermal injury, and electric shock injury. Chain saw operators, metal workers using grinding and polishing wheels, and pneumatic drillers account for most of the cases of vibration-associated Raynaud's phenomenon, also known as vibration white finger. The prevalence of Raynaud's phenomenon is 30% to 50% in these populations.[85-87] The prevalence of vibration white finger also increases with amount of exposure to the trauma. In one survey of shipyard workers, the prevalence was 71% in full-time pneumatic grinders, 33% in part-time pneumatic grinders, and 6% among those with no exposure.[88]

Vibration may induce a local change in the digital arteries which enhances vasoconstriction in response to cold exposure. Arteriography has demonstrated prominent vasospasm, but has not always revealed digital artery occlusions.[89, 90] Merem[91] suggests that the change in arterial wall stress produced by vibration results in endothelial damage. The loss of endothelium-dependent vasodilator function could then be counterbalanced by intrinsic vasoconstrictive forces and contribute to vasospasm. Neurologic abnormalities resulting from vibration have also been proposed as a possible cause, but such abnormalities are not always evident.

In other traumatic vasospastic disorders the presence of vascular injury is more consistent. One such example is the hypothenar hand syndrome, which is a sequela of repetitive hammering with the palm of the hand. In these patients angiography often demonstrates aneurysmal enlargement and thrombosis of the ulnar artery as it crosses the hamate bone, as well as frequent distal artery and palmar arch occlusions.[92-94] Chronic cold injury has also been associated with Raynaud's phenomenon. After 10 years of filleting frozen fish, 90% of these workers had Raynaud's phenomenon.[95]

DRUGS AND TOXINS

A number of drugs and toxins have been associated with the onset of Raynaud's phenomenon (see Table 3). The relationship between *ergot* and digital vasospasm has been evident for centuries. Epidemics of ergotism have occurred following ingestion of contaminated rye. Ergotism is characterized by reports of sustained digital vasospasm resulting in gangrene and intense burning pain known as St. Anthony's fire. Ergot-containing compounds stimulate α-adrenoreceptors and may also stimulate serotonergic receptors. Digital ischemia due to ergot ingestion is characterized by its persistence. *Bromocriptine mesylate* and *methysergide* are two ergot derivatives which have been associated with digital vasospasm during clinical use.[96-99] Methysergide was formerly used in the treatment of migraine. Bromocriptine is currently used in the treatment of hyperprolactinemia, Parkinson's disease, and acromegaly. Vasospasm associated with these compounds is not limited to the digital arteries.

A 50% incidence of Raynaud's phenomenon has been reported in patients using nonselective β *blockers* for control of hypertension.[100] Possible mechanisms for this association include unopposed α-receptor activity, or reflex sympathetic vasoconstriction initiated by the cardiodepressive effect of β-adrenergic blockade.[101, 102] There do not appear to be β-adrenergic receptors in the digital arteries that mediate vasodilation during cold-induced sympathetic stimulation.[103] It is unclear whether cardioselective β-blocking agents or β-blocking agents with α-adrenoreceptor-blocking properties cause less digital vasospasm than nonselective β-blocking drugs.[104–106] Chronic β-blocker therapy does not result in increased vasospastic attacks in patients with Raynaud's phenomenon prior to the initiation of therapy.[107]

Other drugs associated with Raynaud's phenomenon include the chemotherapeutic agents *vinblastine* and *bleomycin*. Raynaud's phenomenon has also been reported with *amphetamines*,[108] the tricyclic antidepressant imipramine,[109 110] and the immunosuppressive agent *cyclosporin*.[111] Cyclosporin increases sympathetic nerve activity, an observation that may be relevant to Raynaud's phenomenon.[112] Industrial exposure to *vinyl chloride* appears to be related to distal phalangeal osteolysis and Raynaud's phenomenon.[113]

BLOOD DYSCRASIAS

Disorders which alter blood rheology are uncommon causes of Raynaud's phenomenon as well as more persistent digital ischemia. These disorders include polycythemia vera, essential thrombocytosis, cryoglobulinemia, cryofibrinogenemia, cold agglutinins, and Waldenström's macroglobulinemia. Episodes of digital pallor in patients with *polycythemia vera* have resolved following phlebotomy.[114] *Cryoglobulinemia* is a rare cause of Raynaud's phenomenon.[115] Cryoglobulins are serum proteins that precipitate in the cold. They are present in monoclonal gammopathy, polyclonal gammopathy, Waldenström's macroglobulinemia, SLE, and rheumatoid arthritis. Their presence is associated with arthralgias, leg ulcers, purpura, renal failure, and Raynaud's phenomenon. Essential cryoglobulinemia refers to those patients with no evident underlying cause. Up to 10% of patients with essential cryoglobulinemia have Raynaud's phenomenon.[116] Both prednisone and alkylating agents have been used to successfully treat cryoglobulinemia.[117] Plasmapheresis has also been used for symptomatic relief.[118] *Cryofibrinogenemia* is a rare disorder that has been associated with Raynaud's phenomenon.[119] In this condition it is the plasma rather than the serum which precipitates at 4° C.

Raynaud's phenomenon is occasionally present in *cold agglutinin* disorders.[120, 121] Cold agglutinins usually include IgM antibodies which occur spontaneously or in association with infectious or lymphoproliferative disorders. They are commonly associated with mycoplasmal pneumonia, and are more common in men than in women.[122] Treatment of patients with cold agglutinins requires the avoidance of cold.

NEUROLOGIC DISORDERS

Raynaud's phenomenon may be present in 10% of patients with median nerve entrapment in the carpal tunnel.[123, 124] *Carpal tunnel syndrome* is associated with typing, tenosynovitis, trauma, amyloidosis, hypothyroidism, and pregnancy. Symptoms of paresthesias in the median nerve distribution can be reproduced on physical examination by wrist flexion or by tapping on the volar surface of the wrist. Nerve conduction studies are abnormal in the median nerve at the wrist. Neurologic disorders resulting in limb immobility have also been associated with Raynaud's phenomenon. Hemiplegic stroke, spinal cord tumors, poliomyelitis, intervertebral disk disease, and syringomyelia have been reported to cause secondary Raynaud's phenomenon.

DIAGNOSIS

Some tests are useful when considering secondary causes of Raynaud's phenomenon. These include: the erythrocyte sedimentation rate, testing for antinuclear antibody, rheumatoid factor, cryoglobulins, and cold agglutinins, and serum protein electrophoresis. The erythrocyte sedimentation rate is often normal in patients with primary Raynaud's phenomenon. Its utility is limited by the fact that it is falsely elevated in the elderly and it is low in one third of patients with scleroderma.[125] In the young, antinuclear antibody titers are typically less than 1:16. They can be elevated to levels of greater than 1:40 in the elderly without systemic disease being present. In general, the titer correlates with the number of organ systems affected by connective tissue disease.[126] The presence of rheumatoid factor is also not a specific finding. Elevated titers are found in patients with rheumatoid arthritis, scleroderma, SLE, dermatomyositis, sarcoidosis, Waldenström's macroglobulinemia, pulmonary fibrosis,

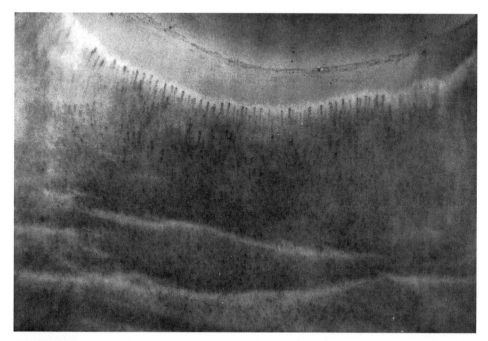

FIGURE 4.
Normal nail-fold capillaroscopy. (Courtesy of H. Maricq, Charleston, SC.)

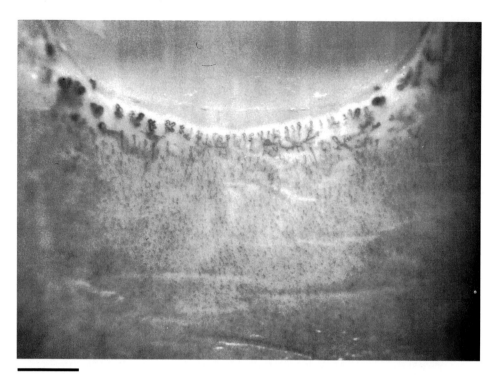

FIGURE 5.

Nail-fold capillaroscopy in a patient with scleroderma. Avascular areas and elongated, tortuous capillary loops are present. (Courtesy of H. Maricq, Charleston, SC.)

endocarditis, tuberculosis, leprosy, and hepatitis. It can also be falsely positive in the elderly. Testing for cryoglobulins is indicated in the presence of weakness, arthralgias, and purpura. Serum protein electrophoresis should be performed in subjects with elevated total serum protein.

Nail-fold capillaroscopy is useful to look for evidence of a connective tissue disorder. Nail-fold capillaroscopy is performed using a magnifying glass, ophthalmoscope, or a compound microscope with a magnification of ×10 to view the clean nail fold covered with immersion oil. Normally the superficial capillaries are regularly spaced hairpin loops (Fig 4). The capillary pattern is blurred when edema is present, and hemorrhages are a nonspecific finding. Capillary abnormalities of scleroderma are often seen first in the nail-fold areas[127] and consist of four- to tenfold enlargement of the loops and avascular areas (Fig 5). The findings on nail-fold capillaroscopy reflect measurable histologic changes within the tissue.[128] Enlarged, deformed capillary loops surrounded by avascular areas are also seen in dermatomyositis and mixed connective tissue disease.[129] In SLE the subpapillary venous plexus may be prominent, deformed capillaries are present, and avascular areas are absent.[129, 130]

Arterial blood supply to the digits can be assessed using a number of techniques. These include systolic pressure measurements, digital plethysmography to measure pulse volume and flow, and Doppler flow mapping. None of these tests, however, are diagnostic of Raynaud's phenomenon since they are neither sensitive nor specific. There is considerable overlap in digital systolic pressure measurements between normal persons and patients with Raynaud's phenomenon. When exposed to environmental or local cooling, digital systolic pressure falls dramatically and at times to zero in patients with Raynaud's phenomenon.[131, 132] Downs and colleagues[133] reported that finger systolic blood pressures, when measured in a warm environment, were useful to predict the presence of arterial occlusive disease. Finger systolic blood pressures less than 70 mm Hg, a gradient of greater than 30 mm Hg from the wrist to the finger, and a difference of more than 15 mm Hg between fingers were predictive of occlusion of digital arteries as proved by arteriography. Digital pulse volume recordings provide qualitative information about blood flow. Plethysmographic techniques are used to evaluate changes in digital volume with each pulse. Pulse waves in the fingers of patients with cold sensitivity have been described as "peaked" with a rapid ascending limb and the dicrotic notch high on the downstroke.[53] The finger pulse volume is diminished during cold-induced vasoconstriction and in the presence of digital artery occlusion. After warming, pulse volume increases if there is no fixed arterial occlusion. Patients with Raynaud's phenomenon tend to have a greater reduction in pulse volume or systolic pressure after cooling than normal subjects. The typical color changes do not

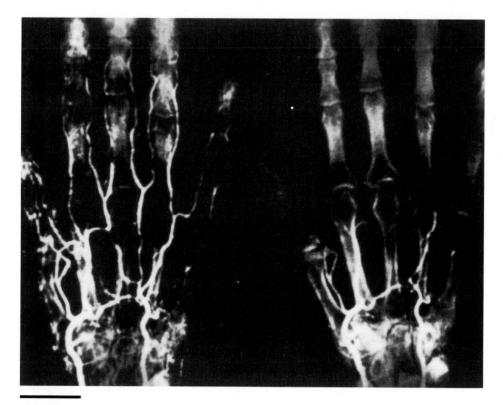

FIGURE 6.

Angiograms before (*left*) and after (*right*) local cold exposure in a patient with Raynaud's phenomenon. (From Creager MA: Vasospastic diseases, in Loscalzo J, Creager MA, Dzau V (eds): *Vascular Medicine.* Boston, Little, Brown, 1992, p 978. Used by permission.)

necessarily accompany the hemodynamic changes. These tests can detect fixed digital arterial obstruction, but do not otherwise distinguish primary from secondary Raynaud's phenomenon.

Angiography has a very limited role in making the diagnosis of Raynaud's phenomenon (Fig 6). It may be indicated in patients with persistent digital ischemia and suspected digital artery occlusions. The anatomic information derived from angiography is used to plan revascularization procedures when digital ischemia occurs secondary to atherosclerosis, thromboangiitis obliterans, or emboli from a subclavian artery aneurysm.

TREATMENT

The symptoms of Raynaud's phenomenon can be treated with nonpharmacologic measures, pharmacologic intervention, and surgical sympathectomy. Treatment must be planned for the individual patient according to the severity of his or her symptoms. In patients with secondary Raynaud's phenomenon, the treatment plan needs to address the underlying cause. For example, treatment of a hypertensive patient who develops Raynaud's phenomenon after initiation of β-blocker therapy should begin with discontinuation of that drug and initiation of another antihypertensive agent.

The diagnosis of Raynaud's phenomenon should be followed by a careful discussion with the patient of the prognosis. The mainstay of therapy for patients with Raynaud's phenomenon is education regarding precipitating factors. Patients should avoid both environmental and local cold exposure in order to decrease digital vasospastic attacks. Directly touching or grasping cold objects should be avoided. Sudden drops in environmental temperature will often precipitate attacks. For example, the decrease in temperature found with air conditioning may exacerbate symptoms. Hands and feet need to be kept warm and dry. In cold climates this may require thermally lined socks and gloves and even measures such as the use of battery-powered hand warmers. Clothing should be loose and warm. An explanation of reflex sympathetic vasoconstriction often helps the patient to understand the need to keep the head and trunk warm in order to decrease symptoms. Cigarette smoking causes cutaneous vasoconstriction and should be strictly avoided.[134] Moisturizer applied to dry skin will help to prevent drying and cracking, which is associated with skin infection.

PHARMACOLOGIC THERAPY

Calcium channel blockers and sympathetic nervous system inhibitors are often effective in the treatment of Raynaud's phenomenon. Other classes of vasoactive medications such as topical nitrates, angiotensin-converting enzyme inhibitors, thromboxane inhibitors, and direct smooth muscle relaxants are probably not beneficial. In fact, many vasodilators reduce vascular resistance and actually divert blood away from the affected digit.

Calcium channel blockers act to decrease the inflow of calcium through the slow channels, resulting in decreased smooth muscle contractractility. Nifedipine may also affect digital circulation through an antiplatelet effect[135] or through blockade of postsynaptic α_2-adrenoreceptors.[136] Of the available calcium channel blockers, nifedipine has been the mainstay of pharmacologic therapy for symptoms of Raynaud's phenomenon.[137] In patients with Raynaud's phenomenon, nifedipine decreases digital vascular resistance during environmental cold exposure.[138] It also increases finger systolic blood pressure and skin temperature during local cold exposure in patients with primary and secondary Raynaud's phenomenon.[139, 140] In a number of placebo-controlled trials, treatment with nifedipine decreased the number and severity of vasospastic attacks.[137, 141, 142] Therapy with nifedipine is initiated at 10 mg orally three times a day, or 30 mg/day of the long-acting preparation. The dose is increased as tolerated until therapeutic effect is achieved. Side effects of nifedipine include hypotension, peripheral edema, and indigestion. The incidence of side effects increases at higher doses.[143] The calcium channel blockers diltiazem, felodipine, nicardipine, and isradipine may also decrease the number and severity of vasospastic attacks in Raynaud's phenomenon. In two small placebo-controlled trials,[144, 145] diltiazem decreased symptoms of digital ischemia. Felodipine decreased the number and duration of vasospastic attacks in a ten-patient study.[146] Nicardipine decreased the frequency of vasospastic attacks only slightly in a multicenter, double-blind placebo-controlled trial.[147] Isradipine therapy resulted in increased finger systolic pressure and subjective improvement in one placebo-controlled trial.[148] Verapamil, on the other hand, has not been shown to be effective therapy for this disorder.[149]

Inhibitors of the sympathetic nervous system such as reserpine, prazosin, methyldopa, guanethidine, phenoxybenzamine, and tolazoline have been evaluated in the treatment of Raynaud's phenomenon. Reserpine decreases the accumulation of norepinephrine in arterial walls.[150] In patients with primary and secondary Raynaud's phenomenon, reserpine increases total fingertip blood flow in both warm and cool environments[151] and attenuates vasoconstrictor responses to cooling.[12] Uncontrolled studies of reserpine in doses up to 0.5 mg have demonstrated symptomatic improvement.[12, 151, 152] The usefulness of reserpine is limited by its side effects of depression, lethargy, nausea, nasal congestion, and peptic ulcers. Guanethidine increases capillary blood flow in patients with Raynaud's phenomenon secondary to scleroderma[153] but its use is accompanied by significant orthostatic hypotension. In 31 patients with primary and secondary Raynaud's phenomenon, a placebo-controlled crossover trial of the α-adrenergic blocker phenoxybenzamine demonstrated improved finger temperatures after cooling.[154] The clinical utility of phenoxybenzamine therapy in Raynaud's phenomenon is unclear.[155, 156] Prazosin blocks α_1-adrenoreceptors and induces a small increase in digital blood flow during intraarterial infusion.[24] A placebo-controlled, double-blind study of prazosin demonstrated decreased frequency of vasospastic attacks in 15 patients with primary Raynaud's phenomenon.[157] However, tachyphylaxis is a common problem with prazosin therapy in Raynaud's phenomenon.[158] Hypotension, headache, and fatigue are common side effects of prazosin therapy. Long-acting α_1-adrenoreceptor antagonists such as terazosin and doxazosin have not been evaluated in patients with Raynaud's phenomenon, but would probably have effects similar to prazosin. Long-term controlled studies of the efficacy of sympathetic nervous system inhibitors in the treatment of Raynaud's phenomenon are unavailable.

Pharmacologic therapy aimed at altering vasoactive arachidonic acid metabolites represent another class of vasodilators which have been evaluated in the treatment of Raynaud's phenomenon. Dazoxiben is a thromboxane synthase inhibitor and may increase production of prostacyclin.[159] In a controlled double-blind trial of dazoxiben and nifedipine in the treatment of Raynaud's phenomenon, dazoxiben was not effective in reducing symptoms.[160] Three double-blind placebo-controlled studies of dazoxiben demonstrated no benefit with this therapy in patients with primary and secondary Raynaud's phenomenon.[161-163]

The efficacy of vasodilator prostanoids have been evaluated in clinical trials. Cicaprost, an oral analog of prostacyclin, was not effective in the treatment of Raynaud's phenomenon secondary to scleroderma.[164] Uncontrolled studies of the intravenous infusion of prostaglandin E_1 have suggested that it may improve healing of ulcers secondary to digital ischemia.[165, 166] Iloprost, a prostacyclin analog with platelet inhibitory effects, was studied in a double-blind placebo-controlled trial for the treatment of severe Raynaud's phenomenon in patients with scleroderma.[167] Iloprost was found to be effective for short-term palliation in these patients. Long-term benefits of prostaglandin therapy have been postulated, but not consistently seen.[168, 169]

Ketanserin, a serotonin receptor antagonist with some α-adrenergic blocking properties, has also been studied as therapy for Raynaud's phenomenon. A placebo-controlled trial in 222 patients with primary and secondary Raynaud's phenomenon found that ketanserin improved symptoms but did not clearly affect digital blood flow.[39] Symptomatic improvement included decreased number of episodes of digital vasospasm, but no change in the duration or severity of the attacks.

SYMPATHECTOMY

Early investigators found lumbar sympathectomy to be useful in treating Raynaud's phenomenon of the lower extremities, but had less success with cervical dorsal sympathectomy.[170] The disparity in the results of cervical dorsal and lumbar sympathectomy was confirmed by Gifford et al.[171] who reviewed the results of sympathectomy in 70 patients with primary Raynaud's phenomenon, and 40 patients with secondary Raynaud's phenomenon. Sympathetic innervation of the lower limbs originates from spinal cord segments T10 to L2, and lower limb sympathectomy is achieved via excision of the second and third lumbar ganglia. During a 15-year period, Janoff and colleagues[172] encountered ten patients with refractory episodic lower extremity vasospasm vs. 600 patients with upper extremity vasospasm. Each of these ten patients underwent lumbar sympathectomy and remained free of symptoms at 4-year follow-up.

Upper limb sympathetic innervation comes from the preganglionic fibers of spinal cord segments T1 to T10 which then synapse in the middle, cervical, and stellate ganglia. Cervical dorsal sympathectomy requires preservation of the upper half of the stellate ganglion in order to prevent the development of Horner's syndrome. The postganglionic fibers travel through the brachial plexus to reach the upper limb. In primary Raynaud's phenomenon and secondary Raynaud's phenomenon due to scleroderma, cervical dorsal sympathectomy is reported to improve outcome in only 60% of the patients initially.[173–175] Relapses do occur, which makes the long-term success of this procedure unclear. Neither the extent of ganglionectomy nor the use of preganglionic section alters operative results.[176, 177] The disappointing results with upper extremity sympathectomy have been attributed to residual sympathetic pathways to the brachial plexus which do not traverse the cervicothoracic sympathetic trunk. For this reason, Baddeley[177] suggested that cervical sympathectomy be reserved for only severe progressive cases with impending digit loss.

More recently, selective digital sympathectomy has been performed in patients with severe Raynaud's phenomenon. The digital artery is stripped of its adventitia over a 3- to 4-mm segment distal to the bifurcation of the common digital artery.[178] More extensive digital sympathectomy is achieved when both common and proximal digital arteries are stripped of their adventitia.[179] Initial results were promising, but limited to patients with Raynaud's phenomenon secondary to trauma. Wilgis[180, 181] further extended this technique by removing adventitia from common digital arteries and the digital arteries distal to the proximal interphalangeal joint. This proved effective in the treatment of both primary Raynaud's phenomenon, and Raynaud's phenomenon following trauma. Results of digital sympathectomy have been much less encouraging in patients with digital vasospasm secondary to scleroderma. Favorable results in patients with scleroderma and Raynaud's phenomenon have been reported with radical distal microarteriolysis. O'Brien and colleagues[182] performed radical microarteriolysis in 13 scleroderma patients suffering from Raynaud's phenomenon. This procedure involves distal adventitiectomy and removal of periarterial scar of the ulnar artery, superficial palmar arch, and digital arteries to the distal interphalangeal joint level. In five cases total occlusion was present and vein bypass grafts were placed. Symptomatic improvement and ulcer healing were reported in all patients at 1-year follow-up. These findings suggest that digital sympathectomy and more extensive radical microarteriolysis may address the "local vascular fault" of Raynaud's phenomenon and improve outcome for patients with primary Raynaud's phenomenon and those with Raynaud's phenomenon secondary to trauma and scleroderma.

REFERENCES

1. Allen EV, Brown GE: Raynaud's disease: a critical review of minimal requisites for diagnosis. *Am J Med Sci* 1932; 183:187–200.
2. LeRoy EC, Medsger TA Jr: Raynaud's phenomenon: A proposal for classification. *Clin Exp Rheumatol* 1991; 10:485–488.
3. Lewis T, Pickering GW: Observations upon maladies in which blood supply to the digits ceases intermittently or permanently and upon bilateral gangrene of the digits: Observations relevant to so-called Raynaud's disease. *Clin Sci* 1934; 1:327–366.

4. Olsen N, Nielsen SL: Prevalence of primary Raynaud's phenomenon in young females. *Scand J Clin Lab Invest* 1978; 37:761–764.

5. Heslop J, Coggan D, Acheson ED: The prevalence of intermittent digital ischemic (Raynaud's phenomenon) in a general practice. *J Coll Gen Pract* 1983; 33:85–89.

6. Maricq HR, Weinrich MC, Keil JE, et al: Prevalence of Raynaud's phenomenon in the general population. *J Chronic Dis* 1986; 39:423–427.

7. Maricq HR, Carpentier PH, Weinrich MC, et al: Geographic variation in the prevalence of Raynaud's phenomenon: Charleston, SC, USA vs Tarentaise, Savoie, France. *J Rheumatol* 1993; 20:70–76.

8. Gifford RW Jr, Hines EA Jr: Raynaud's disease among women and girls. *Circulation* 1957; 16:1012–1021.

9. Clavijo F, Krahenbuhl B: Évolution naturelle du phénomène de Raynaud. *Schweiz Med Wochenschr* 1981; 111:2023–2027.

10. Gerbracht DD, Steen VD, Ziegler GL, et al: Evolution of primary Raynaud's phenomenon (Raynaud's disease) to connective tissue disease. *Arthritis Rheum* 1985; 28:87–92.

11. Peacock JH: Peripheral venous blood concentration of epinephrine and norepinephrine in primary Raynaud's disease. *Circ Res* 1959; 7:821–827.

12. Kontos HA, Wasserman AJ: Effect of reserpine in Raynaud's phenomenon. *Circulation* 1969; 39:259–266.

13. Downey JA, Frewin DB: The effect of cold on blood flow in the hands of patients with Raynaud's phenomenon. *Clin Sci* 1973; 44:279–289.

14. Fagius J, Blumberg H: Sympathetic outflow to the hand in patients with Raynaud's phenomenon. *Cardiovasc Res* 1985; 19:249–253.

15. Lewis T: Experiments relating to the peripheral mechanism involved in spasmodic arrest of the circulation in the fingers, a variety of Raynaud's disease. *Heart* 1929; 15:7–12.

16. Jamieson GG, Ludbrook J, Wilson A: Cold hypersensitivity in Raynaud's phenomenon. *Circulation* 1971; 44:254–264.

17. Freedman RR, Mayes MD, Sabharwal SC: Induction of vasospastic attacks despite digital nerve block in Raynaud's disease and phenomenon. *Circulation* 1989; 80:859–862.

18. Somlyo AP: Sarcoplasmic reticulum and the temperature-dependent contraction of smooth muscle in calcium-free solutions. *J Cell Biol* 1971; 51:722–741.

19. Vanhoutte PM, Shepard JT: Effect of temperature on reactivity of isolated cutaneous veins of the dog. *Am J Physiol* 1970; 218:187–190.

20. Vanhoutte PM, Lorenz RR: Effect of temperature on reactivity of saphenous mesenteric, and femoral veins of the dog. *Am J Physiol* 1970; 218:1746–1750.

21. Rusch NJ, Shepard JT, Vanhoutte PM: The effect of profound cooling on adrenergic transmission in canine cutaneous veins. *J Physiol* 1981; 311:57–65.

22. Vanhoutte PM, Cooke JP, Lindblad LE, et al: Modulation of postjunctional alpha-adrenergic responsiveness by local changes in temperature. *Clin Sci* 1985; 68:121s–123s.

23. Cooke JP, Shepard JT, Vanhoutte PM: The effect of warming on adrenergic neurotransmission in canine cutaneous vein. *Circ Res* 1984; 54:547–553.

24. Coffman JD, Cohen RA: Role of alpha-adrenoreceptor subtypes mediating sympathetic vasoconstriction in human digits. *Eur J Clin Invest* 1988; 18:309–313.

25. Flavahan NA, Cooke JP, Shepard JT, et al: Human postjunctional alpha-1 and alpha-2 adrenoreceptors: Differential distribution in the arteries of the limbs. *J Pharmacol Exp Ther* 1978; 841:361–365.

26. Cooke JP, Creager SJ, Scales KM, et al: Role of digital artery adrenoreceptors in Raynaud's disease. In press.
27. Keenan EJ, Porter JM: Alpha-2-adrenergic receptors in platelets of patients with Raynaud's syndrome. *Surgery* 1984; 94:204–209.
28. Landis EM: Micro-injection studies of capillary blood pressure in Raynaud's disease. *Heart* 1930; 15:247 255.
29. Thulesius O: Methods for evaluation of peripheral vascular function in the upper extremities. *Acta Chir Scand Suppl* 1976; 465:53–54.
30. Cohen RA, Coffman JD: Reduced fingertip arterial pressure in Raynaud's disease. *J Vasc Med Biol* 1989; 1:21–25.
31. Coffman JD, Cohen RA: Plasma levels of 5-hydroxytryptamine during sympathetic stimulation and in Raynaud's phenomenon. *Clin Sci* 1994; 86:7–13.
32. Biondi ML, Marasini B, Bianchi E, et al: Plasma free and intraplatelet serotonin in patients with Raynaud's phenomenon. *Int J Cardiol* 1988; 19:335–339.
33. Vanhoutte PM: 5-Hydroxytryptamine and vascular disease. *Fed Proc* 1983; 42:233–237.
34. Roddie IC, Shepard JT, Whelan RF: The action of 5-hydroxytryptamine on the blood vessels of the human hand and forearm. *Br J Pharmacol* 1955; 10:445–449.
35. Coffman JD, Cohen RA: Serotonergic vasoconstriction in human fingers during reflex sympathetic response to cooling. *Am J Physiol* 1988; 254:H889–H893.
36. Stranden E, Roald OK, Krohg K: Treatment of Raynaud's phenomenon with the 5-HT2 receptor antagonist ketanserin. *Br Med J* 1982; 285:1069–1071.
37. Seibold JR, Terrigino CA: Selective antagonism of S2 serotonergic receptors relieves but does not prevent cold induced vasoconstriction in primary Raynaud's phenomenon. *J Rheum* 1986; 13:337–341.
38. Hechtman DH, Jageneau A: Inhibition of cold induced vasoconstriction with ketanserin. *Microvasc Res* 1985; 30:56–62.
39. Coffman JD, Clement DL, Creager MA, et al: International study of ketanserin in Raynaud's phenomenon. *Am J Med* 1989; 87:264–268.
40. Seibold JR, Jageneau HM: Treatment of Raynaud's phenomenon with ketanserin, a selective antagonist of the serotonin (5-HT$_2$) receptor. *Arthritis Rheum* 1984; 27:139–146.
41. Roald OK, Seem E: Treatment of Raynaud's phenomenon with ketanserin in patients with connective tissue disorders. *Br Med J* 1984; 289:577–580.
42. Lukac J, Rovensky J, Tauchmannova H, et al: Effect of ketanserin on Raynaud's phenomenon in progressive systemic sclerosis: A double-blind trial. *Drugs Exp Clin Res* 1985; 11:659–663.
43. Lopez-Ovejera JA, Saal SD, D'Angelo WA, et al: Reversal of vascular and renal crisis of scleroderma by oral angiotensin converting enzyme blockade. *N Engl J Med* 1979; 300:1417–1419.
44. Coffman JD, Rasmussen HLM: Effect of thromboxane synthetase inhibition in Raynaud's phenomenon. *Clin Pharmacol Ther* 1984; 36:369–373.
45. Gresele P, Volpato R, Migliaci R, et al: Thromboxane does not play a significant role in acute cold-induced vasoconstriction in Raynaud's phenomenon. *Thromb Res* 1992; 66:259–264.
46. Kanno K, Hirata Y, Emori T, et al: Endothelin and Raynaud's phenomenon. *Am J Med* 1991; 90:130–131.
47. Yamane K, Miyauchi T, Suzuki N, et al: Significance of plasma endothelin-1 levels in patients with systemic sclerosis. *J Rheumatol* 1992; 19:1566–1571.
48. Lau CS, Bridges A, Muir A, et al: Further evidence of polymorphonuclear cell activity in patients with Raynaud's phenomenon. *Br J Pharmacol* 1992; 31:375–380.

49. Khan F, Coffman JD: Enhanced cholinergic cutaneous vasodilation in Raynaud's phenomenon. *Circulation* 1994; 89:1183–1188.

50. Lau CS, McLaren M, Belch JJF: Factor VIII von Willebrand factor antigen levels correlate with symptom severity in patients with Raynaud's phenomenon. *Br J Rheumatol* 1991; 30:433–436.

51. DeTakats G, Fowler EF: Raynaud's phenomenon. *JAMA* 1962; 179:1–8.

52. Velayos E, Robinson H, Porciuncula FU: Clinical correlation analysis of 137 patients with Raynaud's phenomenon. *Am J Med Sci* 1971; 262:347–356.

53. Summer DS, Strandness DE: An abnormal finger pulse associated with cold sensitivity. *Ann Surg* 1972; 174:294–298.

54. Blunt RJ, Porter JM: Raynaud's syndrome. *Semin Arthritis Rheum* 1981; 10:282–308.

55. Tuffanelli DL, Winkelman RK: Systemic scleroderma: A clinical study of 727 cases. *Arch Dermatol* 1961; 84:359–373.

56. Falanga V, Medsger TA Jr, Reichlin M, et al: Linear scleroderma. Clinical spectrum, prognosis, and laboratory abnormalities. *Ann Intern Med* 1986; 104:849–857.

57. Masi AT, Rodnan GP, Medsger TA, et al: Preliminary criteria for the classification of systemic sclerosis (scleroderma). *Arthritis Rheum* 1983; 23:581–590.

58. Tan EM, Rodnan GP, Garcia I: Diversity of antinuclear antibodies in progressive systemic sclerosis. *Arthritis Rheum* 1980; 23:617–625.

59. Catoggio LJ, Bernstein RM, Black CM: Serological markers in progressive systemic sclerosis: clinical correlations. *Ann Rheum Dis* 1983; 42:23–27.

60. Medsger TA Jr, Masi AT, Rodnan GP, et al: Survival with systemic sclerosis (scleroderma): A life-table analysis of clinical and demographic factors in 309 patients. *Ann Intern Med* 1971; 75:369–376.

61. Harvey AM, Schulman LE, Tumulty PA, et al: Raynaud's phenomenon associated with lupus erythematosus: A review of the literature and clinical analysis. *Medicine (Baltimore)* 1954; 33:291–322.

62. Hochberg MC, Boyd RE, Ahearn JM, et al: Systemic lupus erythematosus: A review of clinico-laboratory features and immunogenetic markers in 150 patients with emphasis on demographic subsets. *Medicine (Baltimore)* 1985; 64:285–295.

63. Kenamore BD, Levin WC, Ritzman SE: Raynaud's phenomenon as leading sign of lupus erythematosus—report of three cases and classification of cryopathies. *Tex Reports Biol Med* 1968; 26:189–197.

64. Tuffanelli DL: Scleroderma and its relationship to the "collagenoses": dermatomyositis, lupus erythematosus, rheumatoid arthritis, and Sjögren's syndrome. *Am J Med* 1962; 243:133–146.

65. Maricq HR, Spencer-Green G, LeRoy EC: Skin capillary abnormalities as indicators of organ involvement in scleroderma (systemic sclerosis), Raynaud's syndrome, and dermatomyositis. *Am J Med* 1976; 61:862–870.

66. Spencer-Green G, Crowe WE, Levinson JE: Nailfold capillary abnormalities and clinical outcome in childhood dermatomyositis. *Arthritis Rheum* 1982; 25:954–958.

67. Glass D, Soter NA, Schur PH: Rheumatoid vasculitis. *Arth Rheum* 1976; 19:950–952.

68. Scott JT, Hourihane DO, Doyle FH et al: Digital arteries in rheumatoid disease. *Ann Rheum Dis* 1961; 20:224–252.

69. Laws JW, Lillie JG, Scott JT: Arteriographic appearance in rheumatoid arthritis and other disorders. *Br J Radiol* 1963; 36:477–493.

70. Fischer M, Mielke H, Glaefke S, et al: Generalized vasculopathy and finger blood flow abnormalities in rheumatoid arthritis. *J Rheum* 1984; 11:33–37.

71. Birnstingl M: Raynaud's syndrome: Diagnosis and management. *Br J Hosp Med* 1979; 21:602–611.
72. Buerger L: Thromboangiitis obliterans: A study of the vascular lesions leading to presenile spontaneous gangrene. *Am J Med Sci* 1908; 136:567–580.
73. Wessle S, Ming S, Gurewich V, et al: A critical evaluation of thromboangiitis obliterans. *N Engl J Med* 1960; 262:1149–1160.
74. Allen EV, Brown GE: Thromboangiitis obliterans: A clinical study of 200 cases. *Ann Intern Med* 1928; 1:535–550.
75. Adar R, Papa MZ, Mozes M, et al: Cellular sensitivity to collagen in thromboangiitis obliterans. *N Engl J Med* 1983; 308:1113–1116.
76. McKusick VA: Buerger's disease—a distinct clinical and pathological entity. *JAMA* 1962; 181:5–12.
77. Hirai M, Shinoya S: Arterial obstruction of the upper limb in Buerger's disease: Its incidence and primary lesion. *Br J Surg* 1979; 66:124–128.
78. Shinoya S, Ban I, Nakala Y, et al: Diagnosis, pathology and treatment of Buerger's disease. *Surgery* 1974; 75:695–700.
79. Fischer CM: Cerebral thromboangiitis obliterans. *Medicine (Baltimore)* 1957; 36:169–181.
80. Deitch EA, Sikkema WW: Intestinal manifestations of Buerger's disease: Case report and literature review. *Am J Surg* 1981; 47:326–328.
81. Ohno H, Matsuda Y, Takashiba K, et al: Acute myocardial infarction in Buerger's disease. *Am J Cardiol* 1986; 57:690–691.
82. Bouhoutos J, Morris T, Martin P: Unilateral Raynaud's phenomenon in the hand and its significance. *Surgery* 1977; 82:547–551.
83. Urschel HC Jr, Razzuk MA: Management of thoracic outlet syndrome. *Surg Annu* 1973; 5:229–263.
84. Conn J Jr: Thoracic outlet syndromes. *Surg Clin North Am* 1974; 54:155–164.
85. Chatterjee DS, Petrie A, Taylor W: Prevalence of vibration induced white finger in fluorspar mines in Weardale. *Br J Ind Med* 1978; 353:208–218.
86. Theriault G, DeGuire L, Gingras S, et al: Raynaud's phenomenon in forestry workers in Quebec. *Can Med Assoc J* 1982; 126:1404–1408.
87. Brubaker RL, Mackenzie CJ, Eng PR, et al: Vibration white finger disease among tree fellers in British Columbia. *J Occup Med* 1983; 25:403–408.
88. Letez R, Cherniack MG, Gerr F, et al: A cross-sectional epidemiologic survey of shipyard workers exposed to hand-arm vibration. *Br J Ind Med* 1992; 49:53–62.
89. Ashe WF, Cook WT, Old JW: Raynaud's phenomenon of occupational trauma. *N Engl J Med* 1983; 268:281–284.
90. Scatz N: Occlusive arterial disease in the hand due to occupational trauma *N Engl J Med* 1963; 268:281–284.
91. Merem RM: Vibration induced arterial shear stress: the relationship to Raynaud's phenomenon. *Arch Environ Health* 1973; 26:105–110.
92. Conn J Jr, Bergen JJ, Bell JL: Hypothenar hammer syndrome: post traumatic digital ischemia. *Surgery* 1970; 68:1122–1128.
93. Vayssairat M, Debure C, Cormier J-M, et al: Hypothenar hammer syndrome: Seventeen cases with long term follow-up. *J Vasc Surg* 1987; 5:838–843.
94. Millender L, Nalebuff EH, Kasdon E: Aneurysms and thromboses of the ulnar artery in the hand. *Arch Surg* 1972; 105:686–690.
95. Mackiewicz Z, Pislorz A: Raynaud's phenomenon following long-term repeated application of a great difference in temperature. *J Cardiovasc Surg* 1977; 18:151–154.
96. Graham JR: Methysergide for prevention of headache: Experience in 500 patients over 3 years. *N Engl J Med* 1964; 270:67–72.

97. Herlache J, Hoskins P, Schmidt CM: Ergotism. *Angiology* 1973; 24:369–374.

98. Quagliarello J, Barakat R: Raynaud's phenomenon in infertile women. *Vertil Steril* 1987; 48:877–879.

99. Crauad D, Noel G, Daumont M: Syndrome de Raynaud provoque par la bromoergocriphre. *Nouv Presse Med* 1977; 6:2693.

100. Marshall AJ, Roberts CJC, Baritt DW: Raynaud's phenomenon as a side effect of beta-blockers in hypertension. *Br Med J* 1976; 1:1498–1499.

101. White CB, Udwadia BP: Beta adrenoreceptors in the human dorsal hand vein and the effects of propanolol and practolol on venous sensitivity to noradrenaline. *Br J Clin Pharmacol* 1975; 2:99–105.

102. Heck I, Trubestein G, Stumpe KO: Effects of combined beta and alpha receptor blockade on peripheral circulation in essential hypertension. *Clin Sci* 1981; 61:429s.

103. Cohen RA, Coffman JD: Adrenergic vasodilator mechanisms in the finger. *Circ Res* 1981; 49:1196–1201.

104. Eliasson K, Lins LE, Sundqvist K: Vasospastic phenomena in patients treated with beta-adrenoreceptor blocking agents. *Acta Med Scand Suppl* 1979; 628:39–46.

105. Eliasson K, Lins LE, Sundqvist K: Raynaud's phenomenon caused by beta receptor blocking drugs. *Acta Med Scand* 1982; 665:109–112.

106. Steiner JA, Cooper R, McPherson K, et al: Effect of alpha-adrenoreceptor antagonists on prevalence of peripheral vascular symptoms in hypertensive patients. *Br J Clin Pharmacol* 1982; 14:833–837.

107. Coffman JD, Rasmussen HM: Effect of beta-adrenoreceptor blocking drugs in patients with Raynaud's phenomenon. *Circulation* 1985; 72:466–470.

108. Grau JJ, Grau M, Milla A, et al: Cancer chemotherapy and Raynaud's phenomenon. *Ann Intern Med* 1983; 98:258.

109. Bower JS, Davis GB, Kearney TE, et al: Diffuse vascular spasm associated with 4 bromo-2,5-dimethoxyamphetimine ingestion. *JAMA* 1983; 249:1477.

110. Appelbaum PS, Kapoor W: Imipramine induced vasospasm: A case report. *Am J Psychiatry* 1983; 140:913–915.

111. Deray G, LeHoang P, Achour L, et al: Cyclosporin and Raynaud's phenomenon. *Lancet* 1986; 2:1092–1093.

112. Scherrer U, Vissing SF, Morgan BJ, et al: Cyclosporin induced sympathetic activation and hypertension after heart transplantation. *N Engl J Med* 1990; 323:696.

113. Laplante A, Clavel-Chapelon F, Contassot J-C, et al: Exposure to vinyl chloride monomer: Results of a cohort study after seven year follow-up. *Br J Ind Med* 1991; 49:134–137.

114. Brown GE, Griffin HZ: Peripheral arterial disease in polycythemia vera. *Arch Intern Med* 1930; 46:705.

115. Birnstingl M: The Raynaud syndrome. *Postgrad Med J* 1971; 47:297–310.

116. Invernizzi F, Galli M, Serino G, et al: Secondary and essential cryoglobulinemias. *Acta Haematol* 1983; 70:73–82.

117. Ristow SC, Griner PF, Abraham GN, et al: Reversal of systemic manifestations of cryoglobulinemia. *Arch Intern Med* 1976; 136:467–470.

118. McLeod BC, Sassetti RJ: Plasmapheresis with return of cryoglobulin-depleted autologous plasma (cryoglobulinpheresis) in cryoglobulinemia. *Blood* 1980; 55:866–870.

119. Jager BV: Cryofibrinogenemia. *N Engl J Med* 1962; 266:579–585.

120. Hansen PF, Faber M: Raynaud's syndrome originating from reversible precipitation of protein. *Acta Med Scand* 1947; 129:81–94.

121. Marshall RJ, Shepard JT, Thompson ID: Vascular responses in patients with high serum titres of cold agglutinins. *Clin Sci* 1953; 12:255–264.

122. Oleson H: The cold agglutinin syndrome. *Dan Med Bull* 1967; 14:138–142.

123. Loebe M, Heidrich H: The carpal tunnel syndrome—a disease underlying Raynaud's phenomenon. *Angiology* 1988; 39:891–901.

124. Waller DG, Dathan JR: Raynaud's syndrome and carpal tunnel syndrome. *Postgrad Med J* 1985; 61:161–162.

125. Sox HC, Liang MH: The erythrocyte sedimentation rate. Guidelines for rational use. *Ann Intern Med* 1986; 104:515–523.

126. Kallenberg CGM, Vellenga E, Wouda AA, et al: Platelet activation, fibrinolytic activity and circulating immune complexes in Raynaud's phenomenon. *J Rheumatol* 1982b; 9:878–892.

127. Maricq HR, Weinberger AB, LeRoy EC: Early detection of scleroderma spectrum disorders by in vivo capillary microscopy. *J Rheumatol* 1982; 9:289–291.

128. Thompson RP: Nailfold biopsy in scleroderma and related disorders. *Arthritis Rheum* 1984; 27:97–103.

129. Maricq HR, LeRoy EC, D'Angelo WA, et al: Diagnostic potential of in vivo capillary microscopy in scleroderma and related disorders. *Arthritis Rheum* 1980; 23:183–189.

130. Lee P, Leung F, Alderdice C, et al: Nailfold capillary microscopy in the connective tissue disorders: A semiquantitative assessment. *J Rheumatol* 1983; 10:930–938.

131. Krahenbuhl B, Nielsen SL, Lassen NA: Closure of digital arteries in high vascular tone states as demonstrated by measurement of systolic blood pressure in the finger. *Scand J Lab Clin Invest* 1977; 37:71–76.

132. Hoare M: The effect of local cooling on digital systolic pressure in patients with Raynaud's syndrome. *Br J Surg* 1982; 69:S27–S28.

133. Downs AR, Gaskell P, Morrow I, et al: Assessment of arterial obstruction of vessels supplying the fingers by measurement of the local blood pressures and the skin temperature response test—correlation with angiographic evidence. *Surgery* 1975; 77:530–539.

134. Coffman JD: Effect of propanolol on blood pressure and skin flow during cigarette smoking. *J Clin Pharmacol* 1969; 9:39–44.

135. Rademaker M, Thomas RHM, Kirby JD, et al: The antiplatelet effect of nifedipine in patients with systemic sclerosis. *Clin Exp Rheumatol* 1992; 10:57–62.

136. Timmermans PB, van Meel JCA, van Zwieten PA: Calcium antagonists and alpha receptors. *Eur Heart J* 1983; 4C:11–17.

137. Smith CD, McKendry RVR: Controlled trial of nifedipine in the treatment of Raynaud's phenomenon. *Lancet* 1982; 2:1299–1301.

138. Creager MA, Pariser KM, Winston EM, et al: Nifedipine induced fingertip vasodilation in patients with Raynaud's phenomenon. *Am Heart J* 1984; 108:370–373.

139. Nillson H, Jonasson T, Ringqvist I: Treatment of digital vasospastic disease with the calcium entry blocker nifedipine. *Acta Med Scand* 1984; 215:135–139.

140. Wollersheim H, Thein T, van't Laar A: Nifedipine in primary Raynaud's phenomenon and in scleroderma: Oral versus sublingual hemodynamic effects. *J Clin Pharmacol* 1987; 27:907–913.

141. Rodeheffer RJ, Rommer JA, Wigley F, et al: Controlled double blind trial of nifedipine in the treatment of Raynaud's phenomenon. *N Engl J Med* 1983; 308:880–883.

142. Winston EL, Pariser KM, Miller KB, et al: Nifedipine as a therapeutic modality for Raynaud's phenomenon. *Arthritis Rheum* 1983; 26:1177–1180.

143. Nilsson H, Jonasson T, Leppert J, et al: The effect of the calcium entry

blocker nifedipine on cold induced digital vasospasm. *Acta Med Scand* 1978; 221:53–60.

144. Kahan A, Amor B, Menkes CJ: A randomized double blind trial of diltiazem in the treatment of Raynaud's phenomenon. *Ann Rheum Dis* 1985; 44:30–33.

145. Rhedda A, McCans J, Willan AR, et al: A double blind placebo crossover randomized trial of diltiazem in Raynaud's phenomenon. *J Rheum* 1985; 12:724–727.

146. Kallenberg CGM, Wouda AA, Meens L, et al: Once daily felodipine in patients with primary Raynaud's phenomenon. *Eur J Clin Pharmacol* 1991; 40:313–315.

147. French Cooperative Multicenter Group for Raynaud's Phenomenon: Controlled multicenter double blind trial of nicardipine in the treatment of primary Raynaud's phenomenon. *Am Heart J* 1991; 122:352–355.

148. Leppert J, Jonasson T, Nilsson H, et al: The effect of isradipine, a new calcium channel antagonist, in patients with primary Raynaud's phenomenon: A single blind dose response study. *Cardiovasc Drug Ther* 1989; 3:397–401.

149. Kinney EL, Nicholas GG, Gallo J, et al: The treatment of severe Raynaud's phenomenon with verapamil. *J Clin Pharmacol* 1982; 22:74–76.

150. Burn JH, Rand MJ: Noradrenaline in artery walls and its dispersal by reserpine. *Br Med J* 1958; 1:903–907.

151. Coffman JD, Cohen AS: Total and capillary fingertip blood flow in Raynaud's phenomenon. *N Engl J Med* 1971; 285:259–265.

152. Peacock JH: The treatment of primary Raynaud's phenomenon of the upper limb. *Lancet* 1960; 2:65–71.

153. LeRoy EC, Downey JA, Cannon PJ: Skin capillary blood flow in scleroderma. *J Clin Invest* 1971; 50:930–939.

154. Cleophas TJM, van Lier HJJ, Fennis FJM, et al: Treatment of Raynaud's syndrome with adrenergic alpha-blockade with or without beta-blockade. *Angiology* 1984; 35:29–37.

155. Moser M, Prandoni AG, Orbison JA, et al: Clinical experience with sympathetic blocking agents in peripheral vascular disease. *Ann Intern Med* 1953; 38:1245–1254.

156. Hillestad LK: Dibenzyline in vascular disease of the hands. *Angiology* 1962; 13:169–172.

157. Nielsen SL, Vithing K, Rassmussen K: Prazosin treatment of primary Raynaud's phenomenon. *Eur J Clin Pharmacol* 1983; 24:421–423.

158. Wollersheim H, Thien T: Dose-response study of prazosin in Raynaud's phenomenon: Clinical effectiveness versus side effects. *J Clin Pharmacol* 1988; 28:1089–1093.

159. Cowley AJ, Jones EW, Hanley SP: Effects of dazoxiben, an inhibitor of thromboxane synthetase, on forearm vasoconstriction in response to cold stimulation, and on human blood vessel prostacyclin production. *Br J Pharmacol* 1983; 15:107–112.

160. Ettinger WH, Wise RA, Schaffhauser D, et al: Controlled double blind trial of dazoxiben and nifedipine in the treatment of Raynaud's phenomenon. *Am J Med* 1984; 77:451–456.

161. Coffman JD, Rassmussen HM: Effect of thromboxane synthetase inhibition in Raynaud's phenomenon. *Clin Pharmacol Ther* 1984; 36:369–373.

162. Jones EW, Hawkey CJ: A thromboxane synthetase inhibitor in Raynaud's phenomenon. *Prostaglandins Leuko Essen Fatty Acids* 1983; 12:67–71.

163. Luderer JR, Nicholas G, Meumyer MM, et al: Dazoxiben, a thromboxane synthetase inhibitor, in Raynaud's phenomenon. *Clin Pharmacol Ther* 1984; 36:105–115.

164. Lau CS, McLaren M, Scott N, et al: The pharmacologic effects of cicaprost, and oral prostacyclin analog, in patients with Raynaud's syndrome secondary to systemic sclerosis: A preliminary study. *Clin Exp Rheumatol* 1991; 9:271–273.

165. Baron M, Skrinkas G, Urowitz MB, et al: Prostaglandin E1 therapy for digital ulcers in scleroderma. *Can Med Assoc J* 1982; 126:42–47.

166. Clifford PC, Martin MFR, Sheddon EJ, et al: Treatment of vasospastic disease with prostaglandin E1. *Br Med J* 1980; 281:1031–1034.

167. Wigley FM, Wise RA, Seibold JR, et al: Intravenous iloprost infusion in patients with Raynaud's phenomenon secondary to systemic sclerosis. *Ann Intern Med* 1994; 120:199–206.

168. Mohrland JS, Porter JM, Smith EA, et al: A multicenter placebo controlled study of prostaglandin E1 in Raynaud's syndrome. *Ann Rheumatol* 1985; 44:754–760.

169. Rademaker M, Cooke ED, Almond NE, et al: Comparison of intravenous infusions of iloprost and oral nifedipine in treatment of Raynaud's phenomenon in patients with systemic sclerosis: A double blind randomized study. *Br Med J* 1989; 298:561–564.

170. Adson W, Brown GE: The treatment of Raynaud's disease by resection of the upper thoracic and lumbar sympathetic ganglia and trunks. *Surg Gynecol Obstet* 1929; 48:577–603.

171. Gifford RW, Hines EA, Craig WM: Sympathectomy for Raynaud's phenomenon: Follow-up study of 70 women with Raynaud's disease and 54 women with secondary Raynaud's phenomenon. *Circulation* 1958; 17:5–13.

172. Janoff KA, Phinney ES, Porter JM: Lumbar sympathectomy for lower extremity vasospasm. *Am J Surg* 1985; 150:147–152.

173. Johnston EM, Summerly R, Birnstingl M: Prognosis in Raynaud's phenomenon after sympathectomy. *Br Med J* 1965; 1:962–967.

174. Blain A, Coller FA, Carger GB: Raynaud's disease: A study of criteria for prognosis. *Surgery* 1951; 29:387–397.

175. Farmer RG, Gifford RL, Hines EA: Raynaud's disease with sclerodactyly. *Circulation* 1961; 23:13–15.

176. Kinmonth JB, Hadfield GD: Sympathectomy for Raynaud's disease among men. *Br Med J* 1952; 1:1377–1379.

177. Baddely RM: The place of upper dorsal sympathectomy in the treatment of primary Raynaud's disease. *Br J Surg* 1965; 52:426–430.

178. Flatt AE: Digital artery sympathectomy. *J Hand Surg* 1983; 5:550–556.

179. Egloff DV, Mifsud RP, Verdan C: Superselective digital sympathectomy in Raynaud's phenomenon. *Hand* 1982; 15:110–114.

180. Wilgis EFS: The evaluation and treatment of chronic digital ischemia. *Ann Surg* 1981; 193:693–698.

181. Wilgis EFS: Digital sympathectomy for vascular insufficiency. *Hand Clin* 1985; 2:361–367.

182. O'Brien BM, Kumar PAV, Mellow CG, et al: Radical microarteriolysis in the treatment of vasospastic disorders of the hand, especially scleroderma. *J Hand Surg [Br]* 1992; 17:447–452.

Index

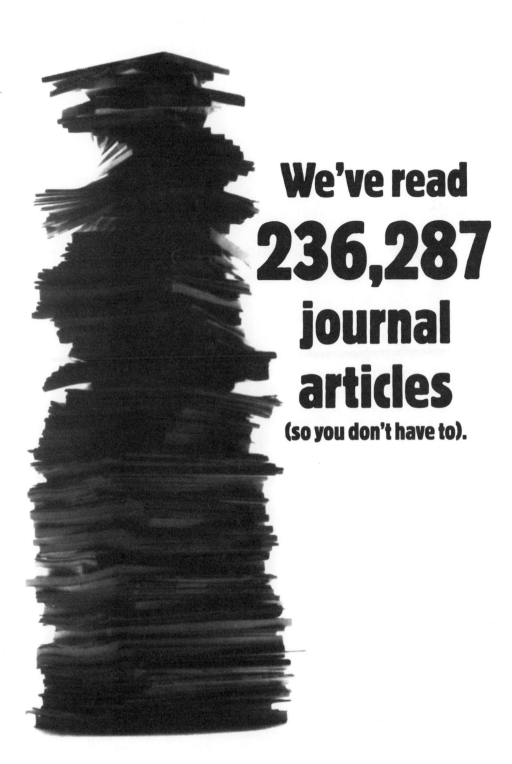

We've read
236,287
journal
articles
(so you don't have to).

The Year Books–
The best from 236,287 journal articles.

At Mosby, we subscribe to more than 950 medical and allied health journals from every corner of the globe. We read them all, tirelessly scanning for anything that relates to your field.

We send everything we find related to a given specialty to the distinguished editors of the **Year Book** in that area, and they pick out *the best*, the articles they feel *every practitioner in that specialty should be aware of.*

For the **1994 Year Books** we surveyed a total of 236,287 articles and found hundreds of articles related to your field. Our expert editors reviewed these and chose the developments you don't want to miss.

The best articles–condensed, organized, and with personal commentary.

Not only do you get the past year's most important articles in your field, you get them in a format that makes them easy to use.

Every article that the editors pick is condensed into a concise, outlined abstract, a summary of the article's most important points highlighted with bold paragraph headings. So you can quickly scan for exactly what you need.

In addition to identifying the year's best articles, the editors write concise commentaries following each article, telling whether or not the study in question is a reliable one, whether a new technique is effective, or whether a particular trend you've head about merits your immediate attention.

No other abstracting service offers this expert advice to help you decide how the year's advances will affect the way you practice.

With a special added benefit for Year Book subscribers.

In 1994, your **Year Book** subscription includes a new added benefit. Access to **MOSBY Document Express**, a rapid-response information retrieval service that puts copies of original source documents in your hands, in a little as a few hours.

With **MOSBY Document Express**, you have convenient, *around-the-clock-access to literally every article* upon which **Year Book** summaries are based. What's more, you can also order journal articles cited in references—or for that matter, virtually any medical or scientific article that can be located. Plus, at your direction, we will deliver the article(s) by FAX, overnight delivery service, or regular mail.

This new added benefit is just one of the enhanced services that makes your **Year Book** subscription an even better value—it's your key to the full breadth of health sciences information. For more details, see **MOSBY Document Express** instructions at the beginning of this book.